Image-Guided
Spine Intervention

Image-Guided Spine Intervention

■ **Douglas S. Fenton, MD**
Assistant Professor of Radiology
Mayo Medical School
Mayo Clinic
Jacksonville, Florida

■ **Leo F. Czervionke, MD**
Associate Professor of Radiology
Mayo Medical School
Mayo Clinic
Jacksonville, Florida

SAUNDERS
An Imprint of Elsevier Science
Philadelphia   London   New York   St. Louis   Sydney   Toronto

SAUNDERS
An Imprint of Elsevier Science

The Curtis Center
Independence Square West
Philadelphia, PA 19106

IMAGE-GUIDED SPINE INTERVENTION ISBN 0–7216–0021–2

Notice

Care has been taken to confirm the accuracy of the information presented and to describe generally accepted practices. However, the authors, editors, publisher, and Mayo are not responsible for errors or omissions or for any consequences from application of the information in this book and make no warranty, expressed or implied, with respect to the currency, completeness, or accuracy of the contents of the publication. Application of this information in a particular situation remains the professional responsibility of the practitioner, who at all times must exercise independent clinical judgment. No endorsement of any company or product is implied or intended.

The authors, editors, and publisher have exerted every effort to ensure that drug selection and dosage set forth in this text are in accordance with current recommendations and practice at the time of publication. However, in view of ongoing research, changes in government regulations, and the constant flow of information relating to drug therapy and drug reactions, the reader is urged to check the package insert for each drug for any change in indications and dosage and for added warnings and precautions. This is particularly important when the recommended agent is a new or infrequently employed drug.

Some drugs and medical devices presented in this publication have Food and Drug Administration (FDA) clearance for limited use. It is the responsibility of the health care provider to ascertain the FDA status of each drug or device planned for use in his or her clinical practice.

Library of Congress Cataloging-in-Publication Data

Fenton, Douglas S. (Douglas Scott)
  Image-guided spine intervention/Douglas S. Fenton, Leo F. Czervionke.
    p.; cm.
  ISBN 0-7216-0021-2
    1. Spine–Imaging. 2. Spine–Surgery. 3. Surgery–Data processing. I. Czervionke, Leo F. II. Mayo
  Foundation for Medical Education and Research. III. Title.
    [DNLM: 1. Spinal Diseases–therapy. 2. Spinal Diseases–surgery. 3. Spine–surgery. 4. Surgery,
  Computer-Assisted. WE 725 F342i 2003]
  RD768.F46 2003
  617.5'6059–dc21   2002075769

Acquisitions Editor: Allan Ross
Developmental Editor: Josh Hawkins
Project Manager: Norman Stellander

RT

Printed in China.

Last digit is the print number: 9   8   7   6   5   4   3   2   1

To Melissa and Jeanne...

To Brooke, Derek, Alec, Eric, Jessica, and Margaret...

Without whose love, support, and patience
this book would not have been possible

Contributors

Joseph T. Alexander, MD

Assistant Professor, Department of Neurosurgery, Wake Forest University School of Medicine; Attending, Wake Forest University Baptist Medical Center, Winston-Salem, North Carolina

Chapters 2 to 10: *A Spine Surgeon's Perspective*

Leo F. Czervionke, MD

Associate Professor of Radiology, Mayo Medical School, Mayo Clinic, Rochester, Minnesota; Consultant, Mayo Clinic, Jacksonville, Florida

Basic Needle Manipulation Techniques; Facet Joint Injection and Medial Branch Block; Facet Denervation; Selective Nerve Root Block; Percutaneous Spine Biopsy; Discography; IntraDiscal ElectroThermal Therapy (IDET™)

Jacques E. Dion, MD

Professor of Radiology and Neurosurgery, Emory School of Medicine, and Head, Interventional Neuroradiology, Emory University Hospital, Atlanta, Georgia

Vertebroplasty

Douglas S. Fenton, MD

Assistant Professor of Radiology, Mayo Medical School, Mayo Clinic, Rochester, Minnesota; Consultant, Mayo Clinic, Jacksonville, Florida

Basic Needle Manipulation Techniques; Facet Joint Injection and Medial Branch Block; Facet Denervation; Selective Nerve Root Block; Percutaneous Spine Biopsy; Vertebroplasty; Discography; IntraDiscal ElectroThermal Therapy (IDET™)

Michael S. Huckman, MD

Professor of Radiology, Rush Medical College; Director of Neuroradiology, Rush-Presbyterian-St. Luke's Medical Center, Department of Radiology and Nuclear Medicine, Chicago, Illinois

Foreword

Mark J. Kransdorf, MD

Professor of Diagnostic Radiology, Mayo Medical School, Mayo Clinic, Rochester, Minnesota; Visiting Professor in Musculoskeletal Radiology, Department of Radiologic Pathology, Armed Forces Institute of Pathology, Washington, DC; Senior Associate Consultant, Department of Radiology, Mayo Clinic, Jacksonville, Florida

Sacroiliac Joint Injection

David A. Miller, MD

Clinical Instructor of Diagnostic Radiology, Mayo Medical School, Mayo Clinic, Rochester, Minnesota; Senior Associate Consultant, Department of Radiology, Mayo Clinic, Jacksonville, Florida

Vertebroplasty

B. Todd Sitzman, MD, MPH

Assistant Professor of Anesthesiology, Mayo Medical School, Mayo Clinic, Rochester, Minnesota; Consultant, Anesthesiology and Pain Management, Mayo Clinic, Jacksonville, Florida

Epidural Injections; Pharmacology for the Spine Injectionist

Foreword

There was a time when the radiologist was an innocent bystander providing fluoroscopic guidance and elucidation of anatomic landmarks to the clinician who would try to put the needle in the right place. It soon became apparent that radiologists had the ability to interpolate an extra dimension to a two-dimensional image based on an understanding of the principles of parallax and magnification. This led to the natural evolution of the idea that the person who understands the radiologic anatomy is also the natural choice to perform the procedure. From the 1940s on, radiology developed the techniques of angiography, myelography, endovascular therapeutic radiology, and the myriad techniques that today comprise the specialties of neuroradiology and interventional radiology. It is therefore not surprising that radiologists have reduced the often draconian techniques of diagnosis and treatment of painful spinal conditions to a set of procedures employing pinpoint targeting of anatomic and pathologic structures using medical imaging techniques and delivering analgesic, ablative, contrast-enhancing, and structure-preserving substances to heretofore remote areas of the body by percutaneous means, usually in an outpatient setting.

Image-Guided Spine Intervention is an incredibly comprehensive volume on image-guided spinal interventions that is certain to become the standard textbook in this rapidly growing field. Drs. Fenton and Czervionke have produced a volume that allows physicians who perform these procedures to "have their cake and also eat it." Not only is it spectacularly illustrated with multicolor photographs and diagrams, but most of the radiologic images are undegraded by intermediate photo processing and lifted straight from the clinical digital image to the textbook page. There is thorough, well-illustrated text on basic principles of needle manipulation and comprehensive discussion of patient selection, caveats, pertinent anatomy, complications, analgesic and therapeutic agents, preoperative and postoperative care, and various commercially available instruments of the trade. That is "having the cake."

What is new in this volume is information that allows the clinician to "eat the cake." Each chapter includes current CPT codes for the procedures discussed and sample dictations with preoperative and intraoperative narrative. These are labor-intensive procedures that are cost effective and likely to produce major reductions in pain and suffering with little or no morbidity. They must be appropriately entered into the patient's medical record and should be fairly reimbursed. The sample dictations and coding information are important factors in helping the physician realize those ends.

Although Drs. Fenton and Czervionke are neuroradiologists, the encyclopedic information contained herein should be of major interest to all physicians and other health professionals involved in the treatment of spinal disorders, whether or not they perform any of the procedures described in this book. In fact, each chapter contains the comments of a spine surgeon on how the procedure under discussion relates to his practice.

It is hard to imagine a more comprehensive textbook on this subject. If history repeats itself in how seminal textbooks are regarded, I suspect that future generations of physicians will refer to Drs. Fenton and Czervionke as the "grandfathers" of this new and burgeoning medical specialty.

Michael S. Huckman, MD

Preface

BOOK OVERVIEW

Our goal when we started this book was to write an instructional text that would have appeal to physicians in a wide variety of specialties, particularly those dealing with the diagnosis and management of spine and paraspinal-related pain disorders. We have made every effort to have each chapter written in a consistent fashion and have attempted to describe all aspects of the procedure. Each chapter begins with a short background of the procedure, followed by the pertinent anatomy, patient selection criteria, and contraindications. The procedural portion of each chapter is written in a cookbook format. It details the equipment necessary for the procedure, including the medications. This book is intended to be a procedural manual and is therefore written in a step-by-step fashion. Each of the procedural steps in the text is augmented by state-of-the-art radiographic images, computed tomographic (CT) images, magnetic resonance (MR) images, pertinent anatomic sections, and/or illustrations. The possible complications related to the procedure are discussed, followed by a section describing our routine postprocedure care and patient follow-up. A typical sample dictation for each procedure is provided, followed by instructive case reports. The most current procedural terminology (CPT) codes for the procedure are listed near the end of the chapter, followed by recent and historical references. The final section is written by a fellowship-trained spine neurosurgeon, who provides a clinical perspective discussing in which situations he finds that these procedures are most beneficial to his patients, in his practice.

EXPERIENCE

By no means should any of these procedures be performed by inexperienced physicians who are unfamiliar with pain-alleviating procedures and needle techniques. Before performing these procedures, the physician should have an excellent understanding of the pertinent gross anatomy and radiologic anatomy, as well as a thorough understanding of the indications for and contraindications to the procedure. The benefit-to-risk ratio for the procedure and radiation safety issues are also important factors to consider before performing these procedures. We strongly recommend that the physician performing these procedures have formal training in these percutaneous needle techniques during his or her residency or fellowship, or has had a training course in which he or she has received hands-on training by an expert proctor. The importance of continuing education for maintaining a current knowledge and level of expertise in performing these procedures cannot be overemphasized.

NEEDLE SYSTEMS AND OTHER EQUIPMENT

Although we specifically mention some of the currently available needle systems and equipment in this text, it is important to keep in mind that other commercially available systems may be perfectly acceptable for performing these procedures. Regardless of the system one uses, we strongly recommend that one **always** use these needle systems or devices according to the manufacturer's guidelines.

PATIENT POSITIONING NOMENCLATURE

Throughout the text, we repeatedly use the terms "left anterior oblique (LAO)" and "right anterior oblique (RAO)" when the patient is prone on the table. As used in this book, these terms refer to positions in which the patient is in contact with the fluoroscopic table top, irrespective of the direction of the x-ray beam. For example, an "LAO radiograph" is one in which the left anterior surface of the patient's torso is in contact with the table top, regardless of the direction of the x-ray beam.

We are confident that, by reading this book, the physician will gain a better overall understanding and appreciation of current percutaneous needle techniques used for the diagnosis and treatment of spine disorders. Furthermore, we hope that this book will prove to be a valuable instructive guide that will assist those physicians who wish to be more proficient in performing these procedures.

Douglas S. Fenton, MD
Leo F. Czervionke, MD

A Spine Surgeon's Perspective

One of the least favorite chief complaints for many clinicians to hear from a patient is "I have neck pain" or "I have back pain." These entities are extremely common in the industrialized world, so much so that almost everyone will have at least one significant episode during his or her lifetime. The advent of readily available magnetic resonance imaging has led to a greater appreciation of the presence of a spectrum of degenerative changes of the spine in *asymptomatic* individuals, rendering the clinical correlation of radiographic "abnormalities" seen in individuals *with symptoms* more challenging. Although severe, the symptoms are often vague and nonlocalizing because of the overlapping innervation of the spine and paraspinal structures. To further complicate matters, the onset of an episode of pain is often intertwined with the legal system if it occurs in an accident or with the Worker's Compensation system if it occurs at the job site, raising the concerns of secondary gain.

By contrast, the evaluation of radicular symptoms in the arms or legs can be more straightforward. Here, a careful clinical evaluation generally gives a better clue to the location of the problem. However, at times a question remains as to the responsible site, and more detailed evaluation is indicated. This is particularly true as we move to more minimally invasive treatment technologies, which will be successful only if directed to the correct target.

There continues to be considerable variation in the evaluation and management of spinal disorders, depending on the training and bias of the treating physician and on less obvious factors such as the region of the country. Many commonly utilized surgical and nonsurgical spine procedures have not been validated by randomized, prospective studies. Although evidence-based medicine is gradually gaining ground, management of spine care remains more art than science at this time.

My role in the commentaries throughout this book is not to make pronouncements regarding the utility of each of these tests or treatments. Rather, it is to foster a better understanding between the physician performing the procedure and the physician ordering the procedure by providing a clinician's perspective as to the rationale for ordering the test in the first place. In the increasingly fragmented manner that spine care is often provided today, it is not unusual for there to be little opportunity for direct interaction or discussion of the nuances of a specific patient between the clinician and the proceduralist. Much of the initial clinical evaluation and nonsurgical treatment of spinal disorders is being directed by nonspecialists; therefore, the proceduralist cannot be certain that the test or treatment ordered is necessarily the one most indicated for the patient. For these reasons, some responsibility for evaluating the appropriateness of the procedure falls on the proceduralist, who should not hesitate to communicate with the clinician if there is any doubt as to the rationale for a planned course of evaluation and treatment.

Joseph T. Alexander, MD

Contents

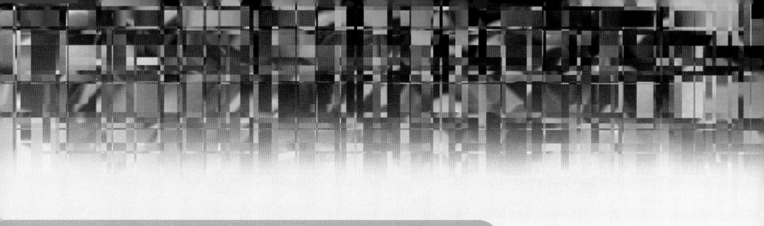

Chapter 1

Basic Needle Manipulation Techniques

- Leo F. Czervionke, MD
- Douglas S. Fenton, MD

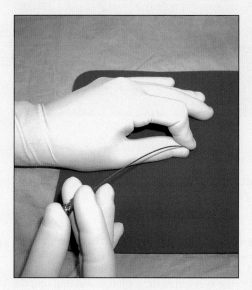

The primary purpose of this book is to describe the techniques necessary to perform accurate, safe, and clinically relevant diagnostic and therapeutic procedures for spine-related pain. The various procedures differ in methodology and purpose, but the common element in all spine interventional procedures is the use of a needle. At first glance, the topic of this chapter may seem simplistic and trivial. However, we have repeatedly observed both novices and experienced spine interventionalists using suboptimal needle manipulation techniques. An understanding of the relatively simple concepts and techniques described in this chapter forms a cornerstone for all the percutaneous needle procedures described in this book.

In general, straight needles have a beveled tip or a pencil-point shaped tip. The focus of this discussion is on beveled needles. Every needle used in our spine procedures is styleted, which means that the needle has two components. The first component is the outer cannula, which serves to deliver medication, accepts smaller needles through it in a coaxial fashion, or is used to perform fine-needle or large-core biopsies (Fig. 1-1). The second component is the inner stylet that seals the cannula so no tissue is able to enter the cannula as the needle is advanced through tissue (Fig. 1-2). **The stylet should always remain entirely within the cannula when there is forward movement of the needle.** The stylet does not necessarily have to be within the cannula when the needle is retracted, although we consider it good practice to stylet the needle during needle removal as well. The outer cannula

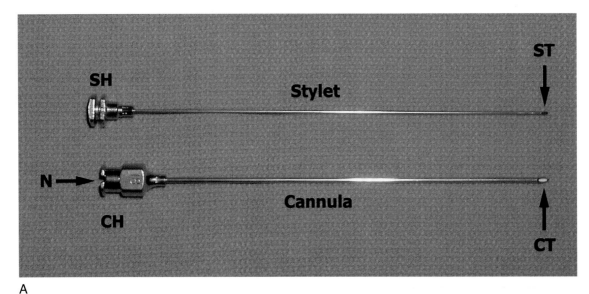

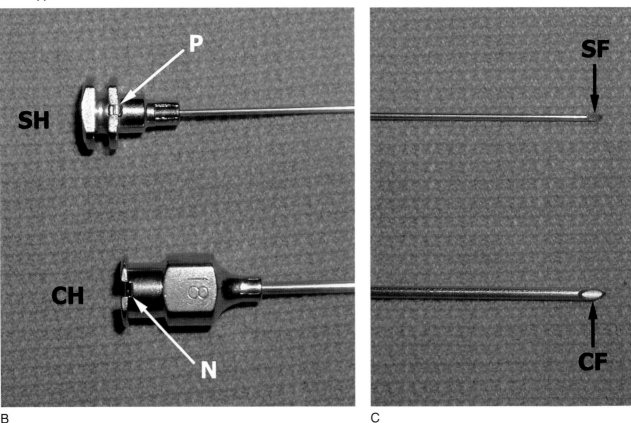

Figure 1-1 ■ Components of an 18-gauge styleted MONOJECT® SENSI-TOUCH needle. *A*, The inner stylet has a beveled tip (ST) that can be inserted into the outer cannula until the bevel of the stylet and the cannula tip (CT) coincide. The cannula hub (CH) has a notch (N) that accepts the corresponding tiny metal protrusion on the stylet hub (SH). *B*, Close-up view of the cannula hub (CH) and the stylet hub (SH). The small protrusion (P) on one side of the stylet hub will fit snugly into the notch (N) on the needle hub. *C*, Close-up view of the distal end of the outer cannula and inner stylet, corresponding to *B*. The needle cannula bevel face (CF) and stylet bevel face (SF) are located on the same side of the needle as the cannula notch in *B*. (MONOJECT® SENSI-TOUCH is a trademark of Sherwood Services AG. Photographed with permission.)

or inner stylet often has a bevel that can aid the physician with needle navigation.

Manipulation of the needle can be a difficult skill to master, especially when working with needles smaller than 20 gauge or longer than 3.5 inches. As needle caliber becomes smaller and needle length is longer, needle navigation becomes more difficult because the needle tends to follow

the path of least resistance, which in the body is dependent on the different densities of the tissues. Therefore, a means must be found to control the direction of the needle.

When any needle is inserted through the skin and into the subcutaneous fat, the needle will go in the direction one would normally anticipate. For example, depressing the needle hub caudad will deflect the needle tip cephalad

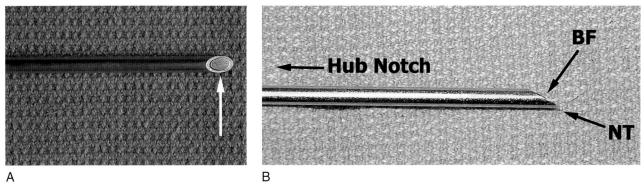

A   B

Figure 1-2 ■ Close-up view of the distal end of a styleted needle. *A*, With the bevel viewed en face, the inner stylet has been inserted into the outer needle cannula so that the stylet face and cannula face coincide (*arrow*). *B*, With the bevel face viewed from the side, the bevel face (BF) faces upward, the same side of the needle as the notch on the hub (*not shown*). Note that the axis of the needle tip (NT) points slightly downward. (The distal end of an Osteo-Site M1 Bone Biopsy Needle photographed with permission of Cook Incorporated, Bloomington, IN.)

regardless of the direction of the bevel. This remains true when the needle is passing through soft, homogeneous, subcutaneous tissues. For some patients with greater amounts of subcutaneous fat or fat-laden muscles, the needle can be directed in this manner. However, in most patients, the advancing needle becomes enveloped by denser tissue or fascia, located beneath the subcutaneous tissue, and the needle no longer moves in the direction one might anticipate. The precise depth this occurs varies depending on the patient, but it becomes apparent while observing the advancing needle at fluoroscopy. When this depth is reached (e.g., 2 or 3 cm below the skin surface), the techniques that follow are useful for directing the course of the needle.

The *first method* uses the needle bevel to control the direction of the needle. The beveled needles widely used in today's practice come in various gauges and lengths. Some needles have plastic hubs, whereas others are entirely metal. A notch usually exists on one side of the hub that corresponds to the side of the bevel face (see Fig. 1-1*B*). It is important to remember that the hub notch is on the same side as the face of the beveled needle tip. The needle tip is pointed on the opposite side of the hub notch (see Fig. 1-1*C*). Because the beveled needle tip is wedge shaped, this facilitates directional needle placement (Fig. 1-3).[1] When advancing a bevel-tipped needle straight into a soft tissue structure, the needle tip will tend to go in a direction slightly

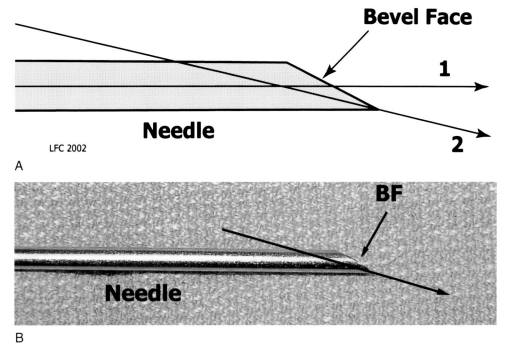

A

B

Figure 1-3 ■ The angle of the needle bevel face is one factor that determines the direction a needle will take when inserted into an object. *A*, The needle bevel face is facing upward. When a needle is inserted into tissue, the needle will have a tendency to move not in the direction of the long axis of the needle shaft (*arrow 1*) but rather in a direction along the axis that bisects the angle formed by the needle tip (*arrow 2*). In reality, depending on the caliber of the needle, the inserted needle generally moves in a direction somewhere between arrows 1 and 2. *B*, The needle, when inserted, will have the tendency to be directed away from the bevel face (BF), along an axis that bisects the angle formed by the needle tip, in the direction of the long arrow, which is the side opposite to the notch on the needle hub. (The distal end of an Osteo-Site M1 Bone Biopsy Needle photographed with permission of Cook Incorporated, Bloomington, IN.)

away from the hub notch (Fig. 1-4).[2] For example, when the bevel face is cephalad, the needle tip is directed caudad. This occurs because there is more surface area on the beveled side, exposing it to greater amounts of tissue and thus forcing the needle in a direction opposite to the bevel face. No amount of needle manipulation will allow one to steer a needle into a desired position if the needle enters the skin too far away from the projection of the target on the skin surface. **To achieve optimal needle placement for all spine procedures, it is important to select an optimal skin entry point and trajectory using fluoroscopic guidance.**

The *second method* for directing a needle is for the operator to place a bend or bow on the needle shaft (Fig. 1-5). This technique works with bevel-tipped or with pencil-point—shaped needles, but the degree of deflection is greatest with bevel-tipped needles. One might think that to deflect the needle tip cephalad, for example, that the needle hub must be pulled caudad. This is true when you move an object (such as a needle) in the air, but this is not observed when advancing the needle into tissue using long, small-caliber needles. This would apply in vivo if needles of large enough gauge (greater than 10 gauge) were used or in the very superficial soft tissues of the body. However, the needles used in spine procedures are usually no larger than 12 gauge, with the majority being 20 gauge or smaller.

The *third method* for directing a needle is to place a small, 5- to 10-degree bend on the needle tip. There are many who advocate the use of placing a "bend" on the needle tip routinely, to facilitate needle placement. We do not advocate this practice. When the needle tip is bent, traversing a large distance in tissue requires that the needle be continually rotated to advance the needle tip or it will stray away from its intended path. This tends to make needle placement actually more difficult and causes more tissue disruption along the path of the advancing needle, resulting in unnecessary discomfort to the patient; therefore we rarely use this technique alone. If a bent needle tip is required for a difficult needle maneuver, we prefer a coaxial technique. A larger, straight needle is inserted with its tip proximal to the target, and then the bent-tipped needle is inserted coaxially through the larger needle. This eliminates the difficulties in advancing the bent-tipped needle by minimizing the distance the bent-tipped needle is in contact with tissue. When the bent-tipped needle emerges from the bore of the larger needle, the bend on the inner needle re-forms and it can be directed in the direction desired.

Regardless of the method used, proper holding of the needle hub is critical in directing the needle to its intended target. The thumb should be placed on top of the needle hub pointing toward the notch, and the index and middle fingers are opposite the thumb at the junction of the hub and the needle so the needle passes between them (Fig. 1-6). To deflect the needle in any direction, the notch should be turned 180 degrees opposite to the desired needle direction. This maneuver will place the sharp edge of the needle tip (oppo-

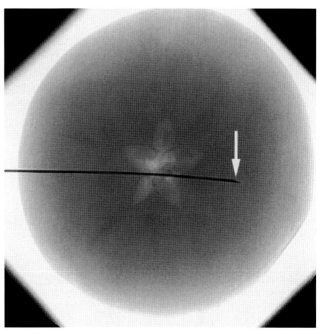

Figure 1-4 ■ Demonstration of the needle deflection technique in a grapefruit with **straight needle insertion**. Radiograph shows a 22-gauge spinal needle inserted perpendicular to the surface of the grapefruit, straight through the grapefruit center, without bending the needle extrinsically. Note that the needle tip deflects slightly downward, in a direction opposite the bevel face (*arrow*).

site to the bevel face) toward the direction you wish the needle to go. The needle should be advanced with short discrete movements using intermittent fluoroscopy. **For safety, the physician should always remember to keep his or her hands out of the primary x-ray beam.**

For directing beveled or nonbeveled needles, with a straight or bowed shaft, it is best to insert the needle by holding the needle hub as just described while at the same time stabilizing the needle shaft at skin surface between the opposite thumb and index finger (Fig. 1-7). The needle cannula and inner stylet are advanced as a single unit with the thumb pushing on the stylet hub. This technique keeps the needle from taking an erratic path. Advancing the needle with the shaft straight will only deflect the needle a small amount. When the needle is confined to the superficial soft tissues, moving the hub cephalad will direct the needle tip in a caudal direction. **However, when the needle is advanced deep to the superficial soft tissues, the opposite actually holds true.** To produce more significant deflection, the portion of the needle external to the patient must be bowed. For example, to optimally deflect a beveled needle tip in a caudal direction, the notch on the hub should be placed cephalad and the needle hub should be bowed caudad (in the direction opposite the notch). This produces a large smooth bow on the needle shaft (Fig. 1-8).

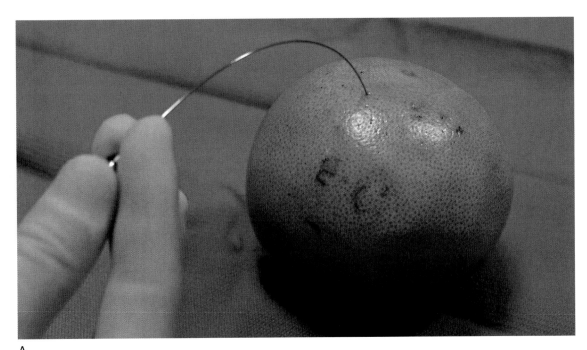

A

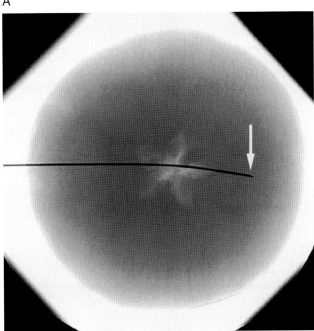

B

Figure 1-5 ■ Demonstration of needle deflection in a grapefruit, with **bowed needle insertion**. *A*, A bend is then placed on the needle, extrinsic to the grapefruit, while inserting the needle into the grapefruit. *B*, After the maneuver demonstrated in *A*, the needle hub was **released** and another radiograph of the grapefruit was obtained. The needle tip is deflected in a downward direction, to a greater degree (*arrow*) than shown in Figure 1-4. Note that the needle shaft is not bowed in passing through the outer portion of the grapefruit until it traverses the tougher tissue near the grapefruit center. This is because the outer, edible portion of the grapefruit is soft and the tissue offers little resistance to the advancing needle. However, when the bowed needle passes through the denser, tougher tissue near the grapefruit center, the needle deflects to a greater degree, because there exists greater resistance to the bowed needle advancement at denser tissue interfaces.

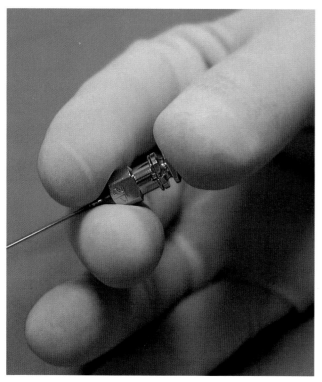

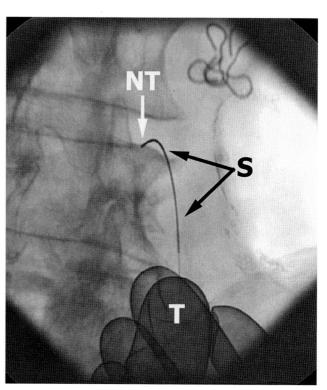

Figure 1-6 ■ Proper technique for holding the needle hub during needle insertion. The thumb is positioned over the stylet hub, and the needle cannula hub is supported between the index and middle fingers. Note that the stylet hub is fitted snugly into the cannula hub, ready for needle insertion. The needle should be inserted with the **thumb** pushing on the stylet hub.

Figure 1-8 ■ Radiograph showing needle bending technique used for insertion of a 22-gauge needle for a medial branch block procedure. Wearing lead-lined gloves covered by sterile gloves, the operator has inserted the needle into the target location, where the needle tip (NT) is positioned. The shaft (S) of the needle is bent during needle insertion to facilitate the desired directional movement of the needle tip. The operator's thumb (T) is pushing the needle hub. We do not advocate or recommend placing one's hands in the primary x-ray beam during needle insertion, as shown here.

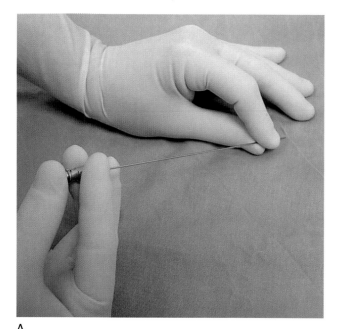

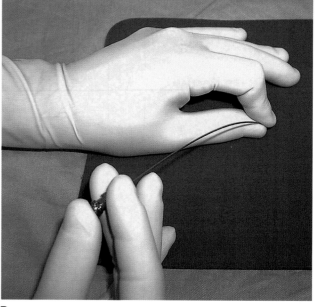

A

B

Figure 1-7 ■ Proper technique for holding the needle with both hands during needle insertion, for a right-handed operator. *A,* **Straight needle insertion technique.** The needle shaft, at the skin surface, is held between the left thumb and index finger. The needle cannula hub is supported between the right thumb and index finger. *B,* **Bent needle insertion technique.** The needle is held in the same fashion as shown in *A,* except that the needle shaft is bowed, with the convexity of the bowed shaft directed cephalad, which is toward the same side as the notch on the needle hub. During needle advancement, the needle tip will tend to move in the direction opposite the side of the needle hub notch.

Once these relatively simple techniques are mastered, even seemingly difficult needle placements become second nature. For example, it will become straightforward for the operator to insert a needle through a small target window of 2 mm in diameter or into a narrowed L5-S1 disc space from a steep, craniocaudad angle.

References

1 Drummond GB, Scott DH. Deflection of spinal needles by the bevel. Anaesthesia 1980; 35:854–857.
2 Sitzman BT, Uncles DR. The effects of needle type, gauge, and tip bend on spinal needle deflection. Anesth Analg 1996; 82:297–301.

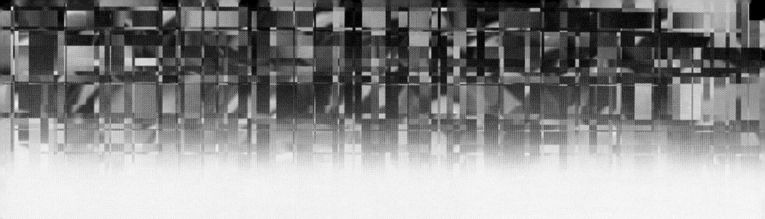

Chapter 2

Facet Joint Injection and Medial Branch Block

- Leo F. Czervionke, MD
- Douglas S. Fenton, MD

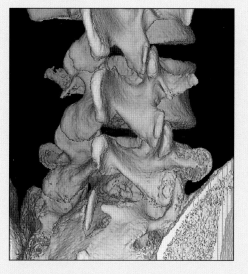

BACKGROUND

Back pain is a complex, often multifactorial condition affecting millions of persons worldwide. The prevalence of lumbar or cervical facet (zygapophysial) joint disease associated with back pain is unknown. Although many technologic, pharmaceutical, and surgical advances for the treatment of back pain have occurred in recent years, the search for the precise cause of back pain in a given patient can be a complex, difficult process. Many factors may contribute to back pain, including vertebral instability, neuromuscular imbalance, disc disease, ligamentous disorders, inflammatory conditions of the nerve roots, facet disease, infections of the vertebrae or discs, and neoplasia. The methods in which diagnostic procedures are performed to localize the source of back pain vary widely. The interpretation and the relevance of these studies continue to be subjects of great controversy.

The facet joint is a true synovium-lined joint allowing the spine to flex, extend, and rotate. Many conditions exist that produce facet disease. However, the major cause of facet joint disease is osteoarthritis, a degenerative condition that results in reduction or loss of facet joint cartilage, erosions of the adjacent bone margins of the facets, bony overgrowth of the facets and articular processes, and, ultimately, instability of the facet joint itself, which may result in vertebral subluxation. The sensory nerve endings innervating the facets and surrounding tissues become irritated by the inflammatory process,

9

resulting in the sensation of pain. Chemical mediators and immunologic factors likely play an important role in pain generation.

In 1963, Hirsch and colleagues demonstrated that pain in the upper back and thigh could be produced by injecting a 10% hypertonic saline solution in the region of the facet joints.[1] Others have demonstrated that the injection of saline or iodinated contrast medium into the cervical or lumbar facets can elicit a pain response in a predictable distribution, depending on the facet joint injected.[2, 3] The intensity of the pain produced is proportional to the volume of fluid injected.[4] The precise manner in which facet arthropathy produces low back pain is still not completely understood.[5] The facet joint is continually subjected to shear, compression, and torsion forces during everyday activity. The shear force on the facet cartilage is greatest with the spine in full flexion. However, maximal pressure in the lumbar facet joints occurs with the spine in extension.[5] Repeated or excessive hyperflexion, hyperextension, or twisting movements may eventually result in facet disease. Disc narrowing may also predispose to facet disease. When the disc becomes narrowed, up to 70% of the compressive force usually applied to the disc is transferred to the facet joints.[6] Developmental anomalies such as facet tropism or spondylolysis may also predispose the facets to disease.

A variety of neurochemical constituents operating at the synapse level and neuropeptides, which have been identified within the facet joint capsule, probably mediate the pain response.[7, 8] Future therapy will undoubtedly be directed at modifying how these chemicals function to alleviate facet-related pain. Certainly, the paraspinal neural interconnections determine which levels will be affected by a facet block.

Unfortunately, facet disease often is not limited to one facet joint, and other degenerative disorders, such as disc disease or spinal instability, contribute to a patient's pain. Therefore, localization of the source of the facet pain can be a challenging process because of referral to anatomic areas remote from the facet joint and because patients with chronic back pain often have other conditions that also contribute to their pain symptom-complex. Psychogenic factors, related to long-standing illness, dependency on drugs, and certain personal relationships in dealing with chronic pain, can make the search for the primary source of back pain elusive. Chronic facet disorders are more common in women.[9]

Imaging studies including radiographs, computed tomography (CT), magnetic resonance (MR) imaging, and bone scanning are often valuable as screening diagnostic tools in the evaluation of back pain and may demonstrate the source of the pain, such as a herniated disc or tumor. These imaging modalities can also detect facet disease even in its early stages. Imaging studies, including radiography, MR imaging, and CT, are unreliable indicators of facetogenic pain.[10] Some patients exhibiting severe facet disease as demonstrated on MR imaging or CT are relatively asymptomatic. Conversely, some patients experiencing severe facetogenic pain have relatively mild facet abnormalities demonstrated on radiographs.

Because imaging cannot be relied on for the diagnosis of facet-related pain, clinical information elicited by a careful history and physical exmination is a vital component of the evaluation. Once the diagnosis of facet syndrome is suggested, a decision is made whether to perform a diagnostic

or therapeutic facet block. We recommend that diagnostic low-volume intra-articular facet injections and/or medial branch blockades be performed initially to confirm the clinical suspicion of facet-related pain and to ascertain which facet joints are involved, because disease in one or more facet joints may be contributing to the patient's pain. We consider a diagnostic facet block positive when the patient experiences 80% pain reduction in the distribution of the nerves that innervate the joint being injected.

It may be necessary to perform facet blocks at other levels or at different times to more accurately determine the likely source of the patient's pain, because back pain can arise from more than one spinal or paraspinal source, and a solitary joint injection may relieve only a portion of the patient's pain.

The production of pain during a facet joint injection does not necessarily mean that the patient's pain is arising from that joint.[6] **Rather, the most important information obtained from a diagnostic facet injection or medial branch block is whether the patient's typical pain was relieved by the injection.**

The facet block is a needle injection procedure in which an anesthetic agent (short- and/or long-acting) is injected into the joint space. A facet block is primarily used as a diagnostic procedure, but it may have short-term therapeutic benefit as well. It is common practice to add a steroidal agent to the anesthetic agent. By doing this, it is assumed that the anesthetic agent will produce rapid pain relief and that the steroid will produce more sustained pain relief response by reducing any inflammation that may exist in the facet joint. The assumption that the steroid will produce a longer period of pain relief has not been proven and has been refuted in the literature.[11, 12] Although unproved, the common thinking in current practice based on uncontrolled studies is that the addition of the steroidal agent is useful and results in no harm to the patient; therefore, this practice is widely accepted.[4, 13-18]

Careful documentation of the procedure, the levels injected, and the patient's response is critical to gain a full appreciation of the patient's pain response pattern. Procedural documentation should include what procedure was performed, what anesthetic was given (e.g., short-acting, long-acting), whether a steroid was given, and, most importantly, a pain diary of the patient's symptoms immediately after the procedure and continuing for 5 to 7 days.

All the information gained should be evaluated by the physician in making an overall assessment of the patient's situation and in deciding whether the patient has facetogenic pain. If the physician believes that facet pain is contributing to the patient's overall pain symptoms, a **therapeutic facet block** can be performed by injecting a larger volume of anesthetic and steroid into the facet joint and/or into the soft tissues surrounding the facets. Repeated therapeutic facet blocks may be necessary to control the patient's pain.

If repeated therapeutic facet blocks are unsuccessful, the patient should be reassessed with imaging or other diagnostic injections to confirm the source of the pain. If the facet joint is again determined to be the source of the pain, then destruction of the facet nerve supply by radiofrequency ablation of the medial branches of the dorsal primary rami of the offending facet should be considered to diminish or eliminate the pain. **Radiofrequency denervation is discussed in detail in Chapter 3.**

The **intra-articular** facet block involves injection of an anesthetic agent into the facet joint. It is believed that this method may be more effective than **extra-articular** (extra-capsular) facet injections.[9] A steroidal agent is usually added to the injection mixture (injectate). This combination is believed to provide a twofold therapeutic effect: the anesthetic dulls the pain from the nerve endings in the synovial lining of the joint space, and the steroid theoretically reduces the inflammation that may exist in the joint and that may be responsible for irritating the nerve endings. With an intra-articular facet block, one usually instills 1 to 3 mL of the injection mixture into the joint. A greater volume of injectate (3 to 5 mL) is often instilled for an extra-articular facet block. Both types of injections may be effective in relieving the patient's pain. Some investigators believe the therapeutic benefit of a low-volume intra-articular injection is negligible and that the therapeutic effect in pain reduction with an intra-articular injection is achieved only with a larger instilled volume (>3 mL) that results in extravasation of the injectate from the facet capsule into the epidural space.[19, 20] Our experience has been that if the patient experienced pain concordant with his or her typical pain when the joint was injected, a therapeutic benefit results even when small injection volumes are instilled into the intact facet joint.

Single, *uncontrolled* diagnostic facet blocks can be unreliable for the diagnosis of facetogenic pain because of the high placebo rate and false-positive rate.[21–23] There is a widely held belief that a single, uncontrolled facet block or a single pair of medial branch blocks is not sufficient to prove that a given patient's pain response is facet related, because there is a high rate of false-positive pain response to facet injection.

Sequential facet injections using *controlled* facet blocks are advocated by some to allow a more accurate assessment of the patient's true pain response. There are two methods of performing controlled facet blocks. In the first method, the suspected facet is injected with a saline placebo on one occasion and with a conventional anesthetic on another occasion. If the placebo control block method is used, informed consent should be obtained from the patient so that he or she clearly understands that one or both of the injections may not provide any therapeutic benefit.

In the second method, *comparative blocks* are performed by injecting a short-acting anesthetic (e.g., 0.3 mL 2% lidocaine) into the facet joint on one occasion and injecting the same facet joint with a long-acting anesthetic (e.g., 0.3 mL 0.5% bupivacaine) on another occasion. In either method, patients should not be told what injection agent is being used and should not be "coached" as to what their response should be. Careful documentation of the injection agent used and the patient's pain response is essential. With comparative controlled blocks, if the offending facet is injected, ideally the patient will report longer relief of his or her pain with the long-acting anesthetic and a shorter duration of pain relief after injection of the short-acting anesthetic. Patients who respond in this ideal fashion to comparative blocks may be candidates for radiofrequency denervation.

Strong advocates of comparative blocks or placebo injections recommend that medial branch radiofrequency denervation not be performed unless the patient responds appropriately to the control injections. Unfortunately, this ideal response to comparative injections does not always occur, but the absence of such a response does not necessarily indicate that the injected facet joint is not the source of the pain, because many factors may be involved. Irrespective of the result of the controlled blocks, the treating physician has the right to proceed with additional diagnostic or therapeutic procedures based on knowledge of the patient and the patient's overall symptom-complex.

We do not perform placebo-controlled facet blocks. We do use comparative blocks in our approach to diagnosing and treating facet disease. We use the following paradigm in our practice. If the patient has an excellent response (complete or near-complete relief of pain) to a diagnostic or therapeutic facet block, we perform a medial branch block with a long-acting anesthetic (0.3 to 0.5 mL of 0.5% bupivacaine) when the patient returns with recurrent pain. If the patient again has an excellent response, we generally recommend medial branch radiofrequency denervation. If the patient reports partial pain relief, we recommend comparative medial branch blocks as described previously. If there is an appropriate response to short- and long-acting anesthetics, respectively, we then recommend a medial branch radiofrequency denervation procedure.

Because the pain response to repeated facet injections can vary widely in the same patient, we prefer medial branch blocks to intra-articular injections when performing comparative blocks. The inconsistent response to repeated facet injections can be related to the relative avascularity of the facet joint, resulting in variable absorption of the anesthetic agent or possibly variable dispersion of the anesthetic agent in the diseased facet joint or into the surrounding perifacetal soft tissues. This is the reason some investigators recommend the injection of water-soluble contrast agent to confirm needle position before instilling the anesthetic agent into the facet joint space for facet blocks. However, we believe contrast medium injection is unnecessary if meticulous attention is given to anatomy and proper needle positioning.

In the case of medial branch blocks, false-negative results can occur if an insufficient amount of anesthetic is deposited at the target point. This may occur because of suboptimal needle positioning, inadequate concentration of the anesthetic agent deposited on the nerve, or inadvertent injection into adjacent vessels that carry the anesthetic agent away from the intended target zone.[24] Injection of a larger volume (more than 0.5 mL) of anesthetic agent for a diagnostic medial branch block can also produce a misleading response to pain, because some of the agent may diffuse into the epidural space.

ANATOMIC CONSIDERATIONS

Lumbar Facet Joints

The articular facet is a conical, bony protuberance with a hyaline cartilage cap located on both ends of the vertebral articular pillar bilaterally. The facets from adjacent vertebrae articulate to form a joint space, which is a true synovium-lined joint. The lumbar facet joints have an arcuate configuration as viewed on axial CT images, with the concavity of the "C"-shaped arc facing inward (Fig. 2-1). The posterior

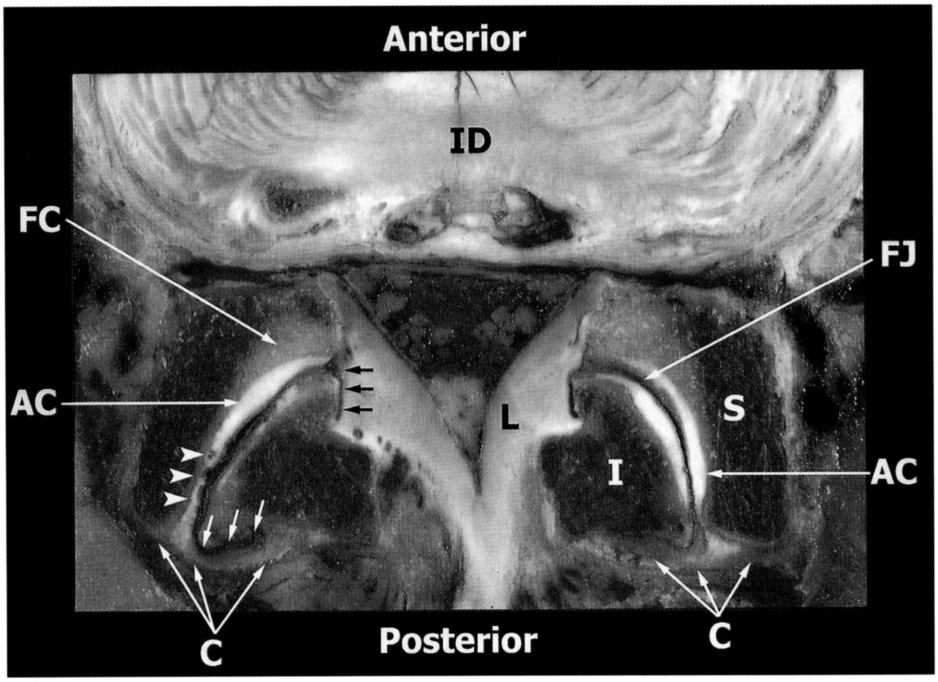

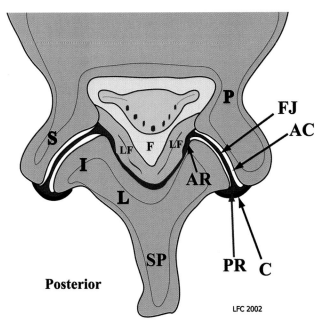

Figure 2-1 ■ Anatomy of the lumbar facets. Axial cryomicrotome image of cadaver specimen at the disc level. The articular facets are the concave surfaces of the superior (S) and inferior (I) articular processes. The articular facets are composed of facet cortex (FC) and overlying white articular cartilage (AC). The synovial-lined facet joint (FJ) is located between the apposing white articular surfaces. Eroded articular cartilage indicated by small white *arrowheads* is secondary to degenerative joint disease (osteoarthritis). Posterior recess facet joint (*small white arrows*) extends posterior to inferior articular process. Anterior recess of facet joint (*small black arrows*) extends between anterior margin of inferior articular process and ligamentum flavum. C = posterior fibrous capsule of facet joint; ID = intervertebral disc; L = ligamentum flavum. (Image from cryomicrotome collection compiled from work by Peter Pech, MD, and Victor M. Haughton, MD, included here with permission of Victor M. Haughton.)

portion of the lumbar facet joint is oriented in a more sagittal plane, whereas the anterior portion of the joint is oriented in a more coronal plane (Fig. 2-2). Because of this arcuate configuration, the joint space may appear "open" at fluoroscopy when the beam is passing tangential to the anterior portion of the "C," when in fact it is not readily accessible from a posterolateral approach (Fig. 2-3).[25] Therefore, it is important to access the posterior portion of the joint, which is oriented in an oblique sagittal plane and is most easily entered with a needle using a shallow approach angle of 10 to 20 degrees from straight anteroposterior (AP). However, depending on the orientation of the facet joint, it may be necessary to use an approach angle of 30 to 45 degrees to enter the joint.

The posterior portion of the facet joint is enveloped by a thick, tough fibrous capsule, but the fibrous capsule is not present anteromedially.[26] A prominent synovium-lined recess does extend anteromedial to the facet joint, where it often extends for a variable distance between the ligamentum flavum medially and the lamina laterally. In some patients, the anterior synovial recess may extend into the ligamentum flavum. This anteromedial synovial recess of the lumbar facet joint is not readily accessible to percutaneous needle placement. It is the inferior portion of this posterior recess that is most accessible to percutaneous needle puncture for facet joint injection.[26, 27] The posterior synovial recess of the lumbar facet joint often extends beyond the articulating surfaces of the lumbar facets into the posterior fibrous capsule. This posterior recess may also extend, to a variable

Figure 2-2 ■ Axial illustration of lumbar facet anatomy at the pedicle level. Synovial-lined facet joint (FJ, *in red*) has an anteromedial recess (AR) bound by a fibrous capsule that may extend beneath the ligamentum flavum (LF) for a variable distance. The posterior recess (PR) is the target site for lumbar facet injection. The needle must penetrate a tough fibrous capsule (C), which can be "felt" as a sensation of increased resistance when traversing the capsule with the needle. AC = facet articular cartilage; S = superior articular process; I = inferior articular process; L = ligamentum flavum; SP = spinous process; P = pedicle; F = posterior epidural fat.

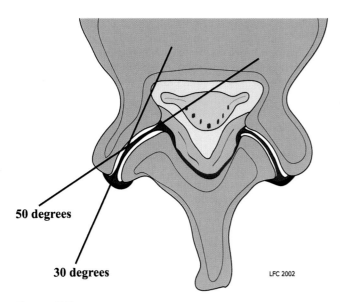

Figure 2-3 ■ Illustration of lumbar facet joint approach angle for percutaneous needle puncture. Starting from straight anteroposterior, the fluoroscope (or patient) is rotated until the facet joint just appears "open" (shown here at 30 degrees), which is the optimal needle trajectory for access into the posterior recess of the joint in this illustration. The facet joint may also appear "open" fluoroscopically at 50 degrees because the x-ray beam at this angle is tangential to the anterior portion of the facet joint, but a needle placed using this trajectory would be impeded by the postero-lateral margin of the superior articular process.

degree, along the posterior surface of either the superior or inferior articular process (see Figs. 2-1 and 2-2).[26]

Fibroadipose pads (menisci) are commonly embedded within the superior and inferior recesses and are covered by synovium, which is in continuity with the synovium of the joint capsule.[28] These menisci are fat-filled synovial reflections that contain fibrous tissue.[29] It has been suggested that synovial villi in these fat pads may become inflamed if the fat pads are somehow trapped by the articular facets.[5, 30] The menisci should not be confused with the tiny fibrofatty "meniscoids" that are embedded in the periphery of the facet cartilage in some patients. The role of these meniscoids is uncertain, but they may function as facet joint stabilizers. A meniscoid that becomes detached could act as a loose body in the joint and theoretically produce pain by "locking" the facet joint.[28]

The inferior portion of the posterior recess of the lumbar facet joint is larger than the superior portion. It is neither necessary nor even desirable to position the needle deep in the joint between the articulating facets, because the portion of the joint space between the articular facets is small in volume and one could argue that needle placement could actually cause damage to the cartilaginous articulating surfaces. The optimal target zone for needle placement is the inferior portion of the posterior joint recess just inferolateral to the inferior articular process (Fig. 2-4). With the needle tip positioned in the inferior recess, the needle tip tends to

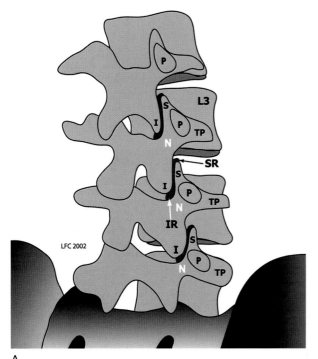

A

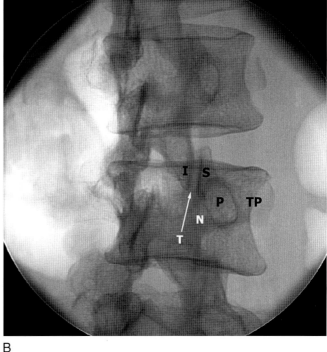

B

Figure 2-4 ■ Optimal entry point for facet joint injection. *A*, Illustration of important bone landmarks in LAO radiograph. Recognition of the "Scotty dog" helps to locate key anatomic structures radiographically, including the pedicle (P, eye), superior articular process (S, ear), inferior articular process (I, front leg/foot) and transverse process (TP, nose). The "neck" (N) of the Scotty dog corresponds to the location of the pars interarticularis. The facet joint may be punctured anywhere in the posterior recess (*red zone*). The optimal puncture site for lumbar facet injection is in the prominent inferior recess (IR) of the facet joint posteriorly, which is located inferolateral to the inferior articular process (I) and above the dog's neck (N). Anatomically, the inferior recess is larger than the posterior portion of the superior recess (SR). *B*, LAO radiograph demonstrating optimal target zone (T) for lumbar facet injection located inferolateral to the inferior articular process (I). S = superior articular process. Facet joint (between I and S) appears wide open at this obliquity. P = pedicle; TP = transverse process; N = neck of Scotty dog (pars interarticularis).

project just superior to the "neck" of the "Scotty dog" fluoroscopically (see Fig. 2-4). Using an x-ray fluoroscopic approach, the presence of this posterior inferior recess allows injected contrast agent to enter the joint even in narrowed, severely osteoarthritic facet joints where the hypertrophic facets appear to obstruct the pathway into the joint space proper (Fig. 2-5). If the facets are overgrown, as a result of osteoarthritis, the hypertrophic bone margins may impede needle access to the joint, even though the joint appears accessible fluoroscopically. In this situation, CT may be helpful in selecting the appropriate needle trajectory (Fig. 2-6).

It is important to understand the innervation of the facets. The **facet block** represents a selective block of nerve endings in the richly innervated joint capsule.[8, 31, 32] These pain-sensing (nociceptive) nerve endings connect with sensory fibers, which join with the medial branch of the dorsal primary ramus (Fig. 2-7). The facet joint synovium is also innervated by sympathetic and parasympathetic fibers,[7] but the presence of nociceptors in the synovium is a subject for debate.[5, 33]

One can achieve a result similar to an intra-articular facet block without entering the facet joint by performing a **medial branch block** by directly injecting a small amount of anesthetic mixture adjacent to the medial branch of the dorsal ramus.[34, 35] A medial branch block is performed both to selectively block a given facet joint to diagnose pain originating from that facet joint and to identify patients who will benefit from medial branch radiofrequency ablation. The medial branch of the dorsal ramus passes through a small foramen in the intertransverse ligament in an antero-posterior direction and then lies against the bone, bound by connective tissue to the periosteum, in a small groove formed where the superior articular process joins the base of the transverse process, which is where the superior and inferior target zones for the medial branch block are located (Fig. 2-8).[36–39]

Slightly more inferiorly, at the level of the caudal margin of the facet joint, the medial branch turns medially and passes through a tiny notch formed between the mamillary and the accessory processes, where the nerve is actually

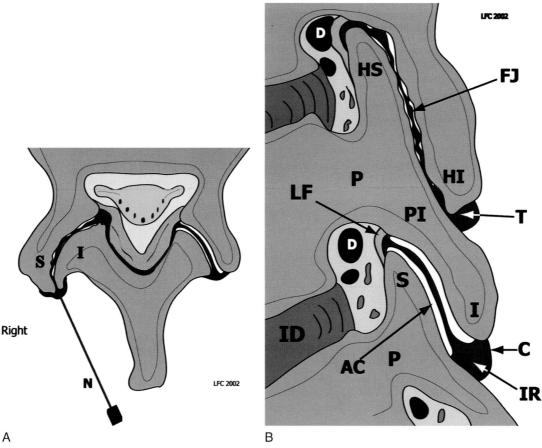

A   B

Figure 2-5 ■ Axial and sagittal illustrations through lumbar facet joints. *A,* Axial illustration of lumbar facet osteoarthritis. Synovial-lined facet joints in *red.* The right inferior articular process (I) and superior articular process (S) show bone overgrowth (facet hypertrophy) while the bony articular facets and articular cartilage are eroded. Interfacetal joint space is narrowed on the right. The right posterior capsule is thickened and redundant. The right posterior recess is smaller than normal but still accessible to needle (N) placement from the trajectory shown. Note that the posterior recess extends more medially along the posterior surface of the inferior articular process for both the normal (left) and abnormal (right) facet joints. *B,* Sagittal illustration directly through the pars interarticularis (PI) showing two contiguous lumbar facet joints. The lower facet joint is normal with intact articular cartilage (AC) and normal-appearing inferior recess (IR) and posterior joint capsule (C). Normal configuration of inferior (I) and superior (S) articular processes. ID = intervertebral disc; D = dorsal root within foramen; LF = ligamentum flavum. The upper facet joint (FJ) is narrowed by facet erosions and articular cartilage damage secondary to osteoarthritis. Hypertrophic superior articular process (HS), thickened ligamentum flavum, and bulging disc cause narrowing of the more superior neural foramen. The hypertrophic inferior articular process (HI) narrows the inferior recess, but needle placement is possible using a posterior trajectory (T) into the inferior recess of the diseased joint.

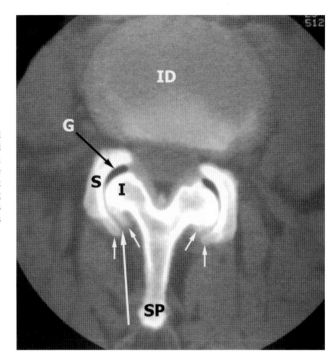

Figure 2-6 ■ Axial CT image demonstrates severely degenerated lumbar facets with gas (G) in the facet joints and hypertrophic inferior and superior articular processes (*short arrows*). S = superior articular process; I = inferior articular process; ID = intervertebral disc. The hypertrophic facets may produce a misleading appearance at fluoroscopy with the facet joint appearing "open" when in fact the hypertropic facets are preventing access to the joint. Optimal needle trajectory, indicated by *long arrow*, is required to access the posterior recess of the right facet joint. SP = spinous process.

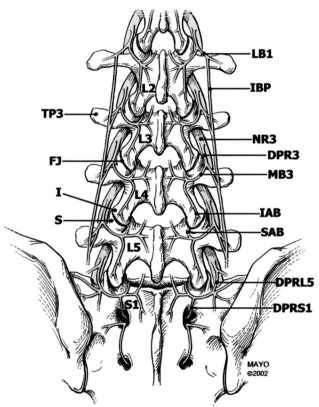

Figure 2-7 ■ Illustration of posterior view of lumbar spine and posterior neural structures. Laminae of L2 through S1 are labeled. *Left*: TP3 = transverse process of L3; FJ = facet (zygapophysial) joint L3-4; I = inferior articular process of L4, S = superior articular process of L5. *Right*: LB1 = lateral branch of dorsal primary ramus of L1; IBP = intermediate branch plexus; NR3 = third lumbar nerve root; DPR3 = dorsal primary ramus of L3; MB3 = medial branch of dorsal primary ramus of L3; IAB = inferior articular branches from L3 medial branch (supplies L4-5 facet joint); SAB = superior articular branches from L4 (supplies L4-5 facet joint also); DPRL5 = dorsal primary ramus of L5; DPRS1 = dorsal primary ramus of S1.

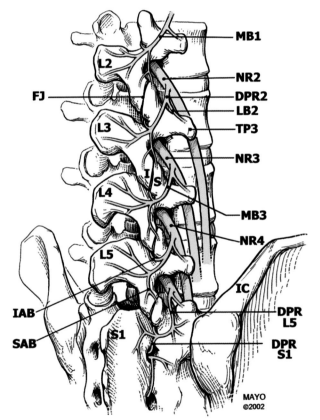

Figure 2-8 ■ Illustration of right posterior view of lumbosacral spine showing key right posterior neural structures. L2 through S1 spinous processes labeled. *Right*: MB1 = medial branch of L1 dorsal primary ramus; NR2 = L2 nerve root; DPR2 = L2 dorsal primary ramus; LB2 = lateral branch of L2 dorsal primary ramus; TP3 = L3 transverse process; NR3 = L3 nerve root; MB = medial branch of L3 dorsal primary ramus that extends around the base of the right superior articular process (S) of L4 and innervates portions of the right L3-4 and L4-5 facet joint capsules; NR4 = L4 nerve root; IC = iliac crest; DPRL5 = L5 dorsal primary ramus; DPRS1 = S1 dorsal primary ramus; I = inferior articular process L3; S = superior articular process of L4. *Left*: FJ = L2-3 facet (zygapophysial) joint, which is innervated by branches of L1 and L2 medial branch nerves; IAB = inferior articular branches from medial branch of L4 dorsal primary ramus; SAB = superior articular branches from medial branch of L4 dorsal primary ramus.

15

held in place within the notch by a tiny ligament called the "mamilloaccessory ligament" (Fig. 2-9).[38] Beyond the ligament, the medial branch sends branches to innervate the zygapophysial joint, multifidus muscle, interspinal muscles, and the interspinous ligaments.[40] There are three branches of the medial branch: the proximal branch, which hooks around the articular process to supply the facet above; the medial descending branch, which courses inferomedially to innervate the superior and medial portions of the facet capsule below, plus muscle and skin; and the ascending branch, which supplies the facet above (see Fig. 2-9).[18] The lateral branch of the dorsal primary ramus supplies the erector spinae muscle group but does not innervate the facets.

A given lumbar facet joint is innervated by nerve fibers from medial branch nerves at two levels. The medial branch nerve at a given level innervates the inferior portion of the facet above and the superior portion of the facet below.[38] For example, the L3 medial branch (which courses over the base of the L4 transverse process) innervates both the **inferior** portion of the L3-4 facet joint and the superior portion of the L4-5 facet joint (see Figs. 2-7 through 2-9). The **superior**

portion of the L3-4 facet is innervated by the L2 medial branch. The L3-4 facet is **not** innervated by the L4 medial branch as one might be tempted to believe. Likewise, the L4-5 facet is innervated by the L3 medial branch superiorly and the L4 medial branch inferiorly.[30] There is evidence that innervation of the lower lumbar facets does not always follow the just-described segmental nerve distribution, that is, the lower lumbar facets may also receive nonsegmental neural contributions from upper lumbar levels by means of sympathetic postganglionic neurons, which can also influence facet pain at lower lumbar levels.[7] This may help to explain why a seemingly well placed medial branch block may relieve only a portion of the patient's pain. However, many other factors may also play a role.

Thoracic Facet Joints

The thoracic facet joints, which are oriented in a near-coronal plane, help protect the spine from shearing force (Fig. 2-10). They are not directly accessible from a straight posterior

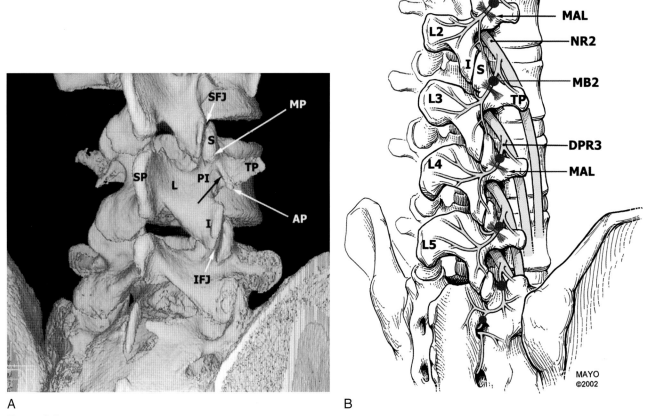

A   B

Figure 2-9 ■ Oblique anatomy of the posterior lumbar spine. *A,* Right posterior view (20 degrees from straight posterior view) of lower lumbar spine on surface rendered three-dimensional CT image. Right L4 posterior vertebral anatomic bone landmarks are labeled, including superior articular process (S), inferior articular process (I), pars interarticularis (PI), lamina (L), and spinous process (SP). The mamilloaccessory ligament overlies a bony ridge (*black arrow*) and extends between the mamillary process (MP) (part of the superior articular process) and the accessory process (AP) (part of the transverse process). The medial branch of the posterior primary ramus (*not shown*) lies deep to the mamilloaccessory ligament. SFJ = superior facet joint (L3-4); IFJ = inferior facet joint (L4-5). *B,* Right posterior oblique illustration of the lumbar spine with pertinent neural structures demonstrated. Medial branch block target zones (*red dots*) are indicated at multiple lumbar levels. MB2 = medial branch block target zone at L2 level; MAL = mamilloaccessory ligament labeled at L2 and L4 levels; NR2 = right second nerve root; DPR3 = dorsal primary ramus of L3; S = superior articular process of L3; I = inferior articular process of L2; TP = transverse process of L3. Spinous processes of L2 through L5 are labeled.

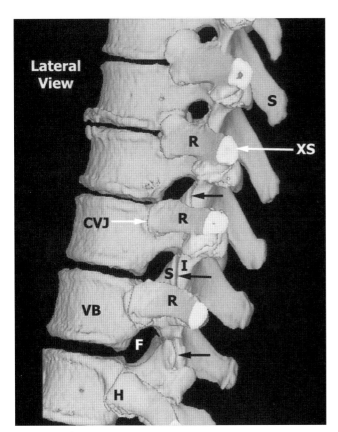

Figure 2-10 ▪ Direct lateral view of the thoracic spine as seen in this three-dimensional volume CT surface-rendered image allows visualization into the thoracic facet joints (*black arrows*) owing to the nearly coronal orientation of the thoracic facet joints. Unfortunately, percutaneous needle access using a direct lateral approach is not feasible because it would require the needle to traverse the pleura and lung. R = anterior surface of the posterior ribs in contact with posterior pleural surface; XS = cross section of rib at limit of image volume; I = inferior articular process; S = superior articular process; CVJ = costovertebral joint; VB = vertebral body; F = neural foramen; H = head of thoracic rib.

approach because of the overlying lamina (Fig. 2-11). This orientation of the thoracic facets makes direct facet joint access extremely difficult from a percutaneous approach, because the lungs prevent access to the thoracic facets from a direct lateral approach and a posterolateral approach would not allow intra-articular needle placement using a single needle. The innervation and numbering for the thoracic medial branch nerves is similar to that in the lumbar region.

Cervical Facet Joints

The cervical facet joints are located between apposing articular facets of adjoining cervical vertebrae. The superior and inferior articular facets are joined by articular pillars of bone, which anatomically correspond to the pars interarticularis in the lumbar region. The cervical facet joint is oriented in a plane 45 degrees from the coronal or sagittal plane (Fig. 2-12) and is also obliquely oriented in the craniocaudal direction (Fig. 2-13), so that only a portion of the facet joint is included on a given axial anatomic or imaging section. A thick fibrous capsule is located lateral to the cervical facet

joint. Synovium-lined recesses of the facet joint extend beneath the capsule adjacent to the lateral margin of the superior and inferior articular facets (Fig. 2-14). The lateral recess of the cervical facet joint is accessible to percutaneous needle puncture for cervical facet joint injections.

The lower cervical medial branch nerves are similar anatomically to the thoracic and lumbar medial branch nerves. The C4-C8 posterior primary rami arise from their respective dorsal root ganglia just lateral to the intervertebral foramen (Fig. 2-15). The medial branch nerve arises from the posterior primary ramus and then passes around the ipsilateral articular pillar. As in the lumbar spine, there is a dual nerve supply to the facet joint. An ascending branch innervates the facet joint above, and a descending branch innervates the facet joint below. However, the numbering of the medial branches is different in the cervical region compared with the thoracic and lumbar spine. In the cervical region, the medial branch nerve that extends around the C4 articular pillar is the C4 medial branch nerve (see Fig. 2-15). For example, at the C5-6 level, the facet joint is innervated by the medial branches of C5 and C6. This numbering applies to the C4 through C7 levels. Because a C8 medial branch exists, the numbering of the thoracic and lumbar facet innervation is different from that of the cervical facets.

The role of the medial branch of C3 differs somewhat from that of the lower cervical nerves. There is a deep medial branch that courses around the articular pillar of C3 similar to the medial branches from C4 through C7. The C3 medial branch has a component that innervates the C3-4 facet joint, but it provides only negligible innervation to the C2-3 facet joint. The primary nerve supply to the C2-3 facet arises from a large superficial medial branch of C3, known as the **third occipital nerve**. This nerve courses around the lateral aspect of the ipsilateral C2-3 facet joint and innervates the C2-3 facet joint, as well as providing cutaneous neural supply for the suboccipital region (see Fig. 2-15). The C2-3 facet also receives supply from small communicating branches arising from the third occipital nerve at its origin.

PATIENT SELECTION

The choice of facet joint to be injected is usually based on clinical findings. The joint selection is usually made by identifying the point of maximal tenderness to palpation and considering the cutaneous distribution of the pain sensation. Radiographs and CT are unreliable in predicting the level of facet pain because facetogenic pain may be associated with normal as well as severely degenerating facets.[10] Primary disorders of the cartilage may also be associated with facet pain.[10]

MR imaging using T2-weighted fast spin echo technique with fat saturation or gadolinium-enhanced MR imaging with fat saturation are relatively new techniques that may identify active inflammation within and/or surrounding the facet joint and aid in diagnosing which facets are likely candidates for a facet block procedure (Fig. 2-16). Patients with facet-related pain often have a history and physical examination consistent with facet syndrome.[41] However, it is important to keep in mind that controversy exists as to what actually constitutes a facet syndrome.[42] The following

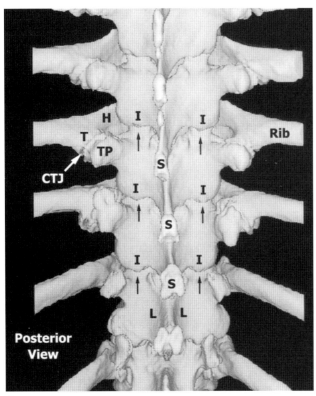

A

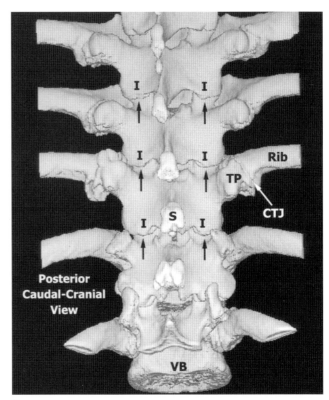

B

Figure 2-11 ▪ Percutaneous approaches to the thoracic facet joint. *A*, Straight posterior view of thoracic spine as seen in this three-dimensional volume CT surface-rendered image. The inferior articular processes (I) shield the upper portions of the superior articular processes (*black arrows*) and the facet joints from view. S = spinous process; H = head of rib; T = tuberosity of rib; TP = transverse process; L = lamina; CTJ = costotransverse joint. *B*, Posterior caudocranial view of thoracic spine in three-dimensional volume CT surface-rendered image. Inferior articular processes (I) still cover the facet joint but superior facets (*arrows*) are now just barely visible. A posterior perifacetal facet block can be performed in this projection with the needle trajectory in a caudocranial trajectory parallel to the long axis of the spinous process (S). *C*, Preferred approach for thoracic facet block: 45-degree right posterior oblique view of the thoracic spine (with slight caudocranial angulation) in three-dimensional volume CT surface-rendered image. The inferior articular process still shields the majority of the thoracic facet joint. The inferolateral margin of the thoracic facets are just visible (*arrows*). The needle is positioned above the transverse process and posterior to the posteromedial aspect of the rib (R). H = head of rib R; I = inferior articular process; S = superior articular process; CVJ = costovertebral joint; CTJ = costotransverse joint.

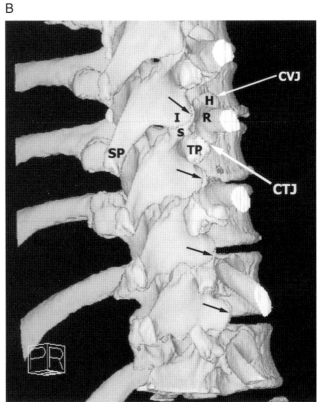

C

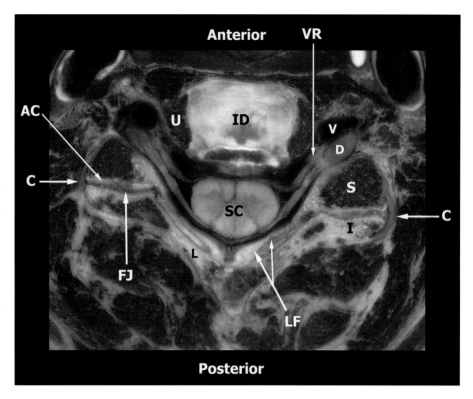

Figure 2-12 ▪ Anatomy of cervical facet joint at intervertebral disc level. Axial cryomicrotome image of cadaver. Cervical facets are oriented in an oblique coronal plane and are readily accessed by a needle using a direct lateral approach. Thick fibrous capsule (C) is located along the lateral aspect of the facet joint. Deep to the fibrous capsule is the lateral recess, which extends along the lateral margin of both the superior (S) and inferior (I) articular process. AC = articular cartilage; LF = ligamentum flavum; L = lamina; SC = spinal cord; ID = intervertebral disc; D = dorsal root ganglion; V = vertebral artery; U = uncinate process; VR = ventral nerve root. (Image from cryomicrotome collection compiled from work by Peter Pech, MD, and Victor M. Haughton, MD, included here with permission of Victor M. Haughton.)

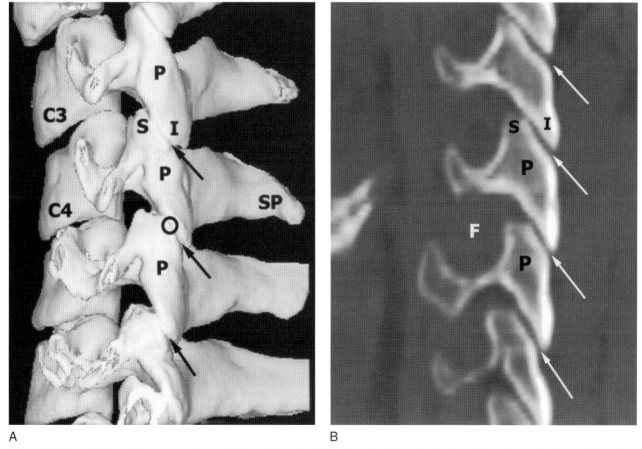

A

B

Figure 2-13 ▪ Radiographic anatomy of facets. *A,* Lateral view of cervical spine: three-dimensional volume CT surface-rendered image. Facet joints (*arrows*) are oriented in oblique coronal plane. Superior articular process (S) of C4 lies anterior to inferior articular process (I) of C3. *Circle* = target point for needle entry site into the C4-5 facet joint; P = articular pillars; SP = spinous process. *B,* Sagittal two-dimensional reformatted CT image through cervical articular pillars (P) and facet joints (*arrows*). S = superior articular process; I = inferior articular process; F = neural foramen.

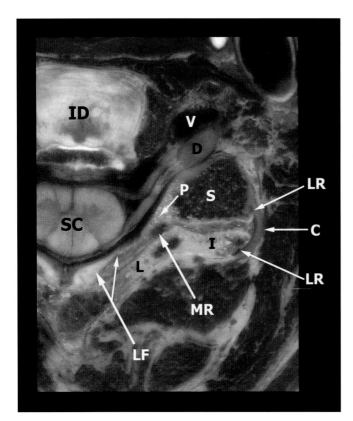

Figure 2-14 ■ Close-up view of axial cryomicrotome image of cadaver cervical facet joint demonstrating fibrous capsule and facet joint recesses. Cervical facet joints are oriented in an oblique coronal plane and readily accessed by a needle using a direct lateral approach. Thick fibrous capsule (C) is located along the lateral aspect of the facet joint. Deep to the fibrous capsule is the lateral recess (LR), which extends along the lateral margin of both the superior (S) and inferior (I) articular process. The medial recess (MR) of the facet joint is bound anteromedially by a bone projection (P) of the superior articular process (S). The ligamentum flavum (LF) (yellow ligament) attaches to this bone projection. Note articular cartilage is very thin in this specimen. L = lamina; SC = spinal cord; ID = intervertebral disc; D = dorsal root ganglion; V = vertebral artery. (Image from cryomicrotome collection compiled from work by Peter Pech, MD, and Victor M. Haughton, MD, included here with permission of Victor M. Haughton.)

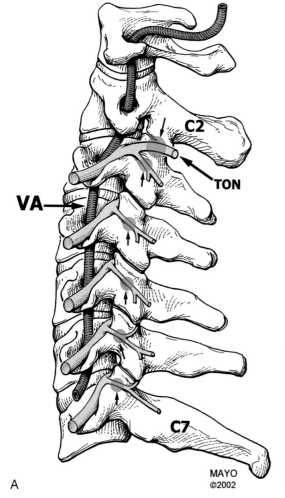

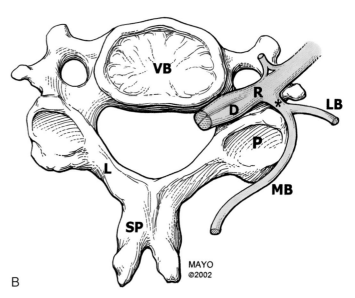

Figure 2-15 ■ Illustrations of cervical medial branch nerves. *A,* Illustration, lateral view of cervical spine. The medial branch nerves extend around the lateral margin of the midportion of the articular pillar at each respective level. The only exception is the C7 medial branch, which extends around the pillar slightly higher, just below the articular facets. The target zones (*small arrows pointing to green dots*) for third occipital nerve (TON) block and medial branch blocks are indicated. C2 = spinous process of C2; C7 = C7 spinous process; VA = vertebral artery. *B,* Axial illustration depicting cervical nerve root (R) and dorsal primary ramus (*asterisk*), which branches into a medial branch (MB) that extends around the articular pillar (P) and innervates adjacent facets and medial posterior paraspinal muscle groups. A lateral branch (LB) innervates the lateral paraspinal muscle groups such as the erector spinae muscle group. VB = vertebral body; SP = spinous process; L = lamina; D = dorsal root ganglion.

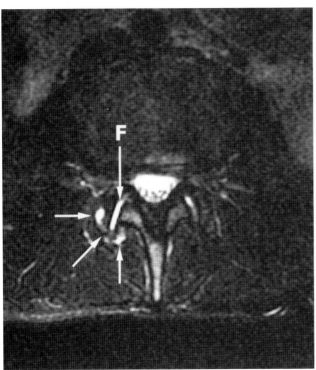
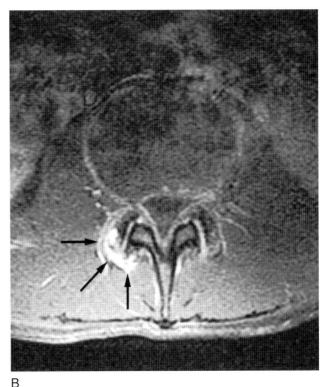

A   B

Figure 2-16 ▪ MR imaging of facet synovitis. *A,* T2-weighted fast spin echo MR image obtained with fat suppression technique reveals increased signal intensity in the tissues (*arrows*) surrounding the right facet joint at L4-5 level and increased amount of fluid (F) within the involved facet joint. *B,* Gadolinium-enhanced T1-weighted spin echo MR image obtained with fat suppression technique reveals enhancing soft tissue (*arrows*) surrounding the right L4-5 facet joint.

are some components of what various investigators have reported as the facet syndrome.

Lumbar Facet Syndrome

- Unilateral or bilateral paravertebral low back pain, which is often aggravated by rest in any posture
- Deep, dull pain that is often limited to the low back, buttock, and hip; the pain can radiate into the thigh and down to the knee in a nondermatomal (nonradicular) distribution. Facetogenic pain does not usually extend below the knee. However, in some patients, referred pain from facet disease, discogenic disease, and other paraspinal disorders may occasionally extend below the knee.[4, 43]
- Pain accentuated by twisting or rotational motion[44]
- More pain on extension than flexion. Pain may be relieved by flexion.[41, 44]
- Pain exacerbated by moving from a sitting to a standing position
- Pain characteristically relieved by standing, walking, rest, or repeated activity
- Morning stiffness
- Normal neurologic examination
- Tenderness to palpation over the affected facet joint
- Radicular pain absent with straight-leg raising

Cervical Facet Syndrome

- Unilateral or bilateral paravertebral neck pain
- Decreased range of motion of the neck
- Local tenderness over the affected facet joint(s)
- Upper cervical facet joints causing not only neck pain but also headaches and cutaneous pain
- Pain frequently referred into the shoulder girdle. Pain can extend to the elbow but rarely distal to the elbow. The pain should follow a nondermatomal (nonradicular) pattern.

CONTRAINDICATIONS

- Coagulopathy (International Normalized Ratio [INR] >1.5 or platelets <50,000/mm^3)
- Pregnancy (because of teratogenic effects of radiation)
- Systemic infection or skin infection over the puncture site
- Severe allergy to any of the medications (relative contraindication)
- Patient has received the maximum amount of steroid, including systemic steroids, allowed for a given time period, unless the injection is to be performed without steroids
- Inability to obtain percutaneous access to the target facet joint or medial branch nerve because of extensive, solid lateral or posterolateral fusion

* Patients with motor weakness, absent reflexes, or long tract signs[13]

PROCEDURE

Equipment/Supplies

Procedural

* Spinal needle, 22-gauge, 3.5-inch (1 per level, lumbar facet block, cervical facet block posterolateral approach, or medial branch block) (Quinke type point, Becton Dickinson & Co., Franklin Lakes, NJ)
* Spinal needle, 25-gauge, 2.5-inch (cervical facet block direct lateral approach) (MONOJECT® SENSI-TOUCH diamond point spinal needles with metal hub, Sherwood Medical Company, St. Louis, MO)
* Luer-lock 3-mL syringe containing injection mixture (1 per level)
* Optional 3-mL syringe containing nonionic iodinated myelographic contrast 300 mg I/mL (Omnipaque [Iohexol] Injection, Nycomed Inc., Princeton, NJ)
* Control 12-mL syringe with 25-gauge, 1.5-inch needle containing 9.5 mL 1% lidocaine for local anesthesia and 0.5 mL 8.4% sodium bicarbonate injectable (1 mEq/mL) to alleviate burning pain associated with anesthetic
* Sterile 4 × 4-inch gauze pads
* Povidone-iodine (Betadine) and alcohol for prepping
* Four sterile towels for draping
* Needle, 18-gauge, 1.5-inch, to draw up lidocaine and medication
* Surgical hat, mask, sterile gloves
* Adhesive bandages

Imaging

* Lead apron
* Multidirectional C-arm fluoroscopy with film archiving capability

Medications (Injection Mixtures)

Facet Block

LUMBAR/THORACIC

Diagnostic: 1.0 to 1.5 mL lidocaine hydrochloride-MPF 2% (Xylocaine-MPF 2%, AstraZeneca LP, Wilmington, DE) (**short acting**)
   or 1.0 to 1.5 mL bupivacaine hydrochloride 0.5%-MPF (Sensorcaine-MPF Injection 0.5%, AstraZeneca LP, Wilmington, DE) (**long acting**)
Therapeutic: Combine
   1. 2.5 mL bupivacaine 0.5%-MPF
   2. 0.5 mL betamethasone sodium phosphate and betamethasone acetate injectable suspension 6 mg/mL (Celestone Soluspan 6 mg/mL, Schering Corporation, Kenilworth, NJ)

CERVICAL

Diagnostic: 0.5 to 1.5 mL lidocaine 2%-MPF
   or 0.5 to 1.5 mL bupivacaine 0.5%-MPF

Therapeutic: Combine
   1. 1.0 mL bupivacaine 0.5%-MPF
   2. 0.5 mL betamethasone 6 mg/mL

Medial Branch Block

LUMBAR/THORACIC/CERVICAL

Diagnostic: 0.3 to 0.5 mL lidocaine 2%-MPF (**short acting**)
   or 0.3–0.5 mL bupivacaine 0.5%-MPF (**long acting**)

Precautions

1. As a general rule, preservative-free medications or compounds (e.g., paraben free, phenol free) are used to prevent flocculation of the steroid compound.[45]
   a. MPF = methylparaben free.
   b. The MPF form is preferable for use in spine intervention procedures because steroid is often given at the same time.
   c. Some preservatives, if they are inadvertently injected intrathecally, can produce arachnoiditis.
2. All medications are used **without** epinephrine because vasoconstrictive properties are neither needed nor wanted, particularly because of the risk of vasospasm in the head and neck region.

Methodology (Facet Block)

General Principles

Facet blocks are performed as outpatient procedures. Patients are instructed to stop using their pain medications on the day of the procedure to allow greater diagnostic accuracy. Patients are also instructed to have a driver with them after the procedure as well as someone who can be responsible for their well-being for the remainder of the day, because sedation may be given, although infrequently, during the examination.

The facet block is both a diagnostic and a therapeutic procedure. There are physicians who believe that, for a therapeutic facet block, it is not necessary to deposit the injection mixture into the facet joint. Instead, they perform an **extra-articular** facet block by injecting a relatively large volume (e.g., 4 to 6 mL of fluid into the extracapsular soft tissues adjacent to the facet joint). This method does indeed have therapeutic benefit in some patients, but we believe the **intra-articular** facet block is most effective when the injectate is delivered directly into the joint space. Injecting a large volume of anesthetic/steroid mixture is not advantageous for a diagnostic facet block for the reason that the patient's reported pain relief may be misleading because more than one level can be affected by a large volume of injectate.

Lumbar Facet Block

X-RAY FLUOROSCOPIC METHOD

Informed consent is obtained. The patient's lower extremity strength is evaluated for comparison with post-procedure strength. We do not routinely use sedation for facet blocks. However, if the clinical situation warrants, a mild intravenous sedative and analgesic (midazolam, 1 to 2 mg, and fentanyl, 75 to 150 µg) may be given. It is important to use appropriate monitoring of the cardiorespiratory status of the patient during the procedure if intravenous sedation is used. It is vital that the patient not be sedated to the point where he or she is not able to fully understand questions or react to the pain produced by the facet block procedure.

We routinely use the following procedure for both diagnostic and therapeutic facet blocks. The patient is placed prone on the fluoroscopy table. The lumbar skin surface is prepared with povidone-iodine (Betadine) and alcohol scrub and draped in a sterile fashion. The puncture site is localized with the patient prone on the table with fluoroscopy in straight AP projection. Beginning from a straight AP radiographic projection, the C-arm is positioned obliquely 10 to 45 degrees until the posterior portion of the facet joint just appears to "open." Because the posterior portion of the facet joint is in a near-sagittal plane, the facet joint can be most easily entered when it is first seen to open as the C-arm is rotated, which is often 10 to 20 degrees from straight AP projection (Fig. 2-17).[25, 46] The upper facet joints, L1-2 and L2-3, can usually be entered with this technique alone. The lower facet joints, L4-5 and L5-S1, are more easily entered when slight caudocranial beam angulation is used (image intensifier above the patient, obliqued toward the patient's head). The ideal point of entry is located inferolateral to the edge of the inferior articulating process, where the posterior joint space recess is largest (Fig. 2-18). However, the joint space can be entered more superiorly as well (Fig. 2-19). Local anesthesia is administered with 1% lidocaine

subcutaneously. The 22-gauge needle is advanced through the facet capsule. A release in resistance to needle advancement is usually "felt" by the operator when the joint capsule has been penetrated.

The patient often experiences pain just before the facet joint capsule is entered and while entering the capsule with the needle. If the patient's pain response is identical to his or her typical pain, it is said to be concordant. We find this to be a good indicator that the subsequent facet block will be effective. One may optionally confirm appropriate positioning of the needle in the joint by injecting 0.25 to 0.5 mL of contrast agent (Iohexol-300) into the joint space. Ideally, the contrast agent will flow into the interfacetal joint space and into the superior recess in a linear or arc-like configuration, depending on the beam angle (Fig. 2-20). Occasionally, the contrast agent will extravasate from the posterolateral aspect of the joint where articular branches penetrate the facet joint capsule. Anteromedial extension of contrast agent may occur in the medial recess adjacent to the ligamentum flavum. In patients with spondylolysis, the contrast commonly extends into the pars defect when the adjacent facet joint is injected, which is not surprising because the pars interarticularis is located just below the inferior recess of the facet joint.[27, 47] A facet block may relieve symptoms associated with spondylolysis.[27] We do not routinely confirm needle placement with contrast medium because injecting a contrast agent may theoretically limit the amount of injectate that can be placed in the joint.

The normal lumbar facet joint will accept 1.0 to 1.5 mL of fluid. For diagnostic injections, the anesthetic is injected

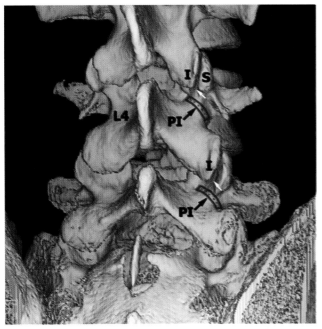

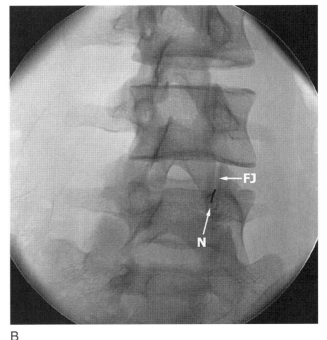

A

B

Figure 2-17 ▪ Ideal target for accessing the lumbar facet joint. *A,* Right posterior view of the spine 10 degrees from straight posterior shows the right L4-5 joint just "open" enough to allow placement of the needle into the inferior portion of the facet joint inferior recesses (*red areas indicated by white arrows*). At a given level, the inferior recesses are located inferolateral to the inferior articular process (I) and above the pars interarticularis (PI) (represented as the *brown collar* around the neck of the "Scotty dog." S = superior articular process of L4. *B,* LAO radiograph of right L4-5 facet block. In this patient, a 10-degree obliquity was sufficient to open the right L4-5 facet joint (FJ) just enough to allow passage of the needle (N) into the inferior aspect of the joint space. In a given patient, depending on the anatomy of the facets, the optimal angle of entry may vary from 0 to 45 degrees.

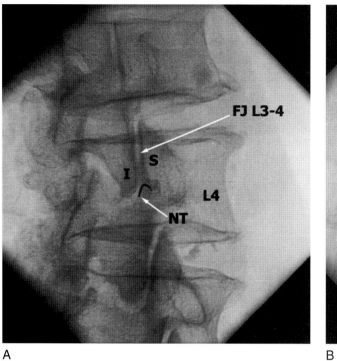

A

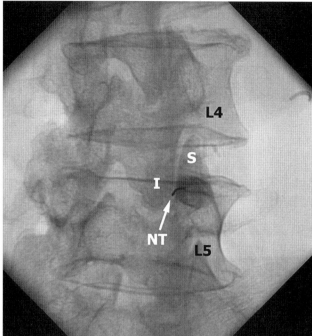

B

Figure 2-18 ▪ Facet blocks at three lumbar levels in the same patient. *A,* Right L3-4 facet injection: LAO radiograph, 35-degree obliquity. Needle tip (NT) projects over inferior recess of facet joint (FJ), which projects inferolateral to the inferior process (I) of L3 (foot of "Scotty dog") that overlies the L4 vertebral body. S = superior articular process of L4. *B,* Right L4-5 facet injection: LAO radiograph, 30-degree obliquity. Inferior portion of facet L4-5 facet joint appears narrowed on radiograph. Needle tip (NT) is positioned inferolateral to the inferior articular process (I) of L4. S = superior articular process of L5. *C,* Right L5-S1 facet injection. Needle tip (NT) is positioned inferolateral to tip of inferior articular process (I) of L5, even though midportion of facet joint (FJ) appears "open" on radiograph.

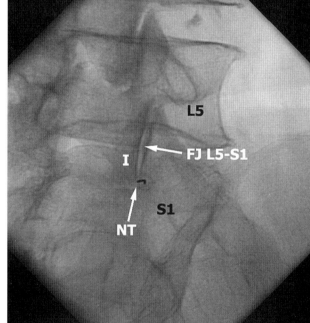

C

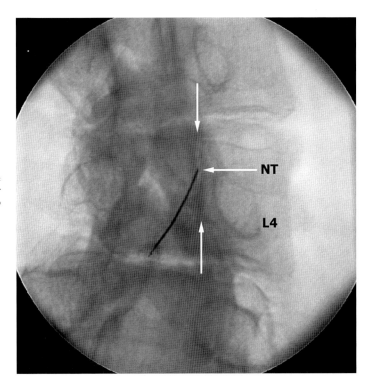

Figure 2-19 ▪ Needle enters facet more superiorly than the usual ideal target. L3-4 facet joint (*between arrows*) projects over the L4 vertebral body on 45-degree LAO radiograph. Needle tip (NT) projects over midportion of facet joint.

only into the joint. The needle is then slowly removed. For therapeutic injections, if the patient reported pain concordant with his or her typical pain before the joint capsule was punctured, a small amount (0.5 to 1.0 mL) of the injectate may also be deposited in the extracapsular soft tissues posterior to the facets.

CT-GUIDED METHOD

Facet blocks may alternatively be performed with the use of CT to guide needle placement,[16] although we rarely use this method in our practice. Otherwise, the technique is the same as that outlined earlier. Because the facet joints are directly visualized in cross-sectional planes with CT, the appropriate angle of approach into the facet joint can be determined precisely. CT guidance can be especially useful when the hypertrophic bony overgrowth of a severely degenerating facet obscures the posterior approach into the facet joint and makes it difficult to determine optimal needle trajectory fluoroscopically. Furthermore, CT allows precise localization of the needle tip without the use of iodinated contrast agent as is sometimes done to confirm needle position when fluoroscopic guidance is used (Fig. 2-21).

Thoracic Facet Block

Requests for thoracic facet blocks are rare. Clearly defined indications for thoracic facet blocks do not exist. Rarely, thoracic facet blocks are performed when the patient has localized tenderness to palpation over a given thoracic facet and the source of the pain cannot be explained. A positive bone scan or abnormal MR image at the level of a painful thoracic facet joint may also guide the physician to the source of the patient's thoracic back pain. Typically, the

patient has had multiple diagnostic imaging procedures, all of which are normal, before a thoracic facet block is even considered. As stated earlier, it is difficult to perform an intra-articular thoracic facet injection because of the coronal orientation of the thoracic facet joints and because the lungs prevent direct lateral access. Although thoracic facet injections may be successfully performed using fluoroscopic guidance, CT guidance is strongly recommended; it allows precise positioning of the needle, while avoiding the lung, nerves, and spinal cord. CT fluoroscopy, if available, is a valuable means of direct visualization during needle placement and is recommended for thoracic facet injections. The thoracic facet injection can be successfully performed by a posterolateral approach, with placement of the needle tip just below the inferior margin of the inferior articular facet and posterior to the superior articular facet (Fig. 2-22). It is not possible or even necessary to position the needle into the interfacetal portion of the joint. The needle positioned just below the lower edge of the inferior articular process penetrates the inferior joint recess, allowing injection into the joint space (Fig. 2-23). Alternatively, the injectate may be deposited in the extracapsular soft tissues posterior to the inferior portion of the facet joint, which is often sufficient to relieve the patient's pain if it is facet related.

A coaxial needle approach can be used with CT guidance to facilitate intra-articular needle placement. An 18-gauge, 3.5-inch spinal needle can be placed by a posterolateral approach so that the tip of the needle is 5 to 10 mm posterior and lateral to the facet joint. The stylet is removed, and a longer 22- or 25-gauge spinal needle, pre-curved 10 to 20 degrees, is then placed in a coaxial fashion through the 18-gauge needle to access the ventrolateral aspect of the facet joint space.

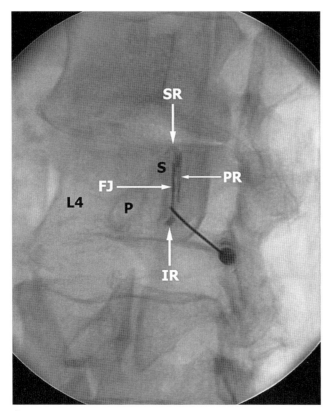

A

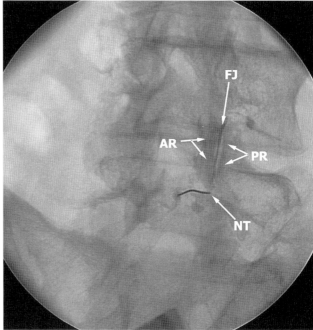

B

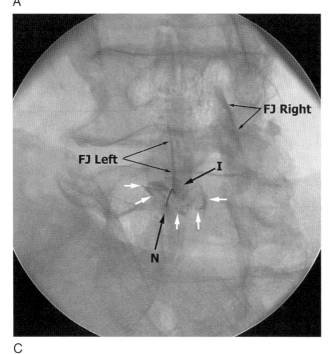

C

Figure 2-20 ■ Lumbar facet arthrography. Appearance of lumbar facet joints after water-soluble contrast agent is injected. *A*, Water-soluble contrast agent has been injected into the interfacetal portion of the left L3-4 facet joint (FJ) shown in RAO radiograph. Superior (SR), inferior (IR) and posterior (PR) recesses of the facet joint are opacified. P = pedicle of L4; S = superior articular process of L4. *B*, Right L4-5 facet block: LAO radiograph. Needle tip (NT) has been positioned in the inferior recess. Contrast agent has been injected opacifying the interfacetal portion of the facet joint (FJ). Anterior (AR) and posterior (PR) recesses of the facet joint are also opacified (*vague dark region on either side of interfacetal contrast*). *C*, RAO radiograph obtained after injection of contrast material into both facet joints (FJ) at the L4-5 level. Note linear configuration of contrast agent in facet joint. Needle (N) has been inserted into the inferior recess (I), which is also opacified with contrast. Note appearance of extravasated contrast material (*white arrows*) into posterior perifacetal soft tissues.

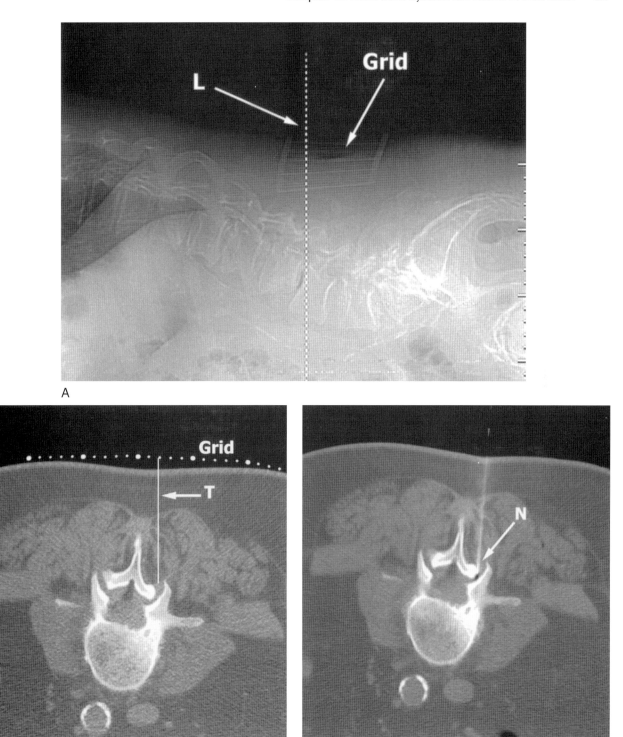

A

B   C

Figure 2-21 ■ CT-guided right L2-3 facet injection. *A*, Lateral scout CT digital radiograph showing surface grid on back and slice location localizer line (L) at the selected L2-3 level. *B*, With surface grid on the back, desired trajectory (T) for the needle is drawn on the image using a straight posteroanterior orientation into the wide-open right L2-3 facet joint. *C*, Needle (N) has been inserted into the right L2-3 facet joint using a near-straight posteroanterior trajectory.

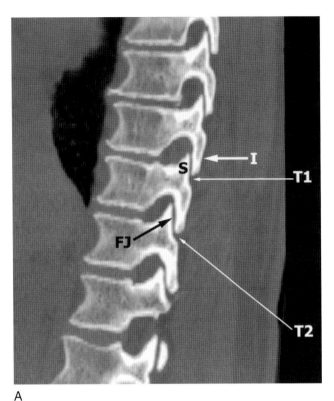

A

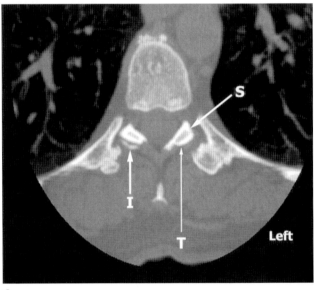

B

C

Figure 2-22 ▪ CT-guided thoracic facet block. *A,* Sagittal two-dimensional reformatted CT image obtained from helical data set. Thoracic facet joint (FJ) is oriented in coronal plane. Inferior articular process (I) prevents needle placement directly into the joint space. A straight parasagittal horizontal needle trajectory (T1) may be used to penetrate the inferior facet capsule or, alternatively, a caudocranial trajectory (T2) may be used. S = superior articular process. *B,* Axial CT image through inferior portion of the inferior process (I) at this thoracic level. Note oblique coronal orientation of facet joint (FJ) in this patient prevents a direct posterolateral approach. Inferior portions of both inferior articular processes are indicated. S = superior articular process. *C,* Axial CT image one level below that shown in *B.* Left inferior articular process is no longer visible. Target point (T) for facet injection is just along posterior margin of superior articular process (S). Lower margin of right inferior articular process (I) is barely visible.

Cervical Facet Block

Cervical facet blocks are usually performed for confirmation of cervical facetogenic pain. Serial controlled (comparative) blocks with single anesthetic agents of varying duration of action are recommended to confirm the diagnosis of cervical facetogenic pain because of the high false-positive rate of pain response and the high placebo rate.[48] When therapeutic cervical blocks are performed, a steroidal agent is usually added to the anesthetic mixture. However, the benefit of

intra-articular steroid deposition to provide a more sustained response has not been proven.[49]

Cervical facet blocks are generally performed with x-ray fluoroscopic guidance. There are two main approaches that can be used to perform the cervical facet block: a *direct lateral approach,* which we prefer, and the *posterolateral approach.* To perform the cervical facet block with the *direct lateral approach,* the painful side is up and the patient is positioned in lateral decubitus position with a folded towel under the head to keep the head parallel to the table. If the

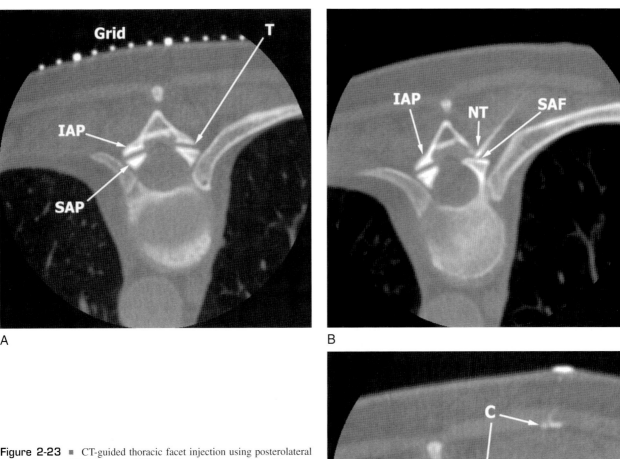

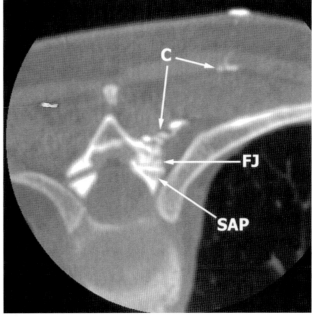

Figure 2-23 ■ CT-guided thoracic facet injection using posterolateral approach at the T7-8 level. *A,* With localizer grid on surface of back, a suitable needle trajectory (T) is chosen to allow needle placement along the inferior edge of the inferior articular facet. IAP = opposite inferolateral edge of the articular process; SAP = superior articular process. *B,* The needle tip (NT) is just inferior to the inferior articular facet until the needle tip just touches the posterior surface of the superior articular facet (SAF). Note ipsilateral inferior articular process is not visible on this CT image. IAP = opposite inferior articular process. *C,* After facet injection, note contrast agent in the facet joint (FJ). The contrast agent (C) is also seen along the needle tract. SAP = superior articular process.

patient's head was flexed laterally toward the suspected facet joint, the joint space would narrow and make intra-articular placement more difficult. When the *direct lateral approach* is used, a neutral lateral decubitus patient position is best, with slight lateral flexion of the spine **away from** the suspected facet joint.

Informed consent is obtained. The patient's upper extremity strength is evaluated for comparison with post-procedure strength. The skin surface on the side of the neck is prepared in sterile fashion and draped. One percent lidocaine is in-

stilled subcutaneously. With the x-ray beam vertical, under fluoroscopic guidance a 25-gauge, 2.5-inch spinal needle is advanced toward the facet joint from a direct lateral approach. Needle depth can be assessed instantly if one has biplane fluoroscopy. With single-plane fluoroscopy, one must advance the needle slowly and evaluate needle position in AP and lateral planes to ensure proper needle position and ascertain that the needle has not passed through the joint space and into the spinal canal (Fig. 2-24). Alternatively, with fluoroscopy in the lateral position, the needle is advanced

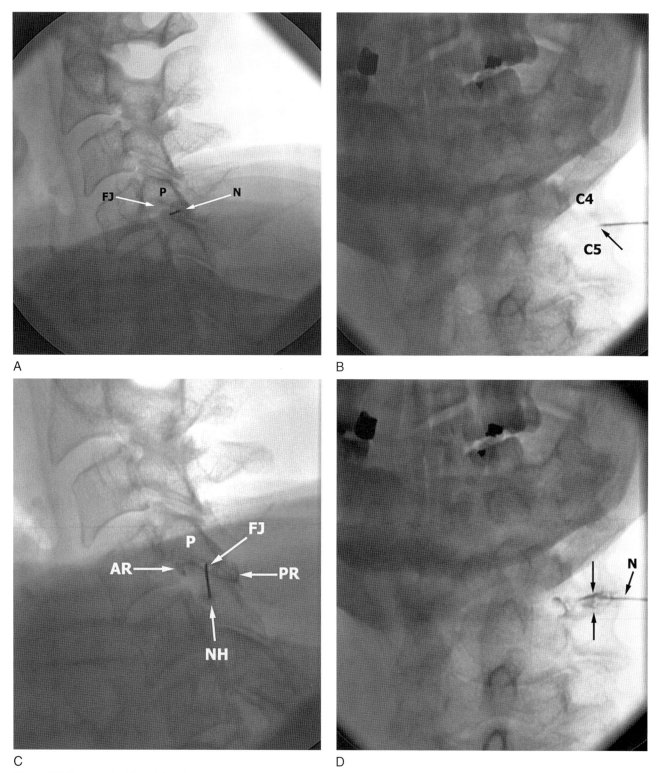

Figure 2-24 ■ Cervical facet joint pain on the right. Right C4-5 facet block. *A*, Lateral radiograph after insertion of the needle (N) into the right C4-5 facet joint (FJ) using a near direct lateral approach. P = C4 pedicle. *B*, AP radiograph confirms needle tip (arrow) in facet joint from right lateral approach. Articular pillars of C4 and C5 are labeled. *C*, Lateral arthrogram with needle in C4-5 facet joint (FJ). AR = anteromedial recess; PR = posterior recess; P = C3 articular pillar; NH = needle hub. *D*, AP radiograph arthrogram shows contrast agent (*arrows*) in right C4-5 facet joint. N = point where needle enters joint.

until it contacts either the superior or the inferior articulating surface of the facet joint. This ensures that the needle position is not too deep. The C-arm fluoroscope is then rotated to AP. The needle is withdrawn a few millimeters and redirected into the facet joint. Water-soluble contrast agent (0.1 to 0.3 mL) can be used to confirm needle tip position in the joint, but this is usually unnecessary (see Fig. 2-24). To perform a diagnostic block, 0.5 to 1.5 mL of short- or long-acting anesthetic is injected into the joint and the patient's pain response is carefully assessed and recorded. It is important to record whether the pain is concordant or discordant, and the intensity of the pain should be assessed and recorded on a scale of 1 to 10. If the patient has a positive response to injection (more than 80% pain reduction in the distribution of the nerves that innervate the joint being injected), comparative medial branch blocks are performed weeks or months later (after the patient's pain has returned) with anesthetic agents of different duration of action, to confirm that the pain is originating from that particular facet, before a radiofrequency ablation procedure is considered. If the patient has no response at the time of the initial procedure, an adjacent facet joint is considered for injection. To perform a therapeutic block, the procedure is the same except that a steroidal agent (e.g., 0.5 mL betamethasone 6 mg/mL) is added to the anesthetic.

The second approach, the *posterolateral approach*[50] to cervical facet block can be used if one does not have a C-arm or biplane fluoroscope, but the greater difficulty with this technique is likely the main reason that cervical medial branch blocks are favored over cervical intra-articular facet blocks. In this technique, the needle puncture site is located along the posterolateral skin surface two or three levels below the intended facet block. A 22-gauge, 3.5-inch spinal needle is advanced in a caudocephalad direction under fluoroscopic guidance to enter the facet joint parallel to its oblique craniocaudal plane. Again, confirmation of needle position by injecting water-soluble iodinated contrast agent is optional. The anesthetic mixture is injected in the same fashion as described previously.

Medial Branch Block Procedure

General Principles

Like facet blocks, medial branch blocks are performed as an outpatient procedure. Patients are instructed to stop using their pain medications on the day of the procedure to allow greater diagnostic accuracy. Patients should be accompanied by a responsible person who can drive them home and who can be responsible for their well-being in the hours after the procedure if sedation is given. In most cases, intravenous sedation is not necessary for routine medial branch blocks.

Lumbar Medial Branch Block

Informed consent is obtained. The patient's lower extremity strength is assessed for comparison before and after the procedure. The patient is placed prone on the fluoroscopy table. The patient's lower back is prepared and draped in a sterile fashion.

ANATOMIC CONSIDERATIONS

The medial branch of the dorsal ramus in the thoracic and lumbar spine (L1 to L4) courses over the base of the transverse process, where it joins the superior articulating process. The primary target zone for the L1 to L4 medial branch lies just caudad to the superior margin of the medial aspect of the transverse process (Fig. 2-25).[51] A secondary target zone is located just below the upper target zone, midway between the superomedial margin of the transverse process and the mamilloaccessory ligament (see Fig. 2-25). A medial branch block placed at the more superior target zone carries an increased risk of a false-negative response if the anesthetic agent is inadvertently injected into the neural foramen or the epidural space.[39]

As previously explained, each facet joint has a dual nerve supply. For example, the L4-5 facet joint synovium is innervated by both the medial branch nerve that courses over the base of the transverse process of L4 (i.e., the L3 medial branch nerve) and the medial branch nerve that courses over the base of the transverse process of L5 (i.e., the L4 medial branch nerve) (see Fig. 2-8). The L5 nerve does not innervate the L4-5 facet. The key point here is that the nerves in the lumbar and thoracic spine are numbered differently than the transverse processes they course over, because each medial branch nerve joins the dorsal primary ramus of the level above.

It is also important to understand the position of the L5 and S1 "medial branch nerves" before undertaking medial branch blocks at these levels. The L5 medial branch is not the medial branch of L5 but rather the dorsal primary ramus of L5, where it lies against the bone along the superomedial aspect of the groove formed by the sacral ala and the superior articulating process of S1 (Fig. 2-26). A secondary target zone is located slightly more inferior to this groove. The dorsal ramus of L5 divides into a medial and lateral branch.[39] The medial branch courses medially around the posterior lumbosacral facet joint, where it innervates the joint and continues more posteriorly to innervate the multifidus muscle. The lateral branch of the L5 dorsal ramus extends caudad, where it communicates with the lateral branch of the S1 dorsal ramus.[37] The target zone for the S1 medial branch nerve is along the superolateral margin of the S1 foramen (Fig. 2-27), although this branch does not significantly contribute to lumbar facet pain.

PATIENT POSITIONING

With maximum fluoroscopic magnification, the junction of the base of the transverse process and the superior articulating process is positioned in the center of the field of view in a straight AP projection. The C-arm is then rotated 10 to 20 degrees from AP toward the side of the back treated (i.e., the C-arm is rotated to the right if the right medial branch is being treated). At this angle, the "Scotty dog" configuration is visible, with the "nose" representing the transverse process, the "eye," the pedicle, and the "ear," the superior articulating process (Fig. 2-28).

NEEDLE PLACEMENT

The following procedure is used for approaching the medial branch nerves for lower thoracic and lumbar levels L1 to L4. The puncture site that permits the optimal approach to the

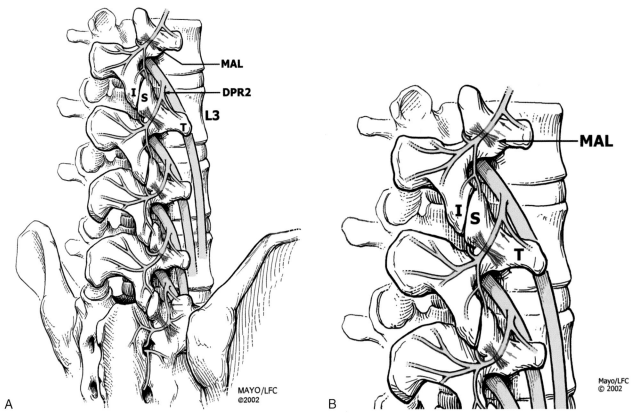

Figure 2-25 ■ Lumbar medial branch block target zones. *A*, Right posterior oblique illustration of lumbosacral spine showing right-sided facet joint innervation from medial branches of the dorsal primary ramus DPR2 of the right second nerve root. Primary medial branch block target zone (*red arrows*) is just superior to the secondary medial branch target zone (*green arrows*) at any given level. Both targets along the medial branch block are located above the mamilloaccessory ligament (MAL). I = inferior articular process of L2; S = superior articular process of L3; T = right transverse process of L3. *B*, Close-up view of *A* centered at L3 level showing primary (*red*) and secondary (*green*) medial branch target zones in the proximal portion of the medial branch nerves located above the mamilloaccessory ligament (MAL).

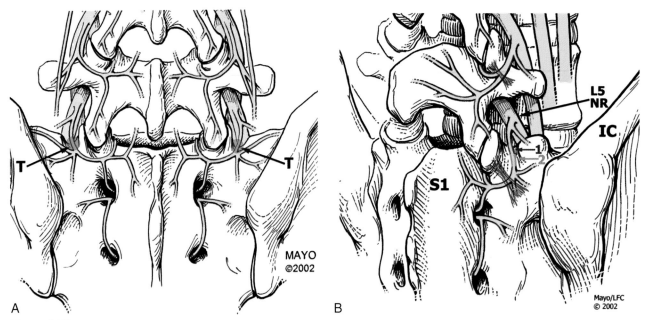

Figure 2-26 ■ L5 dorsal primary ramus block (L5 does not have a true medial branch of the dorsal primary ramus). *A*, Illustration depicting major nerves on posterior view of the lumbosacral junction. Target zones (T) for right and left L5 dorsal primary ramus block are located in a groove along the superior aspect of each sacral wing. *B*, Right posterior oblique illustration of right L5 dorsal primary ramus block primary (*red 1*) and secondary (*green 2*) target zones. L5NR = L5 nerve root; S1 = first sacral vertebra; IC = iliac crest.

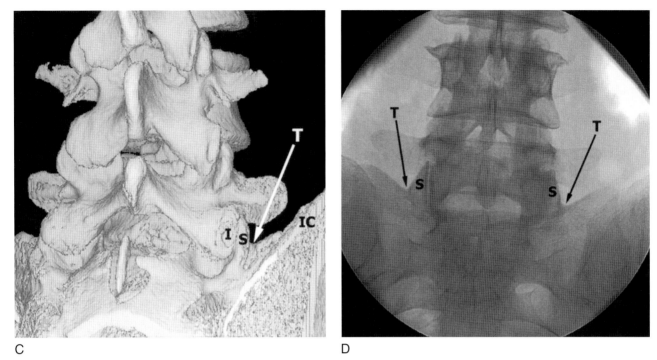

C   D

Figure 2-26 *Cont'd* ■ *C*, Fifteen-degree right posterior oblique view of lumbosacral junction on three-dimensional CT surface-rendered image. Right L5 dorsal primary ramus target (T) is in the groove along the superior aspect of sacral wing located just lateral to the right superior articular process of S1 (S). I = right inferior articular process of L5; IC = right iliac crest. *D,* AP radiograph of lumbosacral junction. Target zones (T) for L5 dorsal primary ramus block are located in the groove along the superior margin of the sacral ala just lateral to the base of the S1 superior articular process (S).

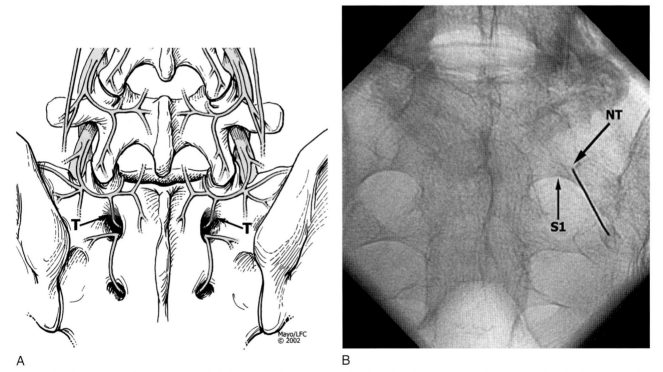

A   B

Figure 2-27 ■ S1 dorsal primary ramus block (S1 "medial branch block"). *A,* Illustration of posterior view of lumbosacral junction. Target zones (T) for the S1 "medial branch block" (actually the dorsal primary ramus of S1) are adjacent to the superior or superolateral margin of the S1 neural foramen. *B,* AP radiograph of upper sacrum after insertion of needle tip (NT) just superolateral to the roof of the right S1 neural foramen elicited pain.

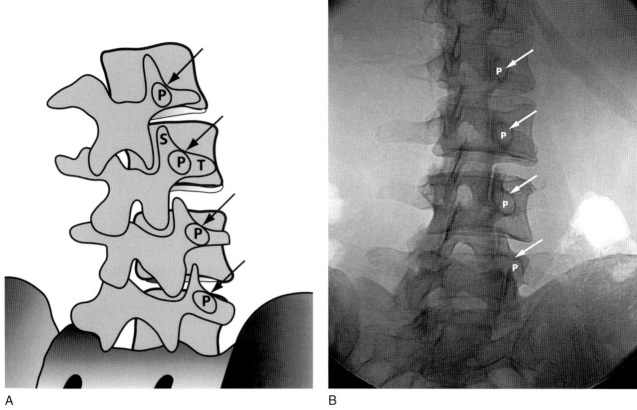

A   B

Figure 2-28 ■ Recognition of "Scotty dog" configuration is used to identify target points for lumbar medial branch block. *A*, Illustration depicting appearance of LAO radiograph demonstrating target points for lumbar medial branch blocks. The target sites (*arrows*) are located in a groove formed where the transverse process (T, nose) joins the superior articular process (S, ear) and the target points project over the superolateral margin of the pedicle (P, eye), which is also approximately at the 1- or 2-o'clock position of the "eye" for this obliquity. *B*, Target points (*arrows*) for medial branch block at various lumbar levels in LAO radiograph of patient. P = pedicle.

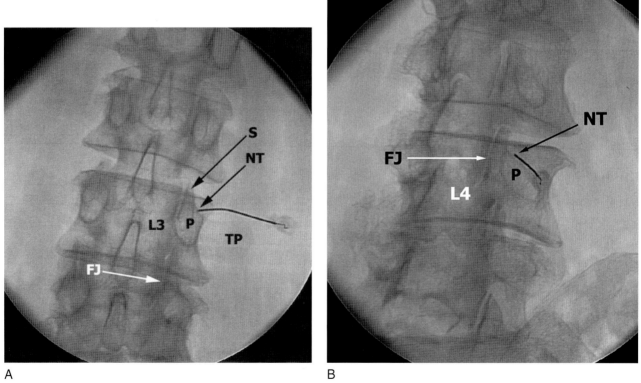

A   B

Figure 2-29 ■ Right L2 and L3 medial branch blocks at the L3 level and L4 level to block innervation of the L3-4 facet joint. *A*, Right L2 medial branch block. Inserted needle tip (NT) projects over superolateral margin of right L3 pedicle (P) in groove between right L3 superior articular process (S) and transverse process (TP). *B*, LAO radiograph after insertion of needle for L3 medial branch block at the L4 vertebral level. Needle tip (NT) projects just superior to L4 pedicle (P). FJ = L3-4 facet joint.

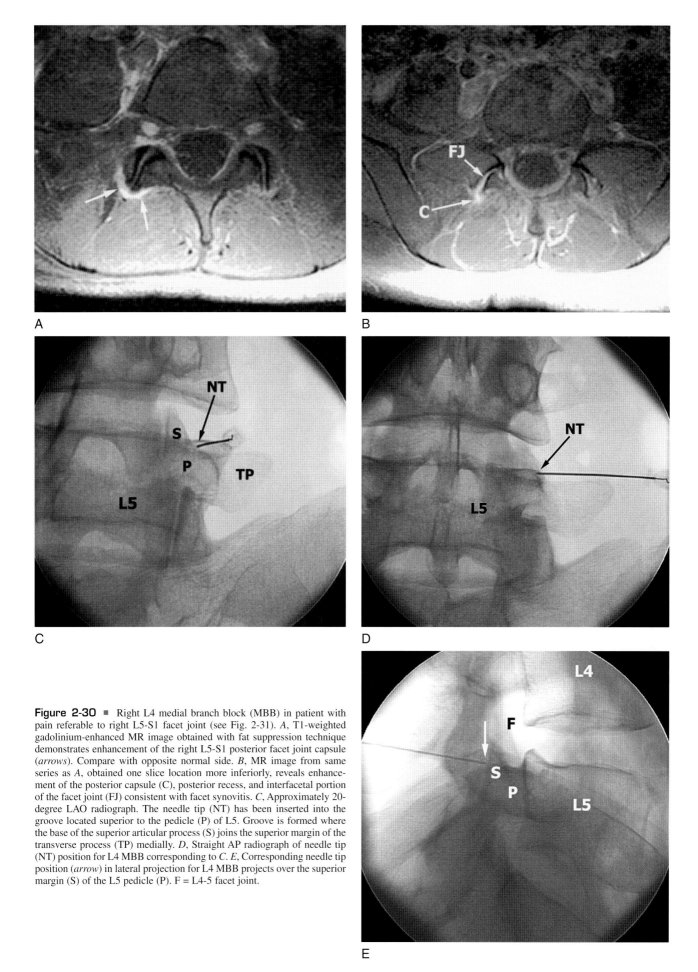

Figure 2-30 ■ Right L4 medial branch block (MBB) in patient with pain referable to right L5-S1 facet joint (see Fig. 2-31). *A*, T1-weighted gadolinium-enhanced MR image obtained with fat suppression technique demonstrates enhancement of the right L5-S1 posterior facet joint capsule (*arrows*). Compare with opposite normal side. *B*, MR image from same series as *A*, obtained one slice location more inferiorly, reveals enhancement of the posterior capsule (C), posterior recess, and interfacetal portion of the facet joint (FJ) consistent with facet synovitis. *C*, Approximately 20-degree LAO radiograph. The needle tip (NT) has been inserted into the groove located superior to the pedicle (P) of L5. Groove is formed where the base of the superior articular process (S) joins the superior margin of the transverse process (TP) medially. *D*, Straight AP radiograph of needle tip (NT) position for L4 MBB corresponding to *C*. *E*, Corresponding needle tip position (*arrow*) in lateral projection for L4 MBB projects over the superior margin (S) of the L5 pedicle (P). F = L4-5 facet joint.

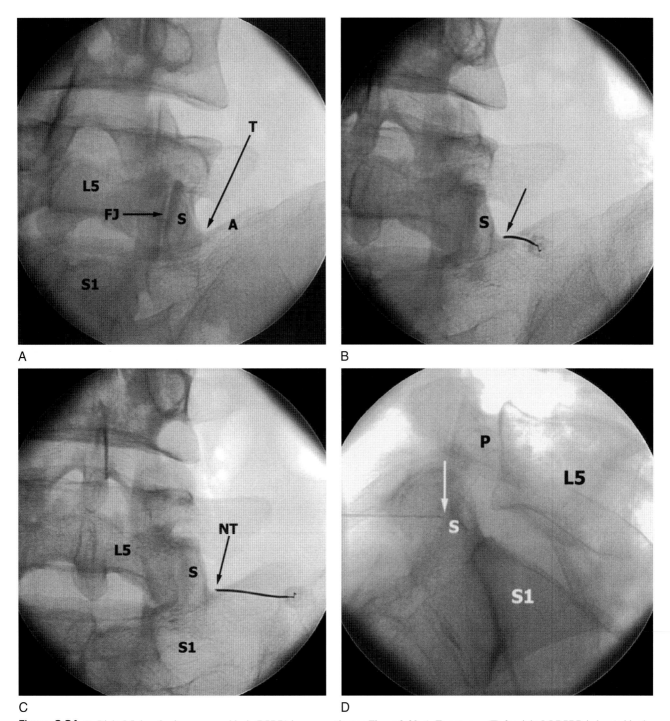

A

B

C

D

Figure 2-31 ■ Right L5 dorsal primary ramus block (DPRB) in same patient as Figure 2-30. *A*, Target zone (T) for right L5 DPRB is located in the groove formed where the superior margin of the sacral ala (A) joins the base of the superior articular process of S1 (S). FJ = L5-S1 facet joint. *B*, Slight LAO radiograph of ideal needle tip position (*arrow*) for right L5 DPRB. S = right superior articular process of S1. *C*, AP radiograph showing ideal needle tip (NT) position for L5 DPRB. S = superior articular process of S1. *D*, Position of needle tip (*arrow*) in ideal position for L5 DPRB in lateral projection corresponding to Figure 2-30B.

medial branch nerve is located at or slightly superior to the level of the transverse process and just lateral to the medial border of the superior articulating process. After sterile preparation of the skin surface, 1% lidocaine is instilled subcutaneously to produce a wide skin wheal for local anesthesia. Skin puncture is made with a 22-gauge, 3.5-inch spinal needle. With the use of intermittent fluoroscopy to minimize the dose of radiation, the needle is advanced anteriorly, medially, and slightly caudad until the needle tip contacts the bone where the base of the transverse process, the superior articulating process, and the pedicle join (Fig. 2-29). The needle is then guided over the superior aspect of the transverse process in short incremental steps until the needle is felt to just slide over the top of the transverse process. At this point, the nerve is oriented in a near horizontal position relative to the needle trajectory, and therefore the nerve is maximally exposed to the needle when it is advanced. A lateral view of the lumbar spine is obtained to demonstrate that the needle is not positioned so far anteriorly that it encroaches on the neural foramen (Fig. 2-30). The needle hub is rotated until the notch of the hub points toward the patient's feet, so that the bevel of the needle tip faces the bone and allows the injectate to be deposited on the medial branch rather than superiorly toward the neural foramen. With the needle thus positioned, the needle tip is located on or immediately adjacent to the medial branch nerve (see Fig. 2-30). To prevent false-negative responses from incorrect needle placement or intravenous needle tip position, some recommend confirmation of needle tip position by the injection of water-soluble contrast medium before instillation of the anesthetic agent.[39] Just before the injection, one should draw back on the syringe to make certain the needle tip is not in a vascular structure, whether or not contrast agent is to be injected. Then 0.3 to 0.5 mL of the anesthetic agent is injected for the medial branch blockade.

The L5 "medial branch nerve" is approached in a similar fashion. The target is at the superomedial aspect of the sacral ala, just lateral to the superior articulating process of S1 (see Fig. 2-26). The needle is advanced under fluoroscopic guidance until contact is made with the bone forming the superior edge of the sacral ala. The needle is then "walked" incrementally over the bone and advanced 2 to 3 mm, where it should lie adjacent to the nerve (Fig. 2-31).

The S1 medial branch is a small nerve that courses over the superolateral aspect of the S1 foramen (see Fig. 2-27). To perform an S1 medial branch block, a straight needle with no bend is passed with a caudocranial trajectory to contact the bone along the superolateral margin of the S1 foramen. In some cases, it can be difficult to optimally position a straight needle adjacent to the S1 medial branch; in this situation, the distal end of the needle tip may be slightly bent so that it lies parallel to the target nerve.

Thoracic Medial Branch Block

Thoracic medial branch blocks are rarely performed, but they can be performed in a manner similar to the lumbar medial branch block procedure. However, it is important to position the needle in close proximity to the lateral margin of the superior articulating process to avoid puncturing the adjacent lung. To avoid the lung, one must visualize on the fluoroscopic image or radiograph the three-line configuration

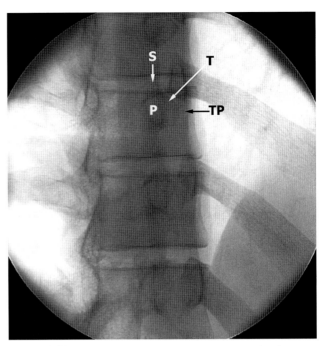

Figure 2-32 ■ LAO radiograph, lower thoracic spine, showing target point (T) for T8 medial branch block. S = superior articular process; P = pedicle; TP = transverse process.

consisting of, from lateral to medial, the anteromedial lung margin, the posterolateral margin of the vertebral body, and the posteromedial lung margin (refer to Fig. 3-8). The radiographic target for a thoracic medial branch block is located just cephalad to the superomedial margin of the transverse process (Fig. 2-32). Cranial or caudal angulation of the C-arm may be necessary to allow optimal separation of the transverse process from the costovertebral junction.

The numbering of the thoracic medial branch nerves is similar to that in the lumbar spine, with one exception. As in the lumbar spine, the medial branches that course over the base of the T2 through T12 transverse processes originate one level higher. The exception is that the C8 medial branch courses over the base of the T1 transverse process.

Cervical Medial Branch Block

Informed consent is obtained. The patient's upper extremity strength is assessed for comparison with post-procedure strength. It is extremely important that the patient not be overly sedated, because he or she must fully understand questions and report an accurate pain response once the needle has been optimally positioned.

ANATOMIC CONSIDERATIONS

Medial branch blocks can be highly specific for the diagnosis of facet-related pain in the cervical region.[52] Cervical medial branch blocks are technically more easily performed than cervical intra-articular facet blocks. As in the lumbar region, high rates of false-positive results have been reported when single, uncontrolled medial branch blocks are performed.[53] Therefore, controlled (comparative) blocks are

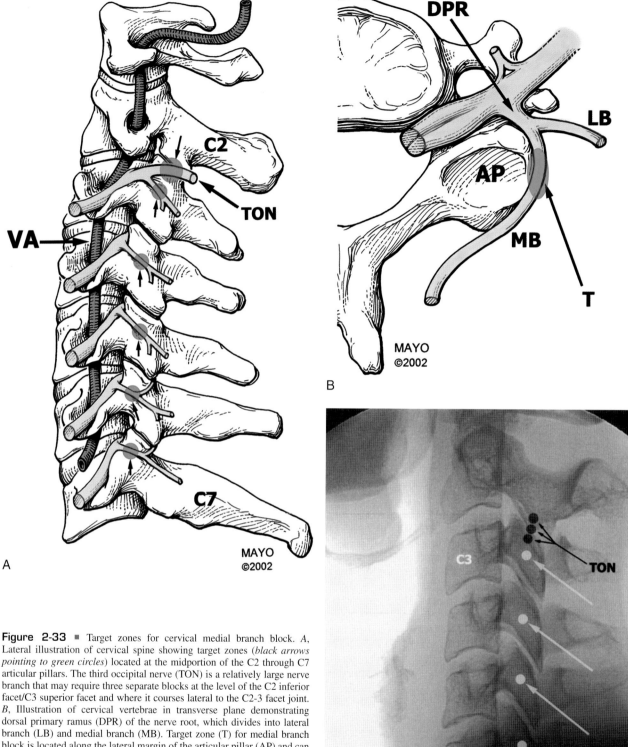

A

B

C

Figure 2-33 ■ Target zones for cervical medial branch block. *A,* Lateral illustration of cervical spine showing target zones (*black arrows pointing to green circles*) located at the midportion of the C2 through C7 articular pillars. The third occipital nerve (TON) is a relatively large nerve branch that may require three separate blocks at the level of the C2 inferior facet/C3 superior facet and where it courses lateral to the C2-3 facet joint. *B,* Illustration of cervical vertebrae in transverse plane demonstrating dorsal primary ramus (DPR) of the nerve root, which divides into lateral branch (LB) and medial branch (MB). Target zone (T) for medial branch block is located along the lateral margin of the articular pillar (AP) and can be approached posterolaterally or from a direct posterior approach so the needle is nearly parallel to the AP orientation of the medial branch at this point. *C,* Lateral radiograph of the spine showing medial branch block target zones at the midarticular pillar levels from C3 to C6 (*white dots*). *White arrows* signify approximate needle trajectory to approach target zone from posterolateral approach. Third occipital nerve (TON) target zones (*black dots*) are also demonstrated.

recommended in which the type of anesthetic used (short-vs. long-acting) is varied to confirm the diagnosis of cervical facetogenic pain. To perform a cervical medial branch block at C3-4 and below, the medial branch nerve is blocked where it crosses the **midportion** of the articular pillar as viewed fluoroscopically in lateral projection (see Fig. 2-8). Injections are performed above and below the level of a given facet joint to block the medial branches crossing the articular pillars above and below the joint.

The C2-3 facet joint nerve supply is blocked by injecting the third occipital nerve where it crosses the posterolateral aspect of the C2-3 joint capsule, with additional injections slightly above and below the facet joint at the level of the articulating facets to block the communicating branches of C3 (Fig. 2-33).

PATIENT POSITIONING

The patient is placed in the lateral decubitus position with the symptomatic side up. A cushion should be placed under the patient's head to keep the neck parallel to the table. With maximum fluoroscopic magnification, the articular pillar (if treating the C3-4 through C7-T1 facet joints) or the C2-3 facet joint is placed in the center of the field of view in a straight lateral plane (Fig. 2-33).

NEEDLE PLACEMENT

With fluoroscopic guidance, the puncture is most easily and safely performed from a posterolateral approach on the side of the patient's pain. With this approach, the needle will pass through muscle and fascia. No major arteries are located along this trajectory. The needle will also remain well posterior to the vertebral artery. Again, one should attempt to

position the needle parallel to the long axis of the medial branch, which, from the posterolateral approach, would be along the articular pillar.

With the use of a lateral fluoroscopic projection, a wide skin wheal of 1% lidocaine is instilled along the posterior border of the sternocleidomastoid muscle at the level of the spinous process related to the target articular pillar. Skin puncture is made with a 22-gauge, 3.5-inch spinal needle. With the help of intermittent fluoroscopy, the needle is advanced ventrally and medially until tangential contact is made with the articular pillar. Either the C-arm can be rotated 10 to 15 degrees left anterior oblique (LAO) or right anterior oblique (RAO) or an AP view can be obtained to ensure that the tip of the needle remains in close relation to the midportion of the articular pillar. The needle position that we try to obtain for the C3 to C6 medial branches is along the ventral aspect of a line that connects the greatest antero-posterior diameter of the articular pillar but remains dorsal to the foramen as seen on lateral imaging (Fig. 2-34).

The transverse process of C7 tends to displace the medial branch more cephalad than the middle of the C7 articular pillar (see Fig. 2-33). To perform a C7 medial branch block, the needle tip is positioned more superiorly than at other cervical levels, so that the needle tip overlies the superior articular process. The C8 medial branch is approached much like the thoracic and lumbar medial branches. For a C8 medial branch block, the needle is placed at the junction of the superior articulating facet and the base of the transverse process of T1.

The third occipital nerve is approached in a fashion similar to that for the other cervical branches. However, because the third occipital nerve is larger than the medial branches,

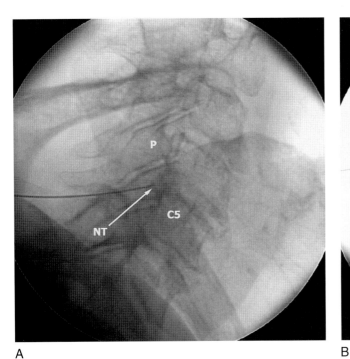
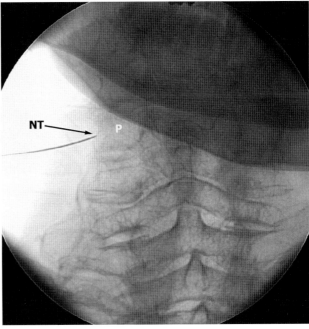

A B

Figure 2-34 ■ C5 medial branch block. *A*, Oblique lateral radiograph. Using a posterolateral approach, the needle has been inserted so that the needle tip (NT) lies against the midportion of the left C5 articular pillar. P = C4 articular pillar. *B*, Corresponding oblique AP radiograph of cervical spine shows needle tip (NT) along the lateral margin of the left C5 articular pillar (P).

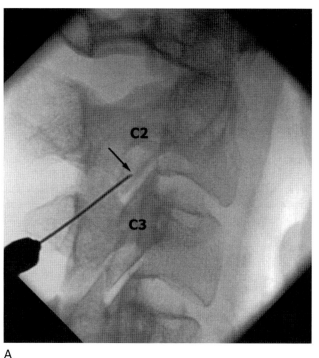

A

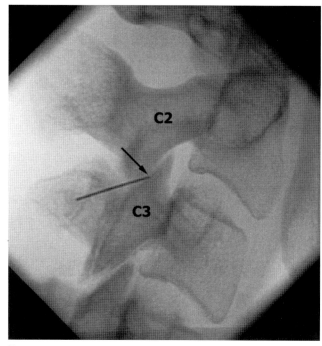

B

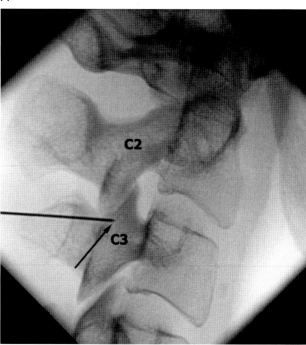

C

Figure 2-35 ■ Lateral radiographs showing third occipital nerve block performed at the C2-3 level using a posterolateral approach. *A,* Upper target zone block. Needle tip (*arrow*) positioned adjacent to inferior articular facet of C2. C2 and C3 indicate respective articular pillars. *B,* Middle target zone block. Needle tip (*arrow*) projects over facet joint at C2-3 level. *C,* Lower target zone block. Needle tip (*arrow*) is positioned adjacent to superior articular facet of C3.

multiple injections are performed. The third occipital nerve courses along the surface of the C2-3 facet joint capsule. The target zone for the needle tip is the anteroinferior margin of the C2 inferior articular facet, the anterosuperior margin of the C3 superior articular facet, and just lateral to the C2-3 facet joint capsule at the level of the joint (Fig. 2-35).

POTENTIAL COMPLICATIONS

* Bleeding
* Infection
* Post-procedural radicular or back pain
* Thecal sac puncture and subsequent headache

- Allergic reactions related to the medications given
- Risk of pneumothorax for thoracic procedures
- Vasovagal reactions and ataxia, especially for cervical procedures

POST-PROCEDURE CARE/FOLLOW-UP

After the facet or medial branch block, the patient is brought to a sitting position and questioned regarding his or her pain response. When the patient feels able to walk, he or she is allowed to stand with two persons assisting, one on each side, in case the patient is weak. Usually, the patient does not have any loss of strength, although this will occasionally occur. If there are no post-procedural complications, the patient can be discharged 15 to 20 minutes after the injection.

If a procedural complication occurs, the patient should be observed until it resolves. A minority of patients will experience severe localized back or neck pain after the procedure, which is usually relieved by an oral analgesic such as Percocet 5/325 (oxycodone HCl and acetaminophen, Endo Pharmaceuticals, Inc., Chadds Ford, PA).

POST-DISCHARGE INSTRUCTIONS

At discharge, the patient should be accompanied by a responsible person who will drive him or her home. Activity should be limited and the referring physician notified if any problems such as excessive back or neck pain, weakness, or fever are experienced. The patient should not operate any heavy machinery or drive a vehicle for the remainder of the day. The following day, the patient is usually able to resume normal activities. The injected steroidal agent may take 3 to 5 days to achieve its anti-inflammatory effect.

The patient should report his or her clinical response to the facet or medial branch block to the referring physician 3 or 4 days after the procedure. Moderate to severe post-procedural pain is usually treated with an oral narcotic analgesic medication. It is recommended that a printed form detailing these instructions be given to the patient at the time of discharge. The patient should be given an appointment for a follow-up visit with the referring physician.

SAMPLE DICTATIONS

Lumbar Spine Facet Block

The procedure and potential complications were explained to the patient, and voluntary informed, signed consent was obtained. The patient was a candidate for intravenous conscious sedation. The patient was placed prone on the table, and the lower back was prepped and draped in a sterile fashion. Subcutaneous lidocaine 1% was instilled into the superficial soft tissues of the patient's lower back for local anesthesia. With the use of fluoroscopic guidance, a 22-gauge, 3.5-inch spinal needle was inserted into the right L4-5 facet joint. After negative aspiration, 2.5 mL of bupivacaine-MPF 0.5% and 0.5 mL betamethasone (6 mg/mL) were instilled in the right L4-5 facet joint and extracapsular

soft tissues. The needle was removed, and the patient was repositioned. A similar procedure was performed on the left L4-5 facet joint. No complications were observed during the procedure or immediately after the procedure.

Lumbar Spine Medial Branch Block

Diagnosis: Right L3-4 facet pain
Procedure: Right L2 and L3 medial branch blocks

The procedure and potential complications were explained to the patient and voluntary informed, signed consent was obtained. The patient was a candidate for intravenous conscious sedation. The patient was placed prone on the table, and the back was prepped and draped in a sterile fashion. Subcutaneous 1% lidocaine was instilled into the superficial soft tissues of the patient's lower back for local anesthesia. A 22-gauge, 3.5-inch spinal needle was advanced along the superior margin of the right L3 transverse process and lateral to the right L3 superior articulating process, and it was directed inferiorly and medially so that the tip struck the junction of the base of the transverse process and the superior articular process of L3. The needle was then walked over the superior aspect of the transverse process and advanced 2 mm along the course of the right L2 medial branch nerve. At this location, 0.5 mL of bupivacaine 0.5% was injected. During the injection, the patient experienced pain concordant with the usual low back and leg pain. The needle was removed. A similar procedure was performed to block the right L3 medial branch nerve. No complications were observed during or immediately after the procedure.

Cervical Spine Facet Block

The procedure and potential complications were explained to the patient, and voluntary informed, signed consent was obtained. The patient was a candidate for intravenous conscious sedation. The patient was placed in the right lateral decubitus position, and the neck was prepped and draped in a sterile fashion. Subcutaneous 1% lidocaine was instilled into the superficial soft tissues of the patient's neck for local anesthesia. With fluoroscopic guidance, a 25-gauge, 2.5-inch spinal needle was placed into the left C3-4 facet joint space. A mixture of 1.0 mL bupivacaine-MPF 0.5% and 0.5 mL betamethasone (6 mg/mL) was instilled into the lateral aspect of the left C3-4 facet joint space. The needle was removed, and the patient was repositioned. A similar procedure was performed on the left C4-5 facet joint. No complications were observed during or immediately after the procedure.

Cervical Spine Medial Branch Block

Diagnosis: Left C4-5 facet pain
Procedure: Left C4 and C5 medial branch blocks

The procedure and potential complications were explained to the patient, and voluntary informed, signed consent was obtained. The patient was a candidate for intravenous conscious sedation. The patient was placed in the right lateral decubitus position on the table, and the neck was prepared and draped in sterile fashion. Subcutaneous 1% lidocaine was instilled into the superficial soft tissues of the patient's neck for local anesthesia. With C-arm fluoroscopic guidance, a left posterolateral approach was used to position a 22-gauge, 3.5-inch spinal needle adjacent to the left C4 articular process. At this point, 0.5 mL bupivacaine-MPF 0.5% was injected. The patient reported pain concordant with the typical left-sided neck pain. The needle was removed. A similar procedure was performed at C5. No complications were encountered during or immediately after the procedure.

CASE REPORTS

CASE 1

Clinical Presentation

A 75-year-old, left-handed man presents with the main complaint of back and bilateral leg discomfort with sitting. The discomfort is relieved with standing or walking. It also bothers him when he is lying down. He describes discomfort in the hamstring region, which, when he straightens his legs, causes some jerking or tingling in his feet. This is always improved with standing up. He denies any weakness or change in his bowel or bladder function.

Imaging and Therapy

There was no instability demonstrated on flexion/extension lumbar spine radiographic series. MR imaging of the lumbar spine demonstrated degenerative disc disease and mild stenosis at L4-5. There was no evidence of any significant stenosis or any root compression.

Bilateral L4-5 Facet Injections (Fig. 2-36)

The procedure and potential complications were explained to the patient, and voluntary informed, signed consent was obtained. His lower back was prepared and draped in usual sterile fashion. Subcutaneous 1% lidocaine was instilled into the superficial soft tissues of the patient's lower back for local anesthesia. With fluoroscopic guidance, a 22-gauge, 3.5-inch spinal needle was placed into the right L4-5 facet joint. After negative aspiration, 1.5 mL of a mixture of 0.75 mL lidocaine 1% and 0.75 mL bupivacaine 0.5% was instilled into the right L4-5 facet joint. The needle was removed, and the patient was repositioned. A similar procedure was performed on the left L4-5 facet joint.

Results

The patient reported relief from his typical bilateral low back pain for a duration of 2 weeks after the bilateral L4-5 facet injections.

Bilateral L3 and L4 Medial Branch Blocks
(Fig. 2-37)

Because of the success of prior, repeated facet injections, medial branch blocks were indicated before possible radiofrequency denervation. The procedure and

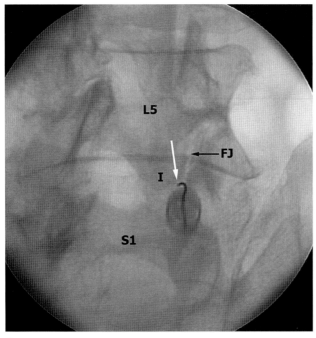
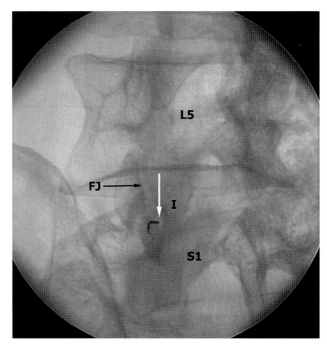

A   B

Figure 2-36 ■ Case 1. Bilateral L5-S1 facet injections. *A,* Slight LAO radiograph. Needle (*white arrow*) has been inserted into inferior recess of the right L5-S1 facet joint inferolateral to the inferior articular process (I) of L5. FJ = facet joint. *B,* Slight RAO radiograph. Needle (*white arrow*) has been inserted into inferior recess of the left L5-S1 facet joint (FJ) inferolateral to the inferior articular process (I) of L5.

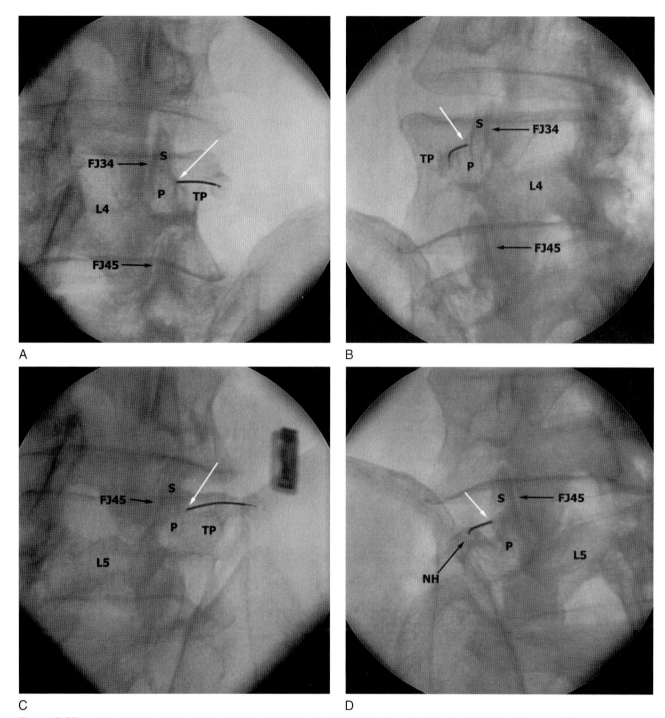

A   B

C   D

Figure 2-37 ■ Case 2. Bilateral L3 and L4 medial branch blocks effectively block pain referable to both L4-5 facet joints. *A*, Right L3 medial branch block: slight LAO radiograph. Needle is inserted along groove formed by junction of right superior articular process (S) and transverse process (TP) of L4 until patient reports pain. Note needle tip (*white arrow*) projects superolateral to the right L4 pedicle (P). FJ34= right L3-4 facet joint, FJ45 = right L4-5 facet joint. *B*, Left L3 medial branch block: RAO radiograph. Needle tip position (*white arrow*) shows where pain was elicited by contact with the left L3 medial branch. S = left superior articular process of L4; P = left pedicle of L4; TP = left transverse process of L4; FJ34 = left L3-4 facet joint; FJ45 = left L4-5 facet joint. *C*, Right L4 medial branch block: LAO radiograph. Needle tip position (*arrow*) shows where pain was elicited by contact with the right L4 medial branch in the groove formed between the right superior articular process (S) and right transverse process (TP) of L5. P = right pedicle of L5; FJ45 = right L4-5 facet joint. *D*, Left L4 medial branch block. Pain elicited with needle position (*white arrow*) in groove superolateral to left pedicle of L5. Needle hub (NH) overlies the left transverse process (P). S = left superior articular process of L5; FJ45 = left L4-5 facet joint.

potential complications were explained to the patient, and voluntary informed, signed consent was obtained. With the patient prone on the fluoroscopic table, his lower back was prepared and draped in usual sterile fashion. Subcutaneous 1% lidocaine was instilled into the superficial soft tissues, and 0.5 mL bupivacaine 0.5% was instilled through the needle for a left L3 medial branch nerve block. This needle was removed. The patient was then repositioned, and medial branch blocks were performed on the right L3 and both L4 medial branch nerves in similar fashion. These nerves innervate the left L4-5 facet joint.

Results

His usual low back pain was relieved for a duration of 3 days after the bilateral medial branch block procedures were performed.

CASE 2

Clinical Presentation

A 75-year-old woman has a history of hypertension, osteoarthritis, and osteoporosis. There is a remote history of cervical trauma from a motor vehicle accident 30 years ago. She has had intermittent headaches since then, and neck pain, which began about 2 years ago and was intermittent, is now constant. She describes an aching pain in the left side of the neck from the mastoid region down to the first rib, which occasionally moves to the shoulder and rarely causes the arm to "go to sleep." Moving her head is painful, and only lying flat gives her complete relief. Turning to the right or left or lateral bending bothers her, as does looking up and down. She is unable to take most anti-inflammatory medications because of gastrointestinal distress.

On physical examination, she is in no acute distress and can heel and toe walk. She is areflexic throughout. Peripheral pulses are full in the arms and legs. Sensation to touch and pin is normal in the arms and legs and in particular C4 through T1. The C3

dermatome is also intact. A strength test is normal for C4 through T1, as is that for the iliopsoas, hamstring, and anterior tibial muscles bilaterally. She has tightness in the left greater than the right scalenes, upper trapezius, and levator muscle of the scapula. Her neck is particularly tender at the C5 segmental level on the left. All motions give her neck pain, but particularly right rotation and lateral bending.

Imaging and Therapy

Bone scan revealed a focus of increased activity in the upper portion of cervical spine on the left.

C2-3 Facet Injection (Fig. 2-38)

Initial facet injection, performed at the C4-5 level, failed to relieve the patient's pain. MR imaging was performed in hopes of better localizing the source of the patient's pain. The MR study revealed multilevel spondylosis and facet osteoarthritis. A region of abnormal signal intensity observed in and adjacent to

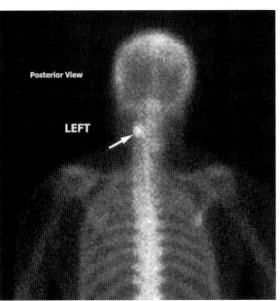
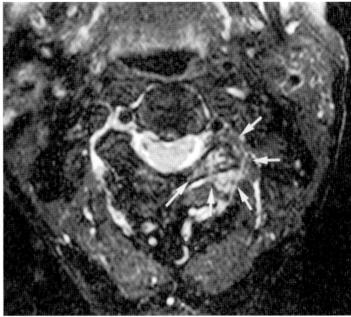

A   B

Figure 2-38 ■ Severe localized left neck pain: C2-3 facet injection. *A,* Technetium-99m radionuclide bone scan indicates focus of increased activity (*arrow*) in upper cervical spine on the left. *B,* Axial T2-weighted fast spin echo MR image with fat saturation technique shows increased signal intensity in the left C2-3 facets, left lamina of C2, and adjacent soft tissues (*arrows*) consistent with facet synovitis.

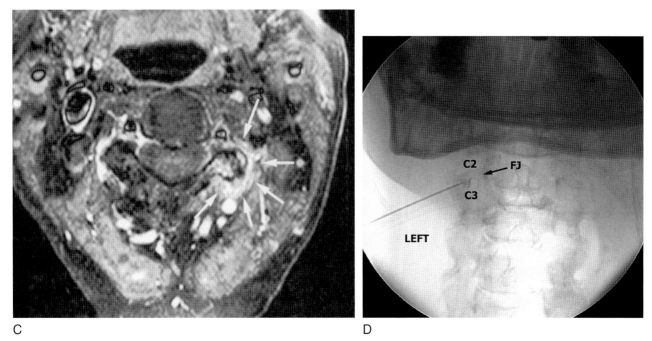

C   D

Figure 2-38 *(Cont'd)* ■ *C*, Axial T1-weighted spin echo MR image with fat saturation after gadolinium enhancement. The left C2-3 facets and perifacetal soft tissues enhance *(arrows)*, which is typical of facet synovitis. *D*, Left C2-3 facet injection. Needle tip positioned in lateral aspect of the left C2-3 facet joint (FJ) in this AP radiograph. Note small amount of water-soluble contrast agent has been injected into the facet joint to confirm needle position before injecting the anesthetic agent into the joint. Patient's pain was relieved by the injection. Follow-up MR image 2 weeks later showed significantly less abnormal contrast agent enhancement in and adjacent to the left C2-3 facets.

the C2-3 facet joint on the left on T2-weighted fast spin echo images and gadolinium-enhanced images obtained with fat suppression technique was consistent with inflammatory facet synovitis. A facet injection was performed at the C2-3 level with 0.3 mL of a mixture of 1 mL bupivicaine 0.5% and 1 mL triamcinolone (40 mg/mL).

Results

The patient had immediate pain relief. Subsequent MR image obtained 2 weeks later showed reduction in the abnormal signal intensity and contrast agent enhancement in and adjacent to the C2-3 facets.

CASE 3

Clinical Presentation

This patient is a male with back pain at the lumbosacral junction with standing and walking and relieved by sitting and lying down. He is only able to walk approximately 15 feet before getting uncomfortable. He has had two prior back surgeries, the first in 1986 for low back pain and right leg pain related to a herniated disc and the second in 1996 for surgical decompression from L2 to L4. On examination, the patient has good mobility. Left lateral bending produces left lumbosacral pain, and right lateral bending produces right lumbosacral pain. Extension produces bilateral low back pain. He has localized tenderness overlying the L5-S1 facets bilaterally.

Imaging and Therapy

CT-Guided Facet injection (Fig. 2-39)

Axial CT was performed to localize the L5-S1 facet joints. Subsequently, a 22-gauge, 3.5-inch spinal needle

was advanced into the left L5-S1 facet joint and confirmed with a small amount of nonionic contrast agent. Subsequently, 1.5 mL of a mixture of 0.5 mL lidocaine 1%-MPF, 1.0 mL of bupivacaine 0.5%, and 0.5 mL of Kenalog (40 mg/mL) was instilled into the left L5-S1 facet joint. The needle was removed. An intra-articular facet block was attempted on the right at L5-S1; however, owing to severe facet hypertrophy related to osteoarthritis, an intra-articular injection was not performed and therefore an extracapsular, periarticular injection was performed. No problems were observed during the procedure or immediately after the procedure.

Results

The patient reported relief of his usual back pain for a duration of 4 weeks after the facet injection procedure.

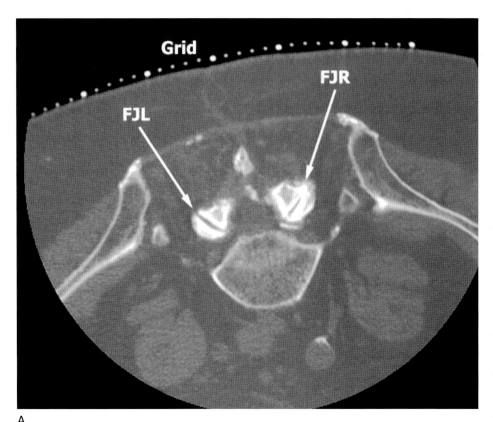

A

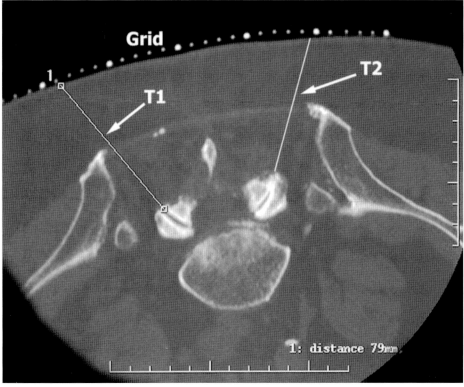

B

Figure 2-39 ■ CT-guided facet injection. *A*, Surface localizer grid on back. Left facet joint (FJL) is open and accessible by percutaneous needle approach from a 45-degree posterolateral approach. Right facet joint (FJR) is severely degenerated owing to osteoarthritis, resulting in facet hypertrophy and closing direct percutaneous access to the facet joint posteriorly. *B*, Needle trajectory lines T1 and T2 are drawn on the CT image for approaching the left and right facet joints, respectively.

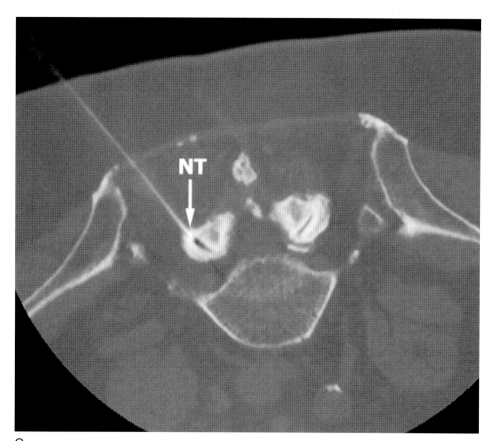

C

Figure 2-39 *(Cont'd)* ■ *C*, Needle tip (NT) has been inserted well into the left L4-5 facet joint. Using CT guidance, it is not necessary or preferable to confirm needle position by injecting contrast agent. *D*, The needle has been inserted using a posterolateral approach, but the needle tip (NT) cannot be placed into the facet joint using this trajectory, because it is impeded by the hypertrophic (H) posterior margin of the right superior articular facet. A better selection would have been trajectory T3, which would have allowed placement of the needle tip through the redundant posterior joint capsule into the posterior recess of the facet joint. Because the injection can be made into the posterior recess it is not necessary to position the needle within the interfacetal portion of the facet joint, which would not have been possible in this case.

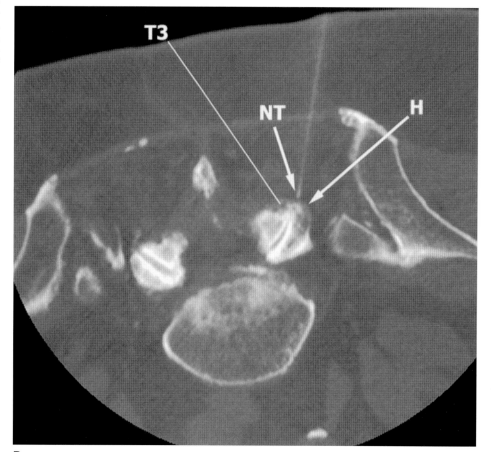

D

CURRENT PROCEDURAL TERMINOLOGY (CPT) CODES

CPT codes for a given procedure can change, and sometimes these codes are only valid in certain states or regions. It is best to consult with CPT coding experts at one's facility to verify that the coding for the procedure is appropriate for your practice and location. Below is a sample of codes that are currently being used for facet injection and medial branch block.[54]

64470 Injection, anesthetic agent and/or steroid, paravertebral facet joint or facet joint nerve; cervical or thoracic, single level

64472 cervical or thoracic, each additional level

(List separately in addition to code for primary procedure)

(Use code 64472 in conjunction with code 64470)

64475 lumbar or sacral, single level

64476 lumbar or sacral, each additional level

(List separately in addition to code for primary procedure)

(Use code 64476 in conjunction with code 64475)

XXXXX-50 Modifier for bilateral procedures

76005 Fluoroscopic guidance and localization of needle or catheter tip for spine or paraspinous diagnostic or therapeutic injection procedures (epidural, transforaminal epidural, subarachnoid, paravertebral facet joint, paravertebral facet joint nerve or sacroiliac joint), including neurolytic agent destruction

76360 CT guidance for needle placement (e.g., biopsy, aspiration, injection, localization device), radiological supervision, and interpretation

99141 Sedation with or without analgesia (conscious sedation); intravenous, intramuscular or inhalation

References

1. Hirsch D, Inglemark B, Miller M. The anatomical basis for low back pain. Acta OrthoScan 1963; 33:1–17.
2. Aprill C, Dwyer A, Bogduk N. Cervical zygapophyseal joint pain patterns: II. A clinical evaluation. Spine 1990; 15:458–461.
3. Dwyer A, Aprill C, Bogduk N. Cervical zygapophyseal joint pain patterns: I. A study in normal volunteers. Spine 1990; 15:453–457.
4. Mooney V, Robertson J. The facet syndrome. Clin Orthop 1976; 140:149–156.
5. Dreyfuss PH, Dreyer SJ, Herring SA. Lumbar zygapophysial (facet) joint injections. Spine 1995; 20:2040–2047.
6. Adams MA, Hutton WC. The mechanical function of the lumbar apophyseal joints. Spine 1983; 8:327–330.
7. Suseki K, Takahashi Y, Takahashi K, et al. Innervation of the lumbar facet joints: Origins and functions. Spine 1997; 22:477–485.
8. Ashton IK, Ashton BA, Gibson SJ, et al. Morphological basis for back pain: The demonstration of nerve fibers and neuropeptides in the lumbar facet joint capsule but not in ligamentum flavum. J Orthop Res 1992; 10:72–78.
9. Lynch MC, Taylor JF. Facet joint injection for low back pain: A clinical study. J Bone Joint Surg Br 1986; 68:138–141.
10. Schwarzer AC, Wang SC, O'Driscoll D, et al. The ability of computed tomography to identify a painful zygapophysial joint in patients with chronic low back pain. Spine 1995; 20:907–912.
11. Lilius G, Laasonen EM, Myllynen P, et al. Lumbar facet joint syndrome: A randomised clinical trial. J Bone Joint Surg Br 1989; 71:681–684.
12. Carette S, Marcoux S, Truchon R, et al. A controlled trial of corticosteroid injections into facet joints for chronic low back pain. N Engl J Med 1991; 325:1002–1007.
13. Carrera GF. Lumbar facet joint injection in low back pain and sciatica: Preliminary results. Radiology 1980; 137:665–667.
14. Carrera GF, Williams AL. Current concepts in evaluation of the lumbar facet joints. Crit Rev Diagn Imaging 1984; 21:85–104.
15. Lau LS, Littlejohn GO, Miller MH. Clinical evaluation of intra-articular injections for lumbar facet joint pain. Med J Aust 1985; 143:563–565.
16. Murtagh FR. Computed tomography and fluoroscopy guided anesthesia and steroid injection in facet syndrome. Spine 1988; 13:686–689.
17. Griffiths HJ, Parantainen H, Olson PN. Diseases of the lumbosacral facet joints. Neuroimaging Clin N Am 1993; 3:567–575.
18. Lippitt AB. The facet joint and its role in spine pain: Management with facet joint injections. Spine 1984; 9:746–750.
19. Moran R, O'Connell D, Walsh MG. The diagnostic value of facet joint injections. Spine 1988; 13:1407–1410.
20. Raymond J, Dumas JM. Intraarticular facet block: Diagnostic test or therapeutic procedure? Radiology 1984; 151:333–336.
21. Schwarzer AC, Derby R, Aprill CN, et al. The value of the provocation response in lumbar zygapophyseal joint injections. Clin J Pain 1994; 10:309–313.
22. Schwarzer AC, Aprill CN, Derby R, et al. The false-positive rate of uncontrolled diagnostic blocks of the lumbar zygapophysial joints. Pain 1994; 58:195–200.
23. Schwarzer AC, Wang SC, Bogduk N, et al. Prevalence and clinical features of lumbar zygapophysial joint pain: A study in an Australian population with chronic low back pain. Ann Rheum Dis 1995; 54:100–106.
24. Kaplan M, Dreyfuss P, Halbrook B, Bogduk N. The ability of lumbar medial branch blocks to anesthetize the zygapophysial joint: A physiologic challenge. Spine 1998; 23:1847–1852.
25. Carrera GF. Lumbar facet joint injection in low back pain and sciatica: Description of technique. Radiology 1980; 137:661–664.
26. Xu GL, Haughton VM, Carrera GF. Lumbar facet joint capsule: Appearance at MR imaging and CT. Radiology 1990; 177:415–420.
27. Maldague B, Mathurin P, Malghem J. Facet joint arthrography in lumbar spondylolysis. Radiology 1981; 140:29–36.
28. Engel R, Bogduk N. The menisci of the lumbar zygapophysial joints. J Anat 1982; 135:795–809.
29. Bogduk N, Engel R. The menisci of the lumbar zygapophyseal joints: A review of their anatomy and clinical significance. Spine 1984; 9:454–460.
30. Destouet JM, Gilula LA, Murphy WA, Monsees B. Lumbar facet joint injection: Indication, technique, clinical correlation, and preliminary results. Radiology 1982; 145:321–325.
31. Beaman DN, Graziano GP, Glover RA, et al. Substance P innervation of lumbar spine facet joints. Spine 1993; 18:1044–1049.
32. Edgar MA, Ghadially JA. Innervation of the lumbar spine. Clin Orthop 1976; 15:35–41.
33. Gronblad M, Korkala O, Konttinen YT, et al. Silver impregnation and immunohistochemical study of nerves in lumbar facet joint plical tissue. Spine 1991; 16:34–38.
34. Schwarzer AC, Derby R, Aprill CN, et al. Pain from the lumbar zygapophysial joints: A test of two models. J Spinal Disord 1994; 7:331–336.
35. Marks RC, Houston T, Thulbourne T. Facet joint injection and facet nerve block: A randomised comparison in 86 patients with chronic low back pain. Pain 1992; 49:325–328.
36. Bogduk N, Colman RR, Winer CE. An anatomical assessment of the "percutaneous rhizolysis" procedure. Med J Aust 1977; 1:397–399.
37. Bogduk N, Long DM. The anatomy of the so-called "articular nerves" and their relationship to facet denervation in the treatment of low-back pain. J Neurosurg 1979; 51:172–177.
38. Bogduk N, Wilson AS, Tynan W. The human lumbar dorsal rami. J Anat 1982; 134:383–397.
39. Dreyfuss P, Schwarzer AC, Lau P, Bogduk N. Specificity of lumbar medial branch and L5 dorsal ramus blocks: A computed tomography study. Spine 1997; 22:895–902.
40. Bogduk N. The innervation of the lumbar spine. Spine 1983; 8:286–293.

41. Eisenstein SM, Parry CR. The lumbar facet arthrosis syndrome: Clinical presentation and articular surface changes. J Bone Joint Surg Br 1987; 69:3–7.
42. Schwarzer AC, Aprill CN, Derby R, et al. Clinical features of patients with pain stemming from the lumbar zygapophysial joints. Is the lumbar facet syndrome a clinical entity? Spine 1994; 19:1132–1137.
43. Bogduk N. Lumbar dorsal ramus syndrome. Med J Aust 1980; 2:537–541.
44. Jackson RP, Jacobs RR, Montesano PX. 1988 Volvo award in clinical sciences: Facet joint injection in low-back pain: A prospective statistical study. Spine 1988; 13:966–971.
45. Physicians' Desk Reference. Montvale, NJ: Medical Economics Company, 2002.
46. Carrera GF. Lumbar facet arthrography and injection in low back pain. Wisc Med J 1979; 78:35–37.
47. Dory MA. Arthrography of the lumbar facet joints. Radiology 1981; 140:23–27.
48. Barnsley L, Lord S, Bogduk N. Comparative local anaesthetic blocks in the diagnosis of cervical zygapophysial joint pain. Pain 1993; 55:99–106.
49. Barnsley L, Lord SM, Wallis BJ, Bogduk N. Lack of effect of intra-articular corticosteroids for chronic pain in the cervical zygapophyseal joints. N Engl J Med 1994; 330:1047–1050.
50. Bogduk N, Marsland A. The cervical zygapophysial joints as a source of neck pain. Spine 1988; 13:610–617.
51. Bogduk N, Long DM. Percutaneous lumbar medial branch neurotomy: A modification of facet denervation. Spine 1980; 5:193–200.
52. Barnsley L, Bogduk N. Medial branch blocks are specific for the diagnosis of cervical zygapophyseal joint pain. Reg Anesth 1993; 18:343–350.
53. Barnsley L, Lord S, Wallis B, Bogduk N. False-positive rates of cervical zygapophysial joint blocks. Clin J Pain 1993; 9:124–130.
54. CPT 2002, CPT Intellectual Property Services. Chicago: American Medical Association, 2002.

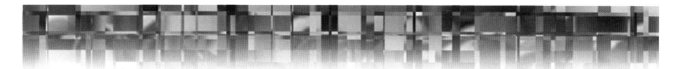

A Spine Surgeon's Perspective

Facet Joint Injection and Medial Branch Block

Joseph T. Alexander, MD

The primary pain generator in patients with axial back pain continues to be debated. In fact, virtually all of the structures in the spinal segment have been demonstrated to contain unmyelinated nerve endings, with the exception of the nucleus pulposus itself. It is likely that in patients with slightly different patterns of spinal deterioration, different structures will be the primary source of discomfort. Facet degeneration, which is commonly seen with aging, may be either the primary event in the degeneration of the motion segment or secondary to ongoing disc degeneration or other processes. In patients with multi-segmental deterioration who are being considered for lumbar stabilization procedures, a facet block or medial branch blocks can provide information similar to that gained from a discogram or a selective nerve block; that is, it can localize which of the abnormal facet complexes being visualized are currently symptomatic. Because I use this procedure as a localizing test, I rarely request injection of multiple facet levels at a single session. It is important to emphasize that temporary relief of symptoms (proportionate to the anesthetic agent infused) is a positive result, because many patients will state that the test "failed" if their symptoms recur before their follow-up visit with the clinician.

One scenario in which a facet block can be of particular diagnostic use is when one is evaluating recurrent pain in a patient with a prior spine fusion. Deterioration of an adjacent segment is increasingly recognized as a source of pain that develops late after a spine fusion. The facet complex adjacent to the fusion is often a pain generator, and yet it may be difficult to visualize because of the presence of metallic fixation hardware. An area of questionable pseudoarthrosis or the tissues around a prominent screw, hook, or rod can also be diagnostically injected in a fashion similar to the facet block.

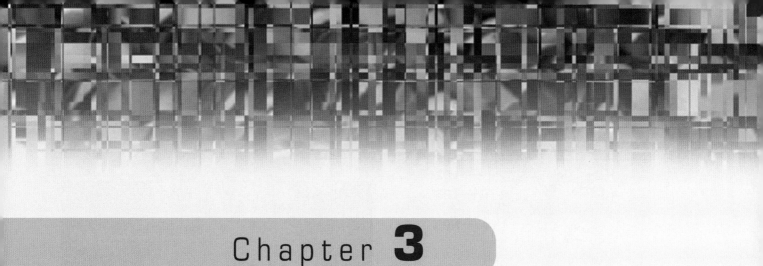

Chapter 3

Facet Denervation

- Douglas S. Fenton, MD
- Leo F. Czervionke, MD

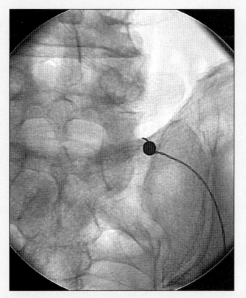

BACKGROUND

The etiology of low back and neck pain is often multifactorial. The facet (zygapophysial) joint is one structure that can cause this pain.[1-4] Although a person can suffer from clinical facet-related pain, imaging studies, including plain radiographs, nuclear medicine bone scans, computed tomography (CT), and magnetic resonance (MR) imaging, may not demonstrate any morphologic abnormality of the facet joint.[5] On the other hand, a gadolinium-enhanced T1- or fat-saturated T2-weighted MR image may demonstrate intrafacetal and/or perifacetal signal abnormalities and the patient may or may not be symptomatic. Because imaging is unreliable for the diagnosis of facet pain, a careful history and physical examination become necessary to support the hypothesis that the patient has facet-related pain. Once the diagnosis of facet syndrome is entertained, diagnostic low-volume intra-articular facet injections and/or medial branch blockades must be meticulously performed. We consider a reduction of at least 80% of the pain that would be attributed to the treated joint or nerve a positive response to these injections. When other sources of back pain have been excluded, multiple facet injections may be necessary to elucidate the source of the pain, because back pain can originate from more than one facet joint and a solitary joint injection may relieve only a portion of the patient's pain. One might then erroneously assume that the response to the injection was not positive, when, in fact,

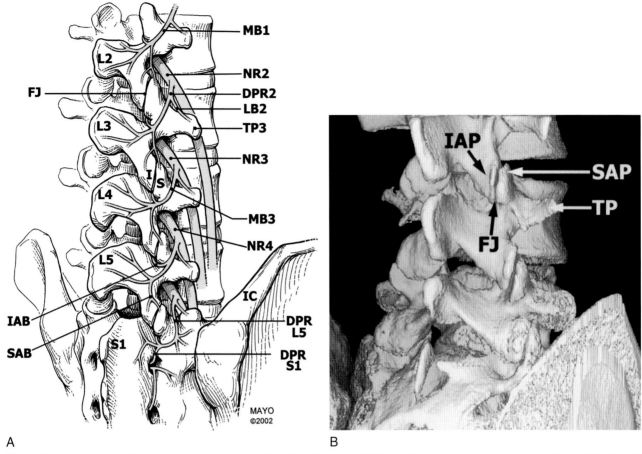

A

B

Figure 3-1 ■ Lumbar medial branch anatomy. *A*, Left anterior oblique illustration. L2 through S1 spinous processes are labeled. *Right*: MB1 = Medial branch of L1 dorsal primary ramus; NR2 = L2 nerve root; DPR2 = L2 dorsal primary ramus; LB2 = lateral branch of L2 dorsal primary ramus; TP3 = L3 transverse process; NR3 = L3 nerve root; MB3 = medial branch of L3 dorsal primary ramus, which extends around the base of the right superior articular process (S) of L4 and innervates portions of the right L3-4 and L4-5 facet joint capsules; NR4 = L4 nerve root; IC = iliac crest; DPRL5 = L5 dorsal primary ramus; DPRS1 = S1 dorsal primary ramus; I = inferior articular process of L3; S = superior articular process of L4. *Left*: FJ = L2-3 facet (zygapophysial) joint, which is innervated by branches of the L1 and L2 medial branch nerves; IAB = inferior articular branches from the medial branch of the L4 dorsal primary ramus; SAB = superior articular branches from the medial branch of the L4 dorsal primary ramus. *B*, LAO three-dimensional CT surface rendering. The medial branch of the dorsal primary ramus (T12-L4) courses over the junction of the base of the transverse process (TP) and the superior articular process (SAP). IAP = inferior articular process; FJ = facet joint.

insufficient levels were studied to determine the source of the pain.

If the physician believes that facet pain is contributing to the patient's overall pain symptoms, destruction of the facet nerve supply should, in theory, diminish or resolve the pain. Radiofrequency denervation has been shown to be effective in the treatment of facet pain, especially in patients who have an excellent response to facet injections and medial branch blocks.[6–11] Shealy performed the first radiofrequency facet denervation procedures.[12] Since that time, there have been several modifications of the radiofrequency technique. The radiofrequency technique is well suited to facet denervation because the lesion size and temperature can be controlled, there is minimal risk to the patient if the person performing the procedure is experienced, and the procedure can be performed on an outpatient basis with very little sedation.

Before performing this procedure, the spine interventionalist must understand the radiographic anatomy of the facet joints, most importantly the nerve supply.[13, 14] Each facet joint (from C3-4 inferiorly) has a dual nerve supply.

The facet joints are innervated by the medial branch of the dorsal ramus, one from the level above the target joint and one from the level below the target joint. It is also important to understand that the nomenclature of the medial branch nerves is different in the cervical and lumbar regions. This will be explained later in this chapter.

The physician and patient both must realize that the effects of the facet denervation procedure are usually not permanent. With proper technique, the patient may have significant pain relief for 1 to 2 years, although some persons will experience shorter or longer pain relief. One must remember that this procedure is performed to spare the patient more invasive procedures. Most patients surveyed would rather have a denervation procedure yearly than surgery once. Also, although the best candidate for denervation is one who has 80% or better pain relief from a series of facet-related procedures (facet injection and/or medial branch block), serious thought should be given to performing radiofrequency denervation in the patient who has less, although undeniably real, pain relief despite technically satisfactory procedures. Although such patients will not be

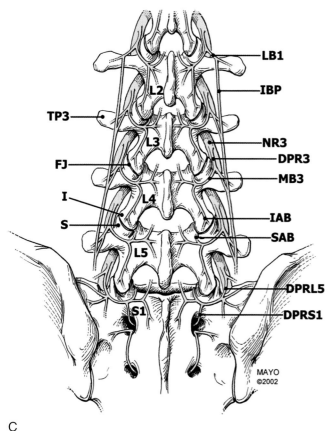

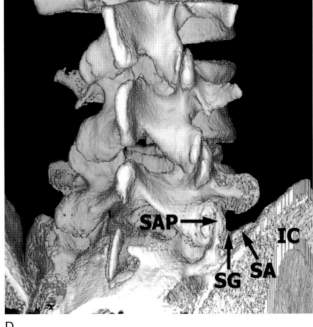

C

D

Figure 3-1 (*Cont'd*) ■ *C*, Posterior illustration of the lumbar spine and posterior neural structures. Laminae of L2 through S1 are labeled. *Left*: TP3 = transverse process of L3; FJ = L3-4 facet (zygapophysial) joint; I = inferior articular process of L4; *S* = superior articular process of L5. *Right*: LB1 = lateral branch of dorsal primary ramus of L1; IBP = intermediate branch plexus; NR3 = third lumbar nerve root; DPR3 = dorsal primary ramus of L3; MB3 = medial branch of the dorsal primary ramus of L3; IAB = inferior articular branches from the L3 medial branch (supplies L4-5 facet joint), SAB = superior articular branches from L4 (supplies L4-5 facet joint also); DPRL5 = dorsal primary ramus of L5; DPRS1 = dorsal primary ramus of S1. *D*, Shallow LAO three-dimensional CT surface rendering. The dorsal primary ramus of L5 lies within the sacral groove (SG) formed by the medial border of the S1 superior articular process (SAP) and the sacral ala (SA). IC = iliac crest.

"cured" of their pain, they may believe that any reduction of their pain would be welcome. Given the procedure's low risk when performed properly, it is hard to deny these patients a chance of obtaining at least partial pain relief that may help with their activities of daily living. There are gray areas regarding who should or should not have the procedure, and each procedure should be individualized to the patient.

ANATOMIC CONSIDERATIONS

Lumbar and Thoracic Spine

The medial branch of the dorsal ramus in the lumbar and thoracic spine courses over the base of the transverse process at the junction of the superior articulating process.[13] Also, with facet denervation, it is important to realize that each facet joint has a dual nerve supply. For example, the left L4-5 facet joint has neural connections with the medial branch nerve that courses over the base of the transverse process of L4 (left L3 medial branch nerve) and the medial branch nerve that courses over the base of the transverse process of L5 (left L4 medial branch nerve) (Fig. 3-1A and B). Note that the medial branch nerves in the lumbar and

thoracic spine are numbered differently from the transverse process they course over, because each nerve arises from the dorsal root ganglia of the **level above**. There is no medial branch of L5, and therefore the target is the dorsal ramus. The position of the L5 dorsal ramus is different from that of the remainder of the nerves. The L5 dorsal ramus lies in the medial aspect of the groove formed by the sacral ala and superior articulating process of S1 (see Fig. 3-1C and D).

Cervical Spine

The lower cervical medial branch nerves are similar anatomically to the lumbar medial branch nerves (Fig. 3-2). The C4 through C8 dorsal primary rami arise from their respective dorsal root ganglia just lateral to the intervertebral foramen. The medial branch nerve arises from the dorsal primary ramus and passes around the ipsilateral articular pillar. As in the lumbar spine, there is a dual supply to the facet joint. An ascending branch innervates the facet joint above, and a descending branch innervates the facet joint below. However, the numbering of the medial branches is different in the cervical spine compared with the lumbar spine. For example, the medial branch nerve that extends around the

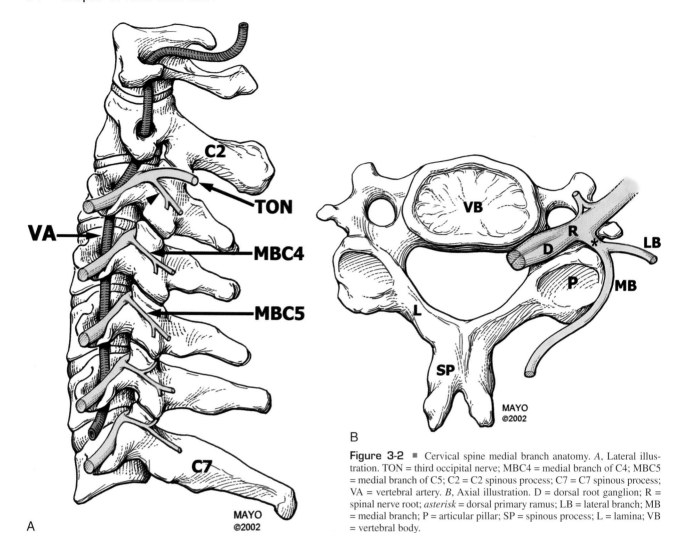

A

B

Figure 3-2 ■ Cervical spine medial branch anatomy. *A,* Lateral illustration. TON = third occipital nerve; MBC4 = medial branch of C4; MBC5 = medial branch of C5; C2 = C2 spinous process; C7 = C7 spinous process; VA = vertebral artery. *B,* Axial illustration. D = dorsal root ganglion; R = spinal nerve root; *asterisk* = dorsal primary ramus; LB = lateral branch; MB = medial branch; P = articular pillar; SP = spinous process; L = lamina; VB = vertebral body.

C4 articular pillar is the C4 medial branch nerve. Thus, the C4 and C5 medial branches innervate the C4-5 facet joint. The medial branch of C3 differs somewhat. There is a deep medial branch that courses around the articular pillar of C3 similar to those of C4 to C8. This C3 medial branch helps innervate the C3-4 facet joint, but it provides little if any neural contribution to the C2-3 facet joint. There is a superficial medial branch of C3 known as the third occipital nerve. This nerve wraps around the lateral aspect of the ipsilateral C2-3 facet joint and supplies the C2-3 facet joint as well as providing a cutaneous supply to the suboccipital region.

In summary, the facet joints inferior to the C2-3 level are denervated by producing a radiofrequency lesion in the tissue adjacent to the articular pillars above and below the joint, and the C2-3 facet joint is denervated by radiofrequency lesioning of the third occipital nerve.[15]

PATIENT SELECTION

The history and physical examination must be consistent with facet syndrome. For the lumbar spine, this involves the following[16]:

- Unilateral or bilateral paravertebral low back pain
- Pain is often limited to the low back, buttock, and hip but can radiate into the thigh and down to the knee in a nondermatomal distribution. The pain is usually not distal to the knee.
- Pain is often associated with twisting or rotational motion.
- More pain occurs on extension than flexion.
- Pain occurs when moving from sitting to standing.
- Pain may be relieved by standing, walking, rest, or repetitive activity.
- Morning stiffness is present.
- Neurologic examination is normal.
- Tenderness is evident over the affected facet joints.
- Radicular pain is absent with straight-leg raising.
- Routine lumbar radiographs may show absent to severe facet degenerative changes.

For the cervical spine, these findings may include the following:

- Unilateral or bilateral paravertebral neck pain
- Decreased range of motion of the neck
- Local tenderness over affected facet joints
- Upper cervical facet joints that cause not only neck pain but also headaches and cutaneous pain

- Pain frequently referred into the shoulder girdle. Pain can extend to the elbow but is rarely distal to the elbow. The pain should not follow a radicular pattern.

The patient must have had relief from at least two facet pain procedures.

- Pain relief must be greater than 80% for the expected distribution of the facet joint.
- Facet pain procedures include two comparative medial branch blocks or a combination of intra-articular facet injection(s) and medial branch block(s). These procedures should be performed at low volume (<1 mL).

Aggressive nonsurgical therapy has been exhausted. Psychosocial factors have been addressed, including emotional problems and addictions. The patient must have realistic goals regarding the outcome and be committed to change those behaviors that negatively affect outcome, both immediate and future.

CONTRAINDICATIONS

- Coagulopathy (International Normalized Ratio [INR] >1.5 or platelets <50,000/mm^3)
- Pregnancy (because of teratogenic effects of radiation)
- Systemic infection or skin infection over the puncture site
- Severe allergy to any of the medications (relative contraindication)
- The patient has received the maximum amount of steroid, including systemic steroids, allowed for a given time period unless the injection is to be performed without steroids
- An extensive solid lateral or posterolateral fusion, which may not allow percutaneous access to the target medial branch nerve
- Patients with motor weakness, absent reflexes, or long tract signs[13]

PROCEDURE

Several radiofrequency generators are on the market. We use the generator and needles from Radionics, Inc. (Burlington, MA) for all our procedures. We have had success with straight-tipped electrodes. Some physicians prefer to make a gentle 5- to 10-degree bend on the distal tip of the straight cannula to facilitate placement along the path of the medial branch. There are also pre-curved electrodes on the market that many physicians prefer. One should try the various needle and electrode types to determine one's preference. The impedances, temperatures, and lengths of times we use for denervation are also only a guideline and may differ among vendors. One should always check with vendors for their denervation guidelines.

Equipment/Supplies

Procedural

Radiofrequency generator
Grounding pad
Sterile connecting cable

SMK electrode (100 mm, lumbar and thoracic; sometimes 145 mm necessary)
SMK electrode (54 mm, cervical)
Disposable SMK styleted needles (1 for each level matching length of probe)
Spinal needle, 22-gauge, 3.5-inch (1 for each level for supplying deep anesthesia) (Quinke type point, Becton Dickinson & Co, Franklin Lakes, NJ)
Control syringe, 12 mL, with 25-gauge, 1.5-inch needle containing 9.5 mL 1% lidocaine for local anesthesia and 0.5 mL 8.4% sodium bicarbonate injectable (1 mEq/mL) to alleviate burning pain associated with anesthetic
Syringe, 6 mL, containing local anesthetic
Syringe, 6 mL, containing steroid
Lead apron
Multidirectional C-arm fluoroscopy with film-archiving capability

Incidentals

Povidone-iodine (Betadine) scrub
Alcohol scrub
Sterile drapes
Sterile gauze
Adhesive bandages
Hats, masks, sterile gloves, and gowns

Medications

Lidocaine-MPF 1% (Xylocaine-MPF 1%, AstraZeneca LP, Wilmington, DE)
Betamethasone sodium phosphate and betamethasone acetate injectable suspension 6 mg/mL (Celestone Soluspan 6 mg/mL, Schering Corporation, Kenilworth, NJ)

Precautions

A preservative-free anesthetic agent is used. MPF means methylparaben free. The MPF form is preferable for use in spine intervention procedures because a steroid is often given at the same time. Many steroid suspensions, when mixed with certain preservatives (e.g., paraben, phenol), may cause flocculation of the steroid.[17] Some preservatives, if they are inadvertently injected intrathecally, may produce arachnoiditis.

No medications should contain epinephrine. Its vasoconstrictive properties are neither needed nor desired, particularly because of the risk of vasospasm in the head and neck region.

Methodology

Facet denervation is performed as an outpatient procedure. Patients are instructed to stop using their pain medications on the day of the procedure to allow greater diagnostic and therapeutic accuracy. They are also instructed to have a driver with them after the procedure as well as someone who can be responsible for their well-being for the remainder of the day because sedation may be given during the examination. As a minimum, electrocardiography, pulse oximetry, and blood pressure monitoring are performed during and immediately after the examination. Facet denervation should not be performed at the same time as a diagnostic facet block or medial branch block, because it is **imperative** that the patient be able to feel concordant pain reproduction during the sensory-testing portion of the denervation procedure. In fact, radiofrequency denervation should not be scheduled if the patient has not been experiencing the facet-related pain symptoms at the usual frequency.

Lumbar Facet Denervation

Informed consent is obtained. The patient is placed prone on the fluoroscopy table. The patient's lower back is prepared and draped in a sterile fashion. An adhesive grounding pad is placed on the patient's upper posterior thigh (shaved if necessary) and connected to the radiofrequency generator. The sterile radiofrequency connecting cable is attached to the radiofrequency generator and the other end is placed on the patient sterile field. The radiofrequency probe is then connected to the connecting cable and clipped to sterile sheets on the patient. Intravenous analgesia/sedation is often necessary. The patient should be monitored by electrocardiography, pulse oximetry, and blood pressure checks. Anesthesia is limited to a mild sedative and analgesic (midazolam, 1 to 2 mg, and fentanyl, 75 to 150 μg). **It is extremely important that the patient not be sedated to**

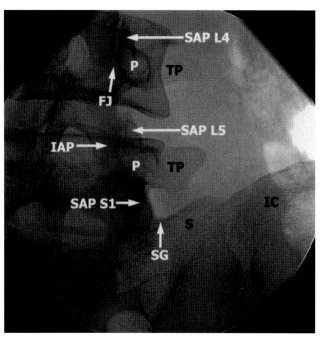

Figure 3-3 ■ Shallow LAO radiograph, partial "Scotty dog" appearance. Ear = superior articular process (SAP); eye = pedicle (P); nose = transverse process (TP); front leg = inferior articular process (IAP); FJ = facet joint; SG = sacral groove; S = sacral ala; IC = iliac crest.

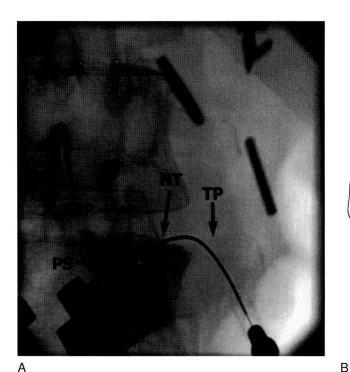

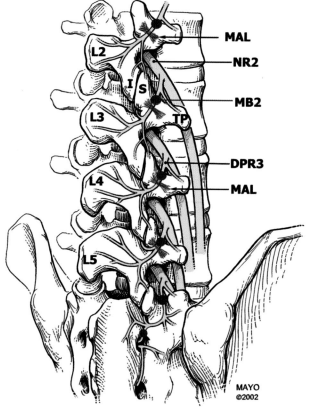

A   B

Figure 3-4 ■ Proper target zone, lumbar medial branch. *A,* Shallow LAO radiograph. The needle tip (NT) is at the superior border of the junction of the superior articular process (SAP) and the transverse process (TP). P = pedicle; PS = pedicle screw. *B,* Shallow LAO illustration demonstrates targets (*red circles*) for denervation. L2 through L5 spinous processes are labeled. MAL = mamilloaccessory ligament; NR2 = second lumbar nerve root; MB2 = medial branch of second lumbar nerve root; DPR3 = dorsal primary ramus of third lumbar nerve root; TP = transverse process; I = inferior articular process; S = superior articular process.

the point that he or she is not able to fully understand questions or to feel pain or sense motor stimulation. When the heating protocol begins, the patient's responses may be the earliest warning that the radiofrequency probe may not be in satisfactory position.

PATIENT POSITIONING

As with all spine procedures, proper patient and/or C-arm positioning can make the procedure straightforward. For the T12 through L4 medial branch nerves, the junction of the base of the transverse process and the superior articulating process is placed in the center of the field of view in a straight anteroposterior plane relative to the patient. The C-arm (image intensifier above the patient) is then rotated 10 to 20 degrees in an oblique angle ipsilateral with respect to the side of the back being treated (i.e., the image intensifier is rotated to the right if the right facet joint is being treated). At this angle, one should begin to see the "Scotty dog" appearance, with the nose being the transverse process, the eye the pedicle, and the ear the superior articulating process (Fig. 3-3).

NEEDLE PLACEMENT

For straight needles, the puncture site that allows easiest access to and greatest exposure of the medial branch nerve is at or slightly craniad to the level of the transverse process and just lateral to the medial border of the superior articulating process. A wide skin wheal of 1% lidocaine is instilled for superficial anesthesia. Skin puncture is then made with a disposable SMK needle (usually SMK-10 in the lumbar region). With the use of intermittent fluoroscopy, the needle is advanced ventral, medial, and slightly caudad until contact is made with the junction of the base of the transverse process, superior articulating process, and pedicle. The needle tip is advanced in small increments by "walking" it over the superior aspect of the transverse process until the needle is just felt to slide over the top of the transverse process (Fig. 3-4). With the needle in this position, it is in close proximity to the medial branch nerve. The nerve at this point has its most horizontal course. Therefore, with this approach, the SMK needle tip and medial branch lie parallel to each other in maximal apposition. A lateral view of the lumbar spine is then obtained to demonstrate that the needle is not too far ventral and not encroaching on the neural foramen (Fig. 3-5).

For curved needles, the puncture site is made at the inferomedial aspect of the transverse process and advanced until the tip contacts the superomedial free edge of the transverse process at the junction of the superior articulating process. The needle is then turned so that the distal tip faces laterally (Fig. 3-6A). The needle is advanced 1 to 2 mm and then turned back so that the distal tip hooks over the transverse process along the path of the medial branch nerve (see Fig. 3-6B).

The L5 dorsal ramus does not have a medial branch nerve. The target for the L5 dorsal ramus is at the superomedial aspect of the sacral ala, just lateral to the superior articulating process of S1. The needle is passed until contact is made with the superior edge of the bone of the sacral ala. The needle is then walked over the bone and advanced 2 to 3 mm, where it should lie close to the nerve (L5 dorsal ramus) (Fig. 3-7).

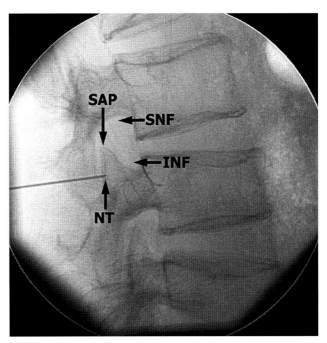

Figure 3-5 ■ Proper needle position, lumbar medial branch. Lateral radiograph. Needle tip (NT) is posterior to the neural foramen and just anterior to the posterior margin of the superior articulating process (SAP). SNF = superior neural foramen; INF = inferior neural foramen.

Thoracic Facet Denervation

Thoracic procedures are performed in a fashion similar to lumbar procedures. The numbering of the nerves innervating the thoracic facets is similar to that in the lumbar region. However, it is important to place the needle close to the lateral border of the superior articulating process to avoid puncturing the adjacent lung. The target for thoracic medial branch denervation is just cephalad to the superomedial aspect of the transverse process (Fig. 3-8). Cranial or caudal angulation of the C-arm may be necessary to separate the transverse process from the costovertebral junction.

Cervical Facet Denervation

It is recommended that cervical facet denervation be performed by experienced, well-trained persons who have a good understanding of the anatomic relationships of the nerves and adjacent spinal structures. Informed consent is obtained. The patient is placed in the lateral decubitus position, pain side up, on the fluoroscopy table. The patient's neck is prepared and draped in a sterile fashion. An adhesive grounding pad is placed on the patient's scapula and connected to the radiofrequency generator. The sterile radiofrequency connecting cable is attached to the radiofrequency generator, and the other end is placed on the patient sterile field. The radiofrequency probe is then connected to the connecting cable and clipped to sterile sheets on the patient. Intravenous anesthesia is often necessary. The patient should be monitored by electrocardiography, pulse oximetry, and blood pressure checks. Anesthesia is limited to a mild sedative and analgesic (midazolam, 1 to 2 mg, and fentanyl, 75 to 150 µg). **It is extremely important that the patient not**

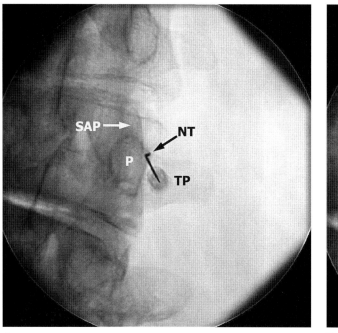

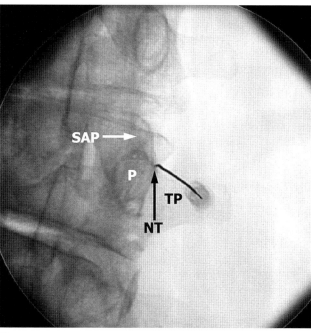

A   B

Figure 3-6 ■ Curved needle technique, shallow LAO radiographs. *A,* The curved needle is seen at the junction of the superior articular process (SAP) and the transverse process (TP) with the needle tip (NT) pointed laterally. *B,* The needle is advanced 1 to 2 mm and turned 180 degrees to face medially along the path of the medial branch. P = pedicle.

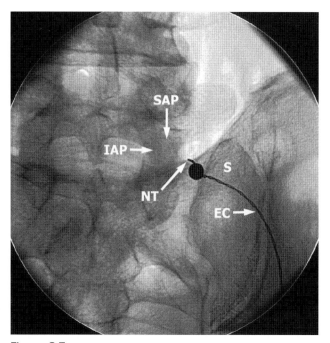

Figure 3-7 ■ Proper needle position, L5 dorsal primary ramus. The needle tip (NT) is in the sacral groove formed by the lateral border of the L5 superior articular process (SAP) and the ipsilateral medial border of the S1 sacral ala (S). IAP = inferior articular process; EC = electrode cable.

be sedated to the point that he or she is not able to fully understand questions or to feel pain or sense motor stimulation. When the heating protocol begins, the patient's responses may be the earliest warning that the radiofrequency probe may not be in a satisfactory position.

PATIENT POSITIONING

The patient is placed in the lateral decubitus position with the symptomatic side up. A cushion should be placed under the patient's head to keep the neck parallel to the table. With the use of maximum fluoroscopic magnification, the articular pillar (if treating the C3-4 through C7-T1 facet joint) or the C2-3 facet joint (if lesioning the third occipital nerve) is placed in the center of the field of view. The target is best visualized if imaging is performed in the straight lateral plane (i.e., the left and right facet joints, articular pillars, and posterior elements are superimposed and appear as a single unit (Fig. 3-9).

NEEDLE PLACEMENT

The puncture is most easily and safely performed from a posterolateral approach, ipsilateral to the side of the pain. With this approach, the needle will pass through muscle and fascial tissues. The needle will also remain well posterior to vascular structures such as the vertebral artery. Again, one should attempt to have the radiofrequency electrode parallel

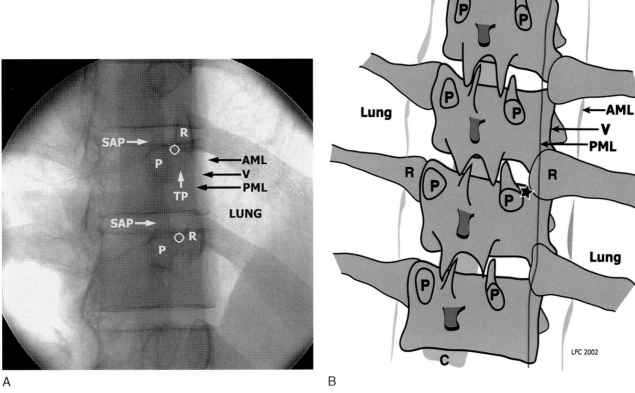

A   B

Figure 3-8 ▪ Proper positioning, thoracic medial branch. LAO radiograph (*A*) and (*B*) illustration. Craniocaudal x-ray beam angulation separates the head of the rib (R) from the target (*white open target*, A; *black star*, B). The superior articular process (SAP) is difficult to visualize in the thoracic region but lies above the pedicle (P). One must be aware of the three-line configuration of the ventral medial lung (VML), vertebral margin (V), and posterior medial lung (PML) to avoid pleural puncture and pneumothorax. AML = anterior medial lung; TP = transverse process; SAP = superior articular process.

Figure 3-9 ▪ Proper positioning, cervical medial branch. Straight lateral radiograph. Left- and right-sided articular pillars (AP) and facet joints (FJ) are aligned to appear as a single unit.

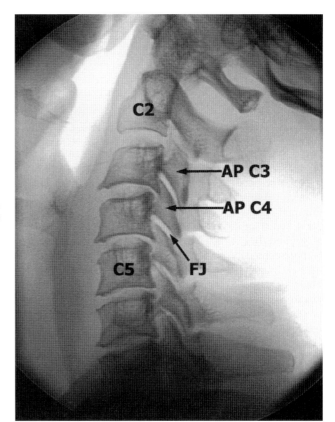

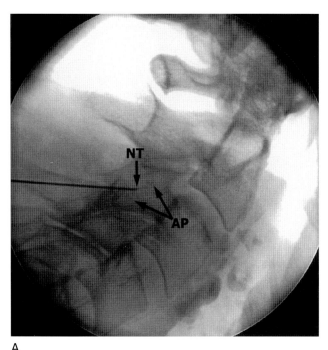

A

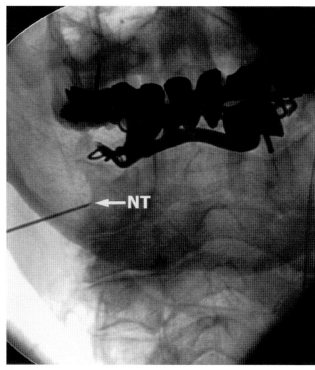

B

Figure 3-10 ■ Proper needle positioning, cervical region. *A,* Lateral radiograph. Needle tip (NT) is seen on the ventral portion of the mid body of the articular pillar (AP). *B,* AP radiograph. Needle tip (NT) is closely apposed to the midvertebral margin.

to the long axis of the medial branch, which, from the posterolateral approach, would be along the articular pillar. With the use of lateral fluoroscopy, a wide skin wheal of 1% lidocaine is instilled along the posterior border of the sternocleidomastoid muscle at the level of the spinous process related to the target articular pillar. Skin puncture is then made with a disposable SMK needle (usually SMK-5 in the cervical region). With the use of intermittent fluoroscopy, the needle is advanced ventrally and medially until tangential contact is made with the articular pillar (Fig. 3-10). The C-arm is rotated 10 to 15 degrees left anterior oblique (LAO) and right anterior oblique (RAO) to ensure that the tip of the needle remains in close relation to the articular pillar.

The first needle position that we try to obtain for the C3 through C6 medial branches is along the ventral aspect of a line that connects the greatest anteroposterior diameter of the articular pillar but remains dorsal to the foramen (Fig. 3-11A and B). For the C7 medial branch, the needle position is more cephalad on the superior articulating facet. The C8 medial branch is approached much like lumbar medial branches. For C8 denervation, the needle is placed at the junction of the superior articulating facet and the transverse process of T1. The third occipital nerve is approached in a fashion similar to that for the other cervical branches. However, because the third occipital nerve is larger than the medial branches, radiofrequency lesions are often produced at several sites along the nerve. This may have to be done at different sessions, as discussed in detail later in this chapter. The third occipital nerve courses along the C2-3 facet joint.

The needles are placed at the anteroinferior aspect of the C2 inferior facet and the anterosuperior aspect of the C3 superior facet (see Fig. 3-11C and D). A third lesion may be delivered along the C2-3 facet joint (see Fig. 3-11E). Because this procedure is performed in the lateral plane, the position of the needle tip can be assessed to ensure that there is no evidence of neural foraminal encroachment.

Assessing Proper Needle Position

Denervation should be considered permanent nerve destruction. Therefore, there are risks to the patient, one of the worst of which is destruction of the dorsal root ganglia or primary ramus. This could lead to denervation of major muscular groups, atrophy, and loss of motor strength and possibly a deafferentation pain syndrome. We believe that with any of the spine procedures, **if it cannot be performed safely or at most with acceptable risk to the patient, it should not be performed at all**. Therefore, it is of utmost importance that strict adherence to **sensory and motor** testing be followed. Some believe that it is superfluous to perform electrical testing before denervation and that it is only necessary to make sure that the needle is in proper anatomic position.[6] We believe differently. Given the serious harm that could be caused to the patient, it is important that the physician performing the procedure test the position of the needle. Also, in our experience, we have seen many cases of anatomic variation. Who is to say that the medial branch in a given patient does not arise close to the dorsal ramus? We see this quite frequently in the cervical spine. In the upper

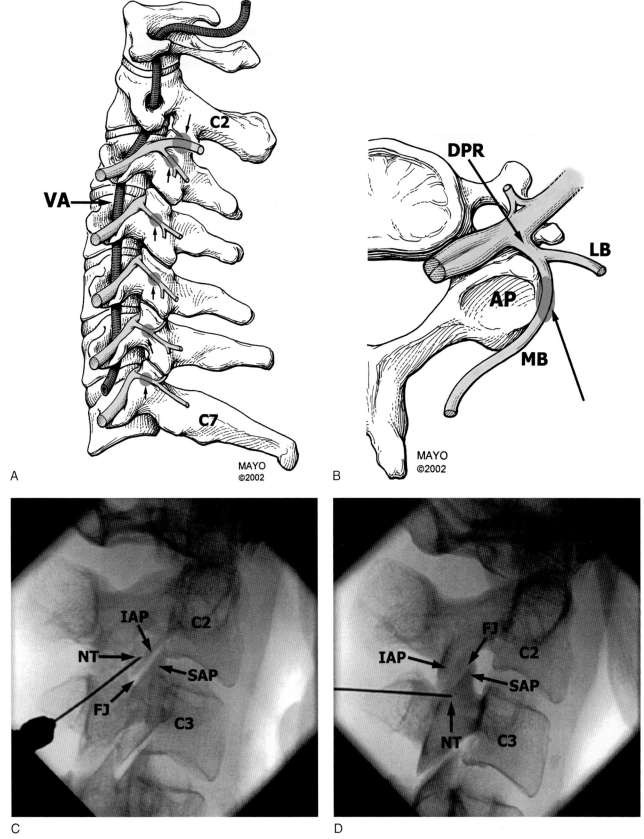

Figure 3-11 ■ Proper needle positioning, cervical region. Lateral radiographs. Lateral (*A*) and axial (*B*) illustrations demonstrate the target zones (*arrows*) for medial branch denervations. C2 = C2 spinous process; C7 = C7 spinous process; VA = vertebral artery; DPR = dorsal primary ramus; LB = lateral branch; MB = medial branch; AP = articular pillar. *C*, Needle tip (NT) contacts the inferior border of the C2 inferior articular process (IAP). *D*, The needle tip (NT) contacts the superior border of the C3 superior articular process (SAP).

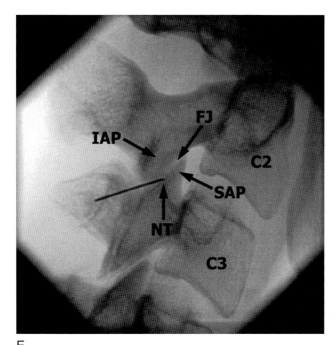

E

Figure 3-11 (*Cont'd*) ■ *E*, The needle tip (NT) overlies the C2-3 facet joint (FJ).

cervical spine, most primary needle positions are acceptable; however, it appears that the medial branch is closer to the dorsal ramus as one proceeds inferiorly. We believe that the minimal additional time expended to test the sensory

and motor responses of the patient is highly beneficial (Fig. 3-12).

When the SMK needle appears to be in satisfactory anatomic position, the stylet is removed and the matching electrode is placed through the needle. The impedance of the tissues surrounding the electrode tip is then checked, followed by sensory and motor stimulation and lastly by creation of the lesion itself.

IMPEDANCE

The tissues of the body have various impedances. For instance, fluid or air has very low impedance and bone has very high impedance. To check the impedance with the Radionics® generator, all mode buttons must be off. For optimal denervation, the impedance should fall within 250 to 500 ohms.

SENSORY TESTING

If impedance falls within the range of normal, sensory testing is performed. Sensory testing is performed at 50 Hz with a range of 0 to 1 volt. The stimulation mode is depressed, and the voltage is gradually increased until the patient experiences symptoms or maximum voltage is reached. The patient is questioned very specifically about any symptoms that are being produced. If, in the lumbar spine, a motor or radicular component is sensed or visualized in the gluteal muscles or extremity during stimulation, or if the patient does not experience any symptoms, the needle must be repositioned. Similarly, if there are motor or radicular symptoms in the upper extremity or face during cervical stimulation, the needle must be repositioned. Needle position should be changed until pain or pressure is elicited that may be con-

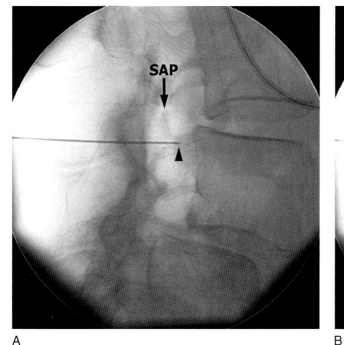

A

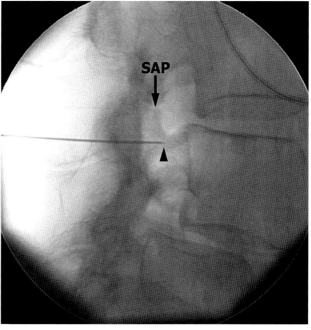

B

Figure 3-12 ■ *A*, Lateral radiograph demonstrates the needle tip (*arrowhead*) 3 mm ventral to the ventral base of the superior articular process (SAP). The patient experienced concordant pain with sensory stimulation but also motor stimulation in the lower extremity. *B*, Lateral radiograph with the needle tip (*arrowhead*) withdrawn to a point 1 mm ventral to the ventral base of the superior articular process (SAP). Patient experienced concordant pain on sensory stimulation and no extremity symptoms with motor stimulation.

cordant with the usual pain without eliciting any radicular or leg pain. Also, the lower the amount of voltage necessary to bring about symptoms, the closer will the needle be positioned adjacent to the actual target. Once sensory stimulation has been completed, the voltage should be turned down to zero and the stimulation mode deselected.

MOTOR TESTING

If impedance falls within the range of normal and sensory testing elicits concordant pain without radicular or extremity pain, motor testing is performed. Motor stimulation is performed at 2 Hz with a voltage range of 1 to 10 volts. The stimulation mode is depressed and the voltage is very gradually increased to at least twice the number of volts to elicit the initial sensory symptoms. The patient is again specifically questioned concerning any pain or pressure felt and its distribution and intensity. It is quite common for the patient to feel a rhythmic thumping sensation in the back or more vigorous thumping in the neck or back. The physician should look for these rhythmic contractions. This thumping sensation represents contractions of the multifidus muscle fibers, which are innervated by the medial branch nerves. These contractions are normal. However, any contractions in the gluteal muscles or lower extremities (in the case of lumbar facet denervation) or in the face and upper extremities (in the case of cervical denervation) must never be considered normal—they indicate too close proximity to the spinal nerve. If contractions like these occur, the needle and electrode must be repositioned and testing must be repeated with impedance checks followed by sensory testing and then motor testing. If the patient does not experience any motor symptoms or has only rhythmic multifidus contractions, we increase the voltage to a maximum of 3 volts, again questioning the patient and evaluating for any abnormal motor contractions. Once the motor stimulation has been completed, the voltage should be turned down to zero and the stimulation mode deselected.

Radiofrequency Lesioning Protocol

The creation of a radiofrequency lesion can be quite painful for the patient. It is recommended that a local anesthetic be administered into the tissue adjacent to the radiofrequency electrode before the procedure to minimize patient discomfort. Most literature on this subject describes a procedure in which the physician removes the radiofrequency electrode, leaving the cannula in place, and injects 0.5 to 1.0 mL of lidocaine directly through the SMK needle and then reinserts the electrode before lesioning. We suggest an alternate approach, similar to that of Dreyfuss and colleagues,[6] which produces excellent results safely and expeditiously. Once the SMK needle is in place and impedance checks and successful sensory and motor testing have been completed, we no longer manipulate the needle. Instead, a 22-gauge, 3.5-inch spinal needle is placed tandem to the SMK needle and advanced, using intermittent fluoroscopy, until the tip is in close proximity to the electrode tip, which is demonstrated by rotating the C-arm back and forth several degrees and visualizing that the needle tips remain in close proximity (Fig. 3-13). This tandem needle approach is recommended because the medial branch nerve is so small and any inadvertent manipulation of the SMK needle may displace the

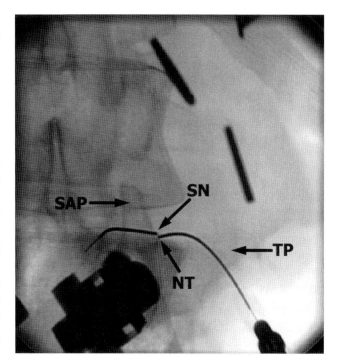

Figure 3-13 ■ Tandem anesthetic needle technique. Shallow LAO radiograph. Electrode needle tip (NT) is at the junction of the base of the transverse process (TP) and the superior articular process (SAP). The tip of the spinal needle (SN) used to deliver deep anesthesia is closely apposed to the electrode needle tip.

electrode from the optimal lesioning position. Because a local anesthetic is given, it would be difficult to determine whether the procedure was entirely successful because of lesioning of the nerve or was merely temporarily effective, because one had inadvertently produced, in effect, a medial branch block. Anesthetic is administered by injecting 0.5 to 1.0 mL of 1% lidocaine-MPF through the spinal needle, depositing it adjacent to the SMK needle tip. After this, the spinal needle is removed. Immediately before lesioning, AP and lateral radiographs of the SMK needle position are obtained for documentation.

The lesion settings are set for 80°C for 90 seconds. The lesion mode button is depressed. The impedance will drop slightly. The electrode temperature is then raised slowly to 80°C, at which point the timer is started. During this procedure, the patient is repeatedly questioned about any symptoms he or she may be feeling, specifically, any pain or contractions in the extremity. If pain or contractions are present in the extremity, radiofrequency lesioning is immediately terminated and consideration must be given to repositioning the needle. **However, once lidocaine has been given, it may be impossible to perform proper sensory and motor testing and therefore this level may have to be abandoned.** If there is no extremity pain, lesioning can continue. The radiofrequency lesioning will terminate automatically when the timer reaches the set time (90 seconds). The electrode is then removed and 2 mg of betamethasone is instilled through the SMK needle before its removal to decrease any inflammation and pain that may occur over the next few days. The remaining levels are treated in identical fashion. After the procedure, the back or neck is cleansed and dried and adhesive bandages are placed over the puncture sites.

Some authors recommend performing multiple lesions along the course of a medial branch to create a greater length of nerve destruction. We reserve this option only if local anesthesia is **not** given to the tissues surrounding the needle tip **and** good sensory and motor testing can be achieved after each needle manipulation. General anesthesia may be necessary if multiple lesioning is to be performed. If anesthetic is injected into the tissues surrounding the needle tip before lesioning, it may be impossible to accurately perform meaningful sensory and motor testing after the needle has been moved. This could lead to serious permanent complications if a denervation was performed. With meticulous sensory and motor testing, an excellent outcome can be achieved, despite the decreased length of the radiofrequency-induced lesion. Patients who have a less than satisfactory outcome can return for a repeat procedure.

POTENTIAL COMPLICATIONS

- Bleeding
- Infection
- Thecal sac puncture and headache
- Allergic reactions pertaining to the medications
- Risk of pneumothorax with thoracic facet denervation
- Vasovagal reactions and ataxia, especially with cervical facet denervation
- **Permanent damage to the spinal nerve**

POST-PROCEDURE CARE/FOLLOW-UP

Immediate[15]

1. The patient should be observed for 2 hours after facet denervation.
2. The patient may sit in a reclining lounge chair; however, if there is significant post-procedure pain or if the patient received intravenous sedation, he or she should be placed at bed rest.
3. Blood pressure, pulse, heart rate, and respiration are evaluated every 30 minutes.

Discharge[15]

1. The patient is discharged into the care of a responsible person.
2. The patient is instructed not to drive or perform any other tasks that require clear thought and quick reactions for the remainder of the day, especially if sedation was given.
3. The patient is given a 2- to 3-day nonrenewable prescription for a narcotic pain reliever and/or a muscle relaxant.
4. Multiple adhesive bandages may be on the patient's back or neck. These should remain dry for at least 24 hours, at which point they can be removed.
5. The patient is instructed to continue taking his or her prescription medication, although pain medication may be tapered as indicated.

6. A discharge sheet should be given to the patient outlining the following:
   a. Which procedure was performed and at what levels
   b. Procedural-related symptoms that typically resolve in 7 to 10 days
      - Pain at the needle puncture site(s)
      - Mild increased back or neck stiffness
      - Deep back or neck pain
   c. Treatment for mild post-procedure symptoms
      - Rest the affected area for 3 to 4 days.
      - Avoid movements that aggravate the pain.
      - Apply cold compresses to the area that hurts.
   d. Signs and symptoms of infection
      - Fever
      - Chills
      - Swelling or drainage from the puncture sites
      - New back or neck pain that is different from the usual pain
   e. Signs and symptoms of possibly more serious problems
      - Stiff neck
      - Increasing pain
      - Motor dysfunction such as difficulty walking or lifting
      - Bowel or bladder dysfunction
   f. Physician name and contact number if the patient has any concerns or if any problems were to arise as a result of the procedure
   g. Advice to schedule a follow-up appointment with the referring physician in 7 to 10 days

SAMPLE DICTATIONS

Lumbar Spine

Procedure:	Facet denervation
Date of Procedure:	Month/day/year
Facility:	Name of facility
Level Treated:	Left L4-5 facet joint (left L3 and L4 medial branches)
Supplies:	SMK-C10 disposable insulated cannulas, 22-gauge (2)
	C112-TC thermocouple cable
	SMK-TC10 thermocouple electrode

The procedure and potential complications were explained to the patient, and voluntary informed, signed consent was obtained. The patient was a candidate for conscious sedation. The patient was placed prone on the table. The patient's back was prepped and draped in usual sterile fashion. Subcutaneous lidocaine was instilled into the superficial soft tissues of the patient's back for local anesthesia. Under fluoroscopic guidance, a 22-gauge, 100-mm SMK needle was advanced percutaneously to the junction of the superior aspect of the left L4 transverse process and the lateral aspect of the left L4 superior articulating facet. The needle was then walked over the transverse process and advanced 2 to 3 mm to lie along the path of the left L3 medial branch nerve. AP and lateral radiographs were obtained to document proper needle position. Sensory and motor stimulation were then performed, which elicited deep local back discomfort but no evidence of motor stimulation in the gluteal muscles or extremities. A tandem needle insertion was performed adjacent to the SMK needle to supply local anesthesia (0.3 mL of 1% lidocaine-MPF) to the tissues around the tip of the SMK needle. Subsequently, a medial branch nerve denervation was performed for 90 seconds at 80°C without complication. The radiofrequency probe was removed with the needle left in place and 0.3 mL of betamethasone (6 mg/mL) was instilled through the needle. The needle was removed and the patient was repositioned. A similar procedure was performed on the left L4 medial branch nerve, without complication. Approximately 2 hours after the procedure, the patient was allowed to ambulate. There was no subjective or objective loss of motor strength. The patient was informed to follow up with his referring physician in 7 to 10 days.

Cervical Spine

Procedure: Facet denervation
Date of Procedure: Month/day/year
Facility: Name of facility
Level Treated: Left C4-5 facet joint (left C4 and C5 medial branches)
Supplies: SMK-C5 disposable insulated cannulas, 22-gauge (2)
                   C112-TC thermocouple cable
                   SMK-TC5 thermocouple electrode

The procedure and potential complications were explained to the patient, and voluntary informed, signed consent was obtained. The patient was a candidate for conscious sedation. The patient was placed in the right lateral decubitus position on the table. The patient's neck, upper chest, and shoulder were prepped and draped in usual sterile fashion. Subcutaneous lidocaine was instilled into the superficial soft tissues of the patient's neck for local anesthesia. Under fluoroscopic guidance, a 22-gauge, 54-mm SMK needle was advanced percutaneously, using a left posterolateral approach, until the needle tip contacted the lateral aspect of the left C4 articular pillar. The needle was then positioned in an orientation tangential to the ventral aspect of the articular pillar, although still remaining in close contact with the bone and along an orientation parallel to the left C4 medial branch nerve. A single spot radiographic image was obtained. Sensory and motor stimulation were then performed, which elicited deep left neck and shoulder discomfort but no evidence of motor stimulation in the extremities or face. A tandem needle insertion was performed adjacent to the SMK needle to supply local anesthesia (0.3 mL 1% lidocaine-MPF) to the tissues around the tip of the SMK needle. Subsequently, a medial branch nerve denervation was performed for 90 seconds at 80°C without complication. The radiofrequency probe was removed with the needle left in place, and 0.3 mL of betamethasone (6 mg/mL) was instilled through the needle. The needle was removed, and the patient was repositioned. A similar procedure was performed on the left C5 medial branch nerve, without complication. Approximately 2 hours after the procedure, the patient's upper extremity strength was tested. There was no subjective or objective loss of motor strength. The patient was informed to follow up with his referring physician in 7 to 10 days.

CASE REPORTS

CASE 1

Clinical Presentation

The patient is an 83-year-old woman with right paraspinal, hip, and proximal thigh pain. She is most comfortable when lying down. The pain is aggravated with prolonged standing and walking. Reflexes are intact. Strength testing is normal bilaterally. Distal pulses are good.

Imaging and Therapy

MR imaging demonstrated advanced facet degenerative changes of L4-5 on the right with fatty atrophy of the right posterior paraspinal musculature (Fig. 3-14A). The patient had excellent pain relief on each occasion after a low-volume right L4-5 intra-articular facet block and low-volume right L3 and L4 medial branch anesthetic blocks. She was a candidate for right L4-5 facet denervation. For needle placement, the superior articular processes of L4 and L5 were positioned approximately 25% from the ventral aspect of their respective vertebral bodies with their respective superior end plates superimposed (see Fig. 3-14B and C). The electrode tip was seen at the junction of the superior articular process and the base of the transverse process at both L4 and L5 (see Fig. 3-14B and C). After successful sensory and motor testing at each level, facet denervation was performed.

Results

During sensory testing, the patient described pain in the back and hip that was similar to her usual pain. During motor testing, the patient felt rhythmic thumping in the back without evidence of sensation or movement in the lower extremity. Three months after the procedure, she stated that she is approximately 90% free of her usual pain.

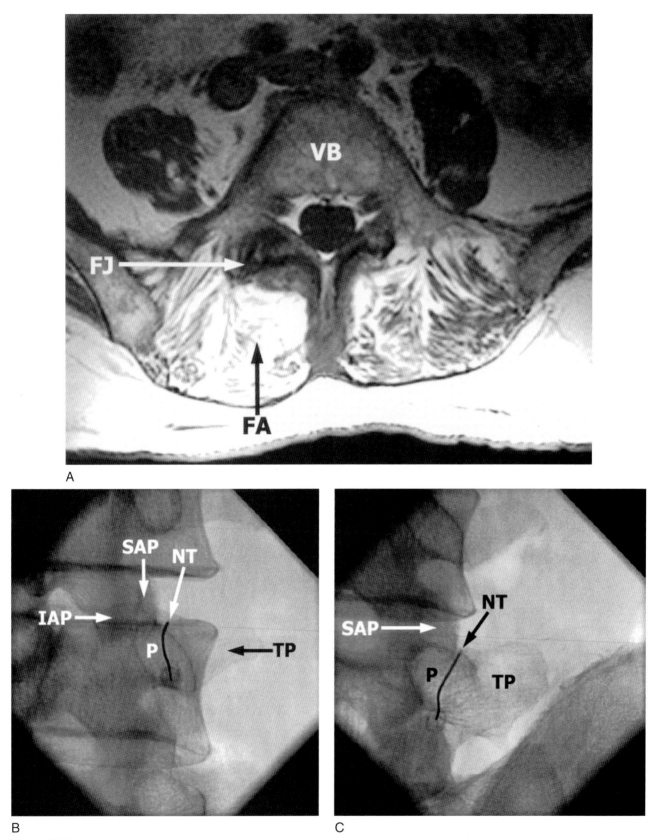

Figure 3-14 ■ *A*, Axial CT image, upper L5 vertebral level (VB). Moderate degeneration and bone overgrowth of the right L4-5 facet joint (FJ) are seen. Note fatty atrophy (FA) of the right posterior paraspinous musculature. *B* and *C*, Shallow LAO radiographs. Needle tips (NT) in proper position for right L3 (*B*) and right L4 (*C*) medial branch denervations. SAP = superior articular process; TP = transverse process; IAP = inferior articular process; P = pedicle.

CASE 2

Clinical Presentation

The patient is a 62-year-old man with right-sided low-back pain of 8 to 9 months duration. The pain radiates into the right paraspinal and hip regions without evidence of lower extremity involvement. It is worst with sitting and first thing in the morning. He has had only minimal improvement with nonsteroidal anti-inflammatory agents and physical therapy. The patient's reflexes and strength are normal. Straight-leg raising and hip motion testing are negative.

Imaging and Therapy

MR imaging demonstrated right L5-S1 facet degenerative change with irregularity of the facet joint and fluid within the joint (Fig. 3-15A). There was also increased signal in the right S1 superior articular

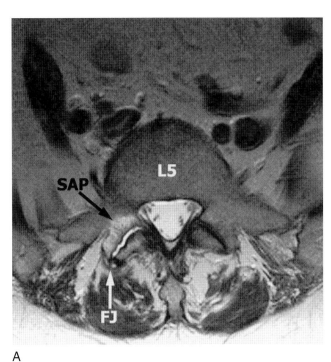

A

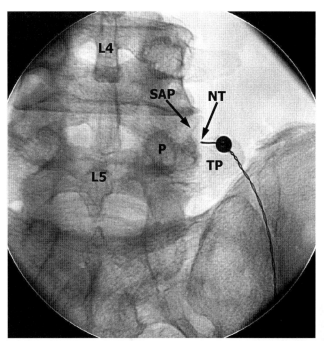

B

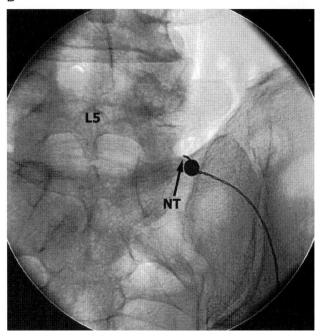

C

Figure 3-15 ■ *A*, Axial MR T2-weighted fast spin echo image, lower L5 vertebral level. Mild irregularity and increased signal intensity are present within the right L5-S1 facet joint (FJ), compatible with degenerative change. Note increased signal intensity involving the right superior articular process of S1 (SAP), compatible with reactive edema. B and C, AP radiographs. The needle tips (NT) are in proper position for a right L4 medial branch denervation (*B*) and a right L5 dorsal primary ramus denervation (*C*). P = pedicle; SAP = superior articular process L5; TP = right L5 transverse process.

process, likely reflecting marrow reactive change owing to chronic inflammation (see Fig. 3-15A). The patient had excellent pain relief on each occasion after a low-volume right L5-S1 intra-articular facet block and low-volume right L4 medial branch and L5 dorsal primary ramus anesthetic blocks. The patient was a candidate for right L5-S1 facet denervation. Slight contralateral obliquity of the C-arm was used for the right L4 denervation. The electrode tip was seen at the junction of the right L5 superior articular process and the base of the L5 transverse process (see Fig. 3-15B). The C-arm was perpendicular to the table for the L5 dorsal primary ramus denervation. The electrode tip was seen at the junction of the superior articular process of S1

and the sacral ala (see Fig. 3-15C). After successful sensory and motor testing at each level, facet denervation was performed.

Results

During sensory testing, the patient described pain in the back and right hip that was similar to his usual pain. During motor testing, the patient felt rhythmic thumping in the back without evidence of sensation or movement in the lower extremity. Three months after the procedure he stated that he is approximately 95% free of his usual pain.

CASE 3

Clinical Presentation

The patient is a 77-year-old man with a 1-year history of right neck, shoulder, and proximal arm pain. The pain is nonradicular. He has significant limitation of neck motion. He has had slight benefit with exercise. The patient's reflexes and strength are normal.

Imaging and Therapy

Bone scan demonstrated abnormal uptake involving the right posterior paramidline cervical spine (Fig. 3-16A). MR imaging demonstrated advanced irregularity and enlargement of the right C4-5 facet joint (see Fig. 3-16B). With the use of a fat suppression, post-contrast T1-

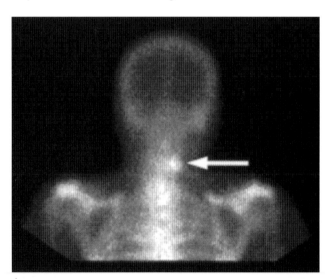

A

Figure 3-16 ■ *A,* Posterior coronal technetium bone scan. There is intense radiotracer uptake in the midcervical spine to the right of the midline (*arrow*), compatible with the region of severe degenerative change. *B,* MR gradient acquisition demonstrates overgrowth and increased signal intensity within right C4-5 facet joint (FJ). *C,* MR fat-saturated post-contrast T1-weighted image at the same level demonstrates enhancement within and surrounding the right C4-5 facet joint (FJ).

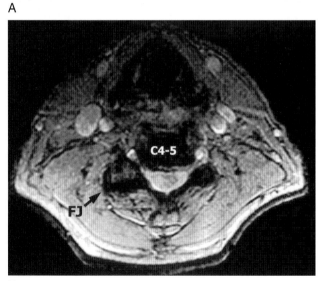

B

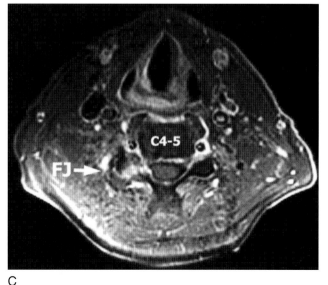

C

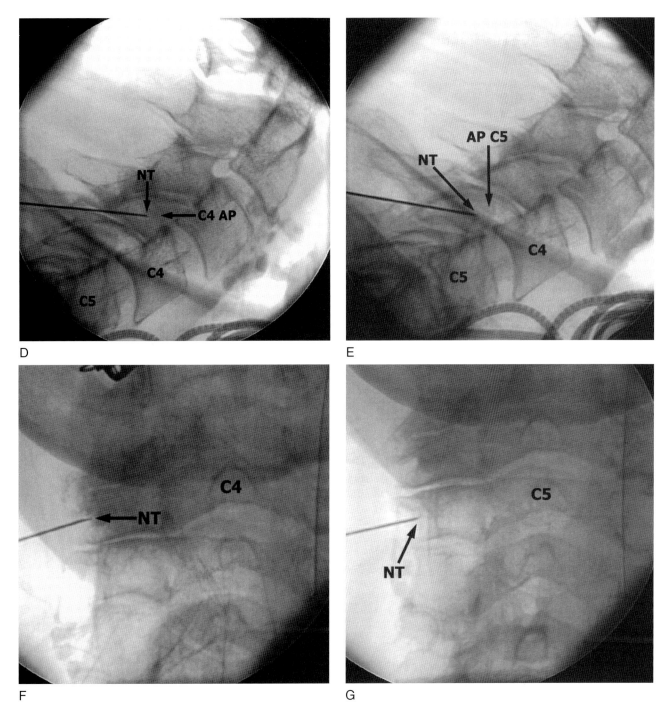

Figure 3-16 *(Cont'd)* ▪ *D* and *E*, Lateral radiographs. Medial branch denervations. The needle tips (NT) are at the mid body of the C4 and C5 articular pillars (AP). AP radiographs F and G demonstrate that the needle tips (NT) are in close contact with the waist of the C4 and C5 articular pillars.

weighted technique, there was considerable intra-articular and periarticular enhancement of the right C4-5 facet joint, which may reflect a localized inflammatory synovitis (see Fig. 3-16C). The patient had complete pain relief on each occasion after a low-volume right C4-5 intra-articular facet block and low-volume right C4 and C5 medial branch blocks. The patient was a candidate for right C4-5 facet denervation. The electrode tips were seen on lateral views to overlie the mid bodies of the C4 and C5 articular pillars (see Fig. 3-16D and E). The corresponding AP views demonstrated that the needle tips were in close contact with the mid bodies of the articular pillars of C4 and C5 (see Fig. 3-16F and G). After successful sensory and motor testing at each level, facet denervation was performed.

Results

During sensory testing, the patient described pain in the right neck and shoulder that was similar to his usual pain. During motor testing, the patient felt rhythmic thumping in the right neck without evidence of sensation or movement in the upper extremity. Six months after the procedure, he stated that he is virtually pain free.

CURRENT PROCEDURAL TERMINOLOGY (CPT) CODES

CPT codes change often and sometimes are valid only for certain states or regions. It is best to consult with coding experts to make sure that coding for one's procedures is legitimate and complete. Below is a sample of codes that are being used for the facet denervation procedure at this writing.[19]

Destruction by Neurolytic Agent (e.g., Chemical, Thermal, Electrical, Radiofrequency or Chemodenervation)

64622 Destruction by neurolytic agent, paravertebral facet joint nerve; lumbar or sacral, single level

64623 lumbar or sacral, each additional level (List searately in addition to code for primary procedure)

(Use 64623 in conjunction with code 64622)

64626 cervical or thoracic, single level

64627 cervical or thoracic, each additional level (List separately in addition to code for primary procedure)

(Use 64627 in conjunction with code 64626)

76005 Fluoroscopic guidance and localization of needle or catheter tip for spine or paraspinous diagnostic or therapeutic injection procedures (epidural, transforaminal epidural, subarachnoid, paravertebral facet joint, paravertebral facet joint nerve or sacroiliac joint), including neurolytic agent destruction

99141 Sedation with or without analgesia (conscious sedation); intravenous, intramuscular or inhalation

XXXXX-50 modifier for bilateral procedures

The injection of local anesthetic and/or steroid either through the SMK needle or by placement of a tandem needle constitutes a medial branch block. Therefore, the following codes may also be valid.

Introduction/Injection of Anesthetic Agent (Nerve Block), Diagnostic or Therapeutic

64470 Injection, anesthetic agent and/or steroid, paravertebral facet joint or facet joint nerve; cervical or thoracic, single level

64472 cervical or thoracic, each additional level (List separately in addition to code for primary procedure)

(Use code 64472 in conjunction with code 64470)

64475 lumbar or sacral, single level

64476 lumbar or sacral, each additional level (List separately in addition to code for primary procedure)

(Use code 64476 in conjunction with code 64475)

XXXXX-50 modifier for bilateral procedures

References

1. Shealy CN. The role of the spinal facets in back and sciatic pain. Headache 1974; 14:101–104.
2. Mooney V, Robertson J. The facet syndrome. Clin Orthop Rel Res 1976; 115:149–156.
3. Fukui S, Ohseto K, Shiotani M, et al. Distribution of referred pain from the lumbar zygapophyseal joints and dorsal rami. Clin J Pain 1997; 13:303–307.
4. Bogduk N, Marsland A. The cervical zygapophysial joints as a source of neck pain. Spine 1988; 13:610–617.
5. Schwarzer AC, Shih-chang W, O'Driscoll D, et al. The ability of computed tomography to identify a painful zygapophysial joint in patients with chronic low back pain. Spine 1995; 20:907–912.
6. Dreyfus P, Halbrook B, Pauza K, et al. Efficacy and validity of radiofrequency neurotomy for chronic lumbar zygapophysial joint pain. Spine 2000; 25:1270–1277.
7. van Kleef M, Barendse GA, Kessels A, et al. Randomized trial of radiofrequency lumbar facet denervation for chronic low back pain. Spine 1999; 24:1937–1942.
8. McDonald GJ, Lord SM, Bogduk N. Long-term follow-up of patients treated with cervical radiofrequency neurotomy for chronic neck pain. Neurosurgery 1999; 45:61–67.
9. Lord SM, Barnsley L, Wallis BJ, et al. Percutaneous radio-frequency neurotomy for chronic cervical zygapophyseal-joint pain. N Engl J Med 1996; 335:1721–1726.
10. Gallagher J, Petriccione Di Vadi PL, Wedley JR, et al. Radiofrequency facet joint denervation in the treatment of low back pain: A prospective controlled double-blind study to assess its efficacy. Pain Clin 1994; 7:193–198.
11. Burton CV. Percutaneous radiofrequency facet denervation. Appl Neurophysiol 1976; 39:80–86.
12. Shealy CN. Percutaneous radiofrequency denervation of the lumbar facets. J Neurosurg 1975; 43:448–451.
13. Bogduk N, Long DM. The anatomy of the so-called "articular nerves" and their relationship to facet denervation in the treatment of low-back pain. J Neurosurg 1979; 51:172–177.
14. Bogduk N. The clinical anatomy of the cervical dorsal rami. Spine 1982; 7:319–330.
15. Lord SM, Barnsley L, Bogduk N. Percutaneous radiofrequency neurotomy in the treatment of cervical zygapophysial joint pain: A caution. Neurosurgery 1995; 36:732–739.
16. Jackson RP. The facet syndrome: Myth or reality? Clin Orthop Rel Res 1992; 279:110–121.
17. Physicians' Desk Reference, 56th ed. Montvale, NJ: Medical Economics Company, 2002.
18. Fenton DS, Czervionke LF. Discography. In Williams AL, Murtagh FR (eds). Handbook of Diagnostic and Therapeutic Spine Procedures. St. Louis: CV Mosby, 2002, pp 187–188.
19. CPT 2002, CPT Intellectual Property Services. Chicago: American Medical Association, 2002.

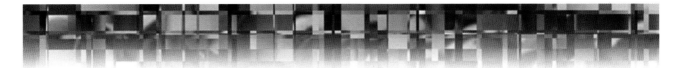

A Spine Surgeon's Perspective

Facet Denervation

Joseph T. Alexander, MD

Despite improvements in surgical technique in recent years, spinal fusion procedures remain major surgical undertakings, at times with significant morbidity and less than ideal outcomes. Some patients with axial pain would rather "try anything" than undergo spine surgery, or they may have widespread, mild degenerative changes that are not amenable to fusion procedures. Other patients with significant degenerative changes might benefit from spine stabilization but are not medically fit for the procedure or have confounding conditions that make surgical success less likely. I have found that, for these patients, facet denervation represents a good option if they have had a positive response to facet and medial branch blocks, as long as they clearly understand that this may not be a permanent solution. In these cases, facet denervation can provide significant improvement in the quality of life.

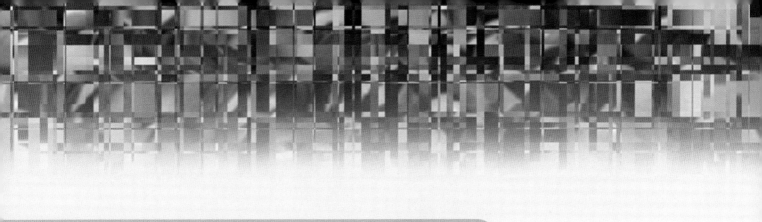

Chapter 4

Selective Nerve Root Block

- Douglas S. Fenton, MD
- Leo F. Czervionke, MD

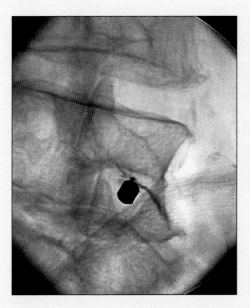

BACKGROUND

The selective nerve root block (SNRB) has both diagnostic and therapeutic potential. SNRB is a minimally invasive percutaneous outpatient procedure that can be performed with minimal or no sedation. The procedure can be performed by fluoroscopic or computed tomographic (CT) guidance, depending on the site of injection. SNRB is often overlooked as a diagnostic tool and as a potential temporizing pain relief therapy.

SNRB is most appropriately used in patients with radicular pain. In many instances, the source of the radicular pain can be diagnosed with imaging procedures (magnetic resonance [MR] imaging, CT) and with a careful neurologic examination. However, there are patients with radicular symptoms for whom results of a neurologic examination may be equivocal and an imaging study may demonstrate nonspecific findings at one or more levels. All too often these patients are sent for epidural injections that produce little or no therapeutic benefit for the patient and provide no diagnostic information to the clinician regarding the specific level from which the pain is originating. The epidural injection is a relatively high volume injection intended to permeate a large area of the epidural space and thereby deliver a small amount of diluted agent to each of multiple vertebral levels. In contrast, SNRB delivers a low volume of concentrated medication directly into the nerve root sleeve in question. The diagnostic potential of SNRB can be of great importance.

Used properly as a diagnostic tool, SNRB will elicit pain in the distribution of the nerve root sheath that has been injected. If the needle contacts the nerve responsible for the pain, the patient will report that the pain is concordant with his or her usual pain. If the patient describes the pain as undeniably discordant, the needle can be withdrawn and either another level can be attempted or the nerve block can be postponed after further review of any imaging studies and clinical findings.

In patients with multilevel imaging abnormalities, or in the case of the postoperative patient, SNRB can help guide the surgeon to the proper level or levels where the pain is originating; this information may help to limit the extent of surgery or in some cases may obviate surgery. Derby et al.[1] demonstrated that the injection of steroids during SNRB had an excellent negative predictive value. Patients with more than 1 year of radicular pain who did not have a long-term response to a selective nerve root steroid injection had a poor surgical outcome, and those with a positive response to injection response had a positive surgical outcome. SNRB can offer more long-term therapeutic relief when steroids are delivered with anesthetic agents if the pain is caused by a potentially reversible inflammatory process.

In the vast majority of patients, a single-level SNRB is sufficient both diagnostically and therapeutically. However, in rare instances, a two-level SNRB may be required. This is most clearly evident in a patient with a posterolateral disc herniation, or an osteophyte, or a combination of these, which can affect both the exiting and the traversing nerve roots. Such a patient will likely present with a complex neurologic examination. Performing a single-level SNRB would demonstrate only a portion of the pain complex. In this scenario, we first perform a one-level SNRB at what is thought, by pain distribution, to be the most affected nerve root. The patient is then placed in a holding area for 1 to 2 hours and reevaluated for any residual pain. The distribution of the residual pain is documented. If necessary, the second level can be injected and then the patient is reevaluated. We recommend that no more than two SNRBs be performed in any one session because the diagnostic information obtained from more numerous injections would be difficult to interpret.

We suggest that the patient receive no more than 40 mg of betamethasone (or other steroid equivalent) and no more than four steroid-containing injections in any 1 year.

PATIENT SELECTION

Patients who are candidates for SNRB generally have radicular pain and should have recent MR or CT imaging to exclude another condition that might be producing radicular pain, such as a herniated disc or neoplasm. Patients with radicular pain who are considered for SNRB include the following:

- Patients with minimal or no definitive imaging findings
- Patients with multilevel imaging abnormalities, to more accurately define the levels for possible surgery
- Postoperative patients with unexplainable or complex recurrent pain
- Patients with equivocal neurologic examinations

- Patients with a known cause for the pain who would benefit from temporary pain relief (e.g., pain caused by disc herniation)

CONTRAINDICATIONS

- Coagulopathy (International Normalized Ratio [INR] >1.5 or platelets <50,000/mm^3)
- Pregnancy (because of teratogenic effects of radiation)
- Systemic infection or skin infection over the puncture site
- Severe allergy to any component of the injectate
- The patient has received the maximum amount of steroid, including systemic steroids, allowed for a given time period, unless the injection is to be performed without steroids

PROCEDURE

Equipment/Supplies

Spinal needle, 22-gauge, 6-inch (or possibly 3.5-inch for some thoracic procedures) (1 per level, lumbar or thoracic) (MONOJECT Special Technique Needle With Stylet, Diamond Point, Sherwood Medical, St. Louis, MO)

Spinal needle, 25-gauge, 3.5-inch (1 per level, cervical) (Quinke type point, Becton Dickinson & Co., Franklin Lakes, NJ)

Syringe, 3 mL, containing injectate (1 per level)

Syringe, 3 mL (optional) containing nonionic iodinated myelographic contrast medium, 300 mg I/mL (Omnipaque [Iohexol] Injection, Nycomed, Inc., Princeton, NJ)

Control syringe, 12 mL, with 25 gauge, 1.5-inch needle containing 9.5 mL 1% lidocaine for local anesthesia and 0.5 mL 8.4% sodium bicarbonate injectable (1 mEq/mL) to alleviate burning pain associated with anesthetic

Sterile gauze

Povidone-iodine (Betadine) scrub

Alcohol scrub

Sterile towels, drapes, gloves, gown, hat, mask

Adhesive bandage

Lead apron

C-arm or biplane fluoroscopy optimal

Medications

Diagnostic Injection Mixture (Injectate)

Lumbar, Thoracic, Cervical

Combine:

1. Lidocaine hydrochloride 1% MPF, 0.5 mL (Xylocaine-MPF* 1%, AstraZeneca LP, Wilmington, DE)*
2. Bupivacaine hydrochloride 0.25% MPF, 0.5 mL (Sensorcaine-MPF Injection 0.25%, AstraZeneca LP, Wilmington, DE)*

---

*Local anesthetics should be from single-use vials and be free of paraben (MPF) and phenol to prevent flocculation of the steroid.[2]

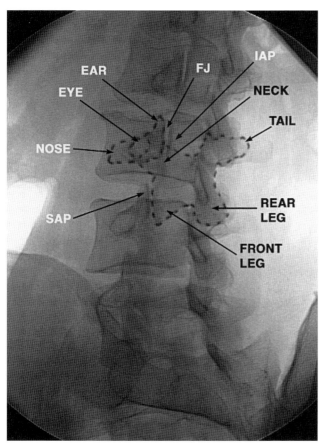

Figure 4-1 ▪ RAO lumbar spine radiograph demonstrating "Scotty dog" (*dashed lines*). EAR = left superior articular process L3; EYE = left pedicle L3; NOSE = left transverse process L3; *SAP* = left superior articular process L4; FRONT LEG = left inferior articular process L3; REAR LEG = superimposed right inferior articular process L3 and right superior articular process L4; TAIL = right transverse process L3; NECK = left pars interarticularis L3; IAP = left inferior articular process L2; FJ = left L2-3 facet joint.

Therapeutic Injection Mixture (Injectate)

LUMBAR OR THORACIC

Combine:

1. Lidocaine hydrochloride 1% MPF, 0.5 mL*
2. Bupivacaine hydrochloride 0.25% MPF, 1.0 mL*
3. 0.5 mL Betamethasone sodium phosphate and betamethasone acetate injectable suspension 6 mg/mL (Celestone Soluspan, Schering Corporation, Kenilworth, NJ)
4. Alternatively, if betamethasone is unavailable, 0.5 mL of triamcinolone acetonide injectable, 40 mg/mL (Kenalog-40, Apothecon, Princeton, NJ)

CERVICAL

Combine:

1. Bupivacaine hydrochloride 0.25% MPF, 1.0 mL*
2. 0.5 mL Betamethasone sodium phosphate and betamethasone acetate injectable suspension 6 mg/mL

*Local anesthetics should be from single-use vials and be free of paraben (MPF) and phenol to prevent flocculation of the steroid.[2]

All medications used should not contain epinephrine because vasoconstrictive properties are neither needed nor desired, particularly because of the risk of vasospasm in the head and neck region.

Methodology

Lumbosacral

Informed consent is obtained. The patient's lower extremity strength is evaluated for comparison with post-procedure strength. The patient is placed prone on the fluoroscopy table. The patient's lower back is prepared and draped in a sterile fashion.

L1 TO L4 LUMBAR NERVE ROOTS

Proper positioning is the key to an effective SNRB. The C-arm (image intensifier above the patient) is rotated in an ipsilateral oblique angle with respect to the suspected nerve root. This will bring into view the "Scotty dog" appearance (Fig. 4-1). The C-arm (or patient) is rotated until the ventral aspect of the superior articulating process (ear of the "Scotty dog"), which has the same vertebral number as the nerve root to be injected, is midway between the anterior and the posterior aspects of the vertebral body superior end plate. Also, the superior end plates of this vertebral body should appear superimposed at fluoroscopy (see Fig. 4-1). The vertebral body serves to limit the depth of needle penetration. The nerve root normally passes a few millimeters inferior to the pedicle (eye of the "Scotty dog") and 1 to 2 mm superficial to the vertebral body (Fig. 4-2).

It is important to realize that the artery of Adamkiewicz (arteria radicularis magna) enters the spinal canal through the neural foramen in close proximity to the dorsal root ganglion. This artery, which is the main supply to the lower two thirds of the spinal cord, arises from a segmental artery from the aorta and enters the spinal canal anywhere from T7 to L4. The typical location of the artery of Adamkiewicz is on the left (approximately 80%) from T9 to L1. The artery usually enters in the superior or middle portion of the neural foramen, slightly ventral and superolateral to the dorsal root ganglion.[3] Therefore, with lower thoracic and upper lumbar SNRBs (and particularly left-sided SNRBs at these levels), we prefer to block the nerve slightly more inferolaterally in relation to the pedicle.

L5 LUMBAR NERVE ROOT

The C-arm is rotated in a similar fashion. Often, the area in which the needle has to be passed is a triangular window formed by the inferior margin of the transverse process of L5, the superior articulating process of S1, and the iliac crest (Fig. 4-3). However, with standard positioning, the iliac crest may completely obstruct one's approach (Fig. 4-4*A*). If one is not able to achieve a position that places the superior articular facet at the midpoint of the vertebral body, one obtains the best possible angle that allows visualization of the upside-down triangle (see Fig. 4-4*B*). In this case, needle insertion is performed from a lateral to medial direction to pass medial to the iliac crest with the tip of the needle projecting inferior to the pedicle (see Fig. 4-4*C*). Once again, the vertebral body forms the backdrop for the triangle so that the vertebral body limits the depth of needle penetration.

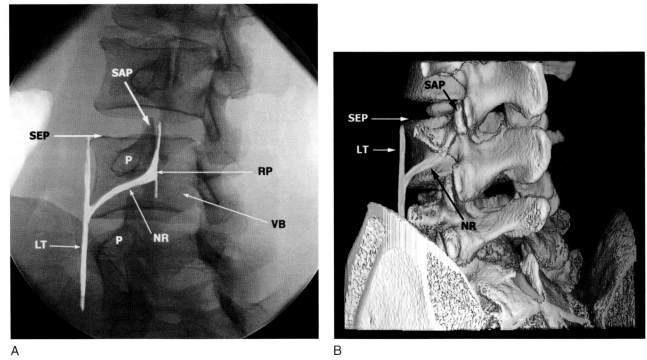

Figure 4-2 ■ RAO lumbar spine radiograph (*A*) and RAO three-dimensional (3D) surface rendering (*B*) depicting anatomy and proper fluoroscopic positioning for left L4 SNRB. Left L4 nerve root/sheath (NR) is the target zone beneath the L4 pedicle (P). At the L4 vertebral body (VB) level, the nerve root arises from the root pouch (RP) and joins other nerves from above to form the lumbosacral trunk (LT). The left superior articular process of L4 (SAP) is positioned midway between the anterior and posterior margins of the L4 vertebral body, and the anterior and posterior portions of the superior end plate of L4 (SEP) should superimpose.

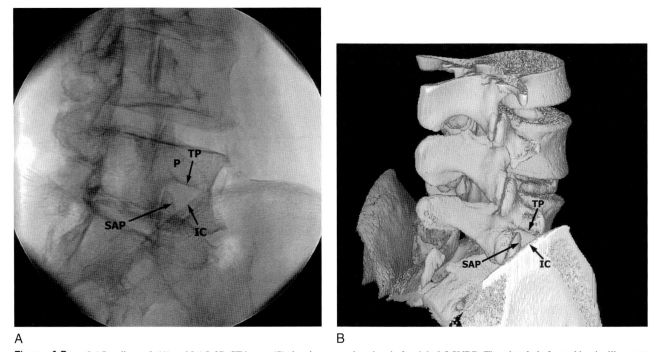

Figure 4-3 ■ LAO radiograph (*A*) and LAO 3D CT image (*B*) showing entry site triangle for right L5 SNRB. The triangle is formed by the iliac crest (IC), the inferior margin of the right L5 transverse process (TP), and the right S1 superior articular process (SAP). P = pedicle.

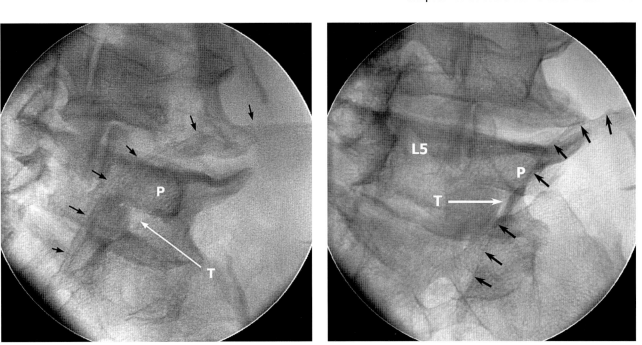

A

B

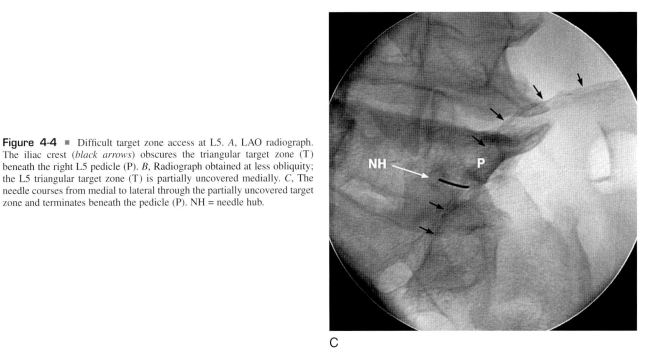

C

Figure 4-4 ■ Difficult target zone access at L5. *A*, LAO radiograph. The iliac crest (*black arrows*) obscures the triangular target zone (T) beneath the right L5 pedicle (P). *B*, Radiograph obtained at less obliquity; the L5 triangular target zone (T) is partially uncovered medially. *C*, The needle courses from medial to lateral through the partially uncovered target zone and terminates beneath the pedicle (P). NH = needle hub.

S1 SACRAL NERVE ROOT

The C-arm can usually remain with the x-ray beam in the straight AP projection or with at most 5 to 10 degrees of ipsilateral lateral angulation. The S1 sacral foramen is seen as a round lucency in the upper sacrum (Fig. 4-5*A*). Slight caudocranial angulation of the x-ray beam (image intensifier above the patient, obliqued toward the patient's head) may help facilitate optimal needle placement (see Fig. 4-5*B*). There is no depth indicator for sacral needle placement. Therefore, one must be careful not to pass through the foramen into the pelvis, and so it is important to monitor the needle trajectory in AP and lateral planes for S1 injections.

It should be noted that for S1 nerve blocks the needle is placed parallel to the nerve sheath. Therefore, there is often epidural spread of injectate and thus this procedure is identical to an S1 transforaminal epidural injection.

ASSESSING PROPER NEEDLE POSITION:
LUMBOSACRAL

Once a good working position has been established by means of appropriate radiographic landmarks, as described earlier, superficial and deep local anesthesia can be delivered. The spinal needle is then passed through the skin parallel to the x-ray beam. For lumbar nerve roots **L3 and L4**, the

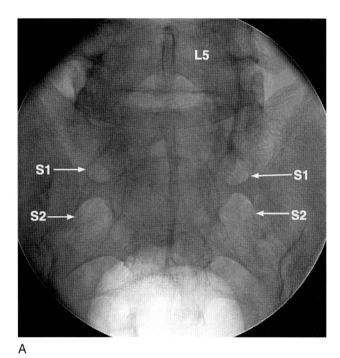

A

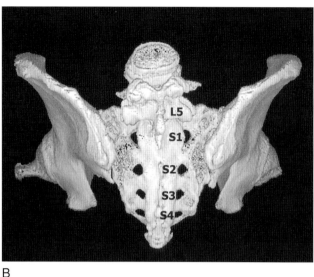

B

Figure 4-5 ■ *A,* AP radiograph at lumbosacral junction. S1 and S2 sacral neural foramina are indicated bilaterally, representing target sites for S1 and S2 nerve blocks. L5 = L5 vertebra. *B,* Prone caudally angulated three-dimensional CT image of sacral foramina. Sacral foramina S1 through S4 are indicated, demonstrating accessibility of the sacral nerve roots with the patient in the prone position. L5 = L5 vertebra.

needle is advanced to a point just inferolateral to the pedicle until radicular pain is elicited (Fig. 4-6). For L1 and L2 (and T9 to T12), the needle is positioned more inferior and lateral in relation to the pedicle (in the inferior neural foramen) to decrease the risk of injury to the artery of Adamkiewicz. Often, the needle must be passed until it makes contact

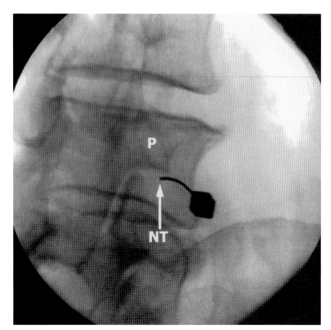

Figure 4-6 ■ LAO radiograph demonstrating proper needle position for right L4 SNRB. The needle tip (NT) is a few millimeters inferior and lateral to the pedicle (P). This position is true for nerve roots L1 through L4.

with the vertebral body. If radicular pain is not elicited, the needle is repositioned a few millimeters away until radicular pain is reported. For the **L5** nerve root, the needle is advanced parallel to the x-ray beam through the center of the triangle until radicular pain is achieved (Fig. 4-7). If radicular pain is not elicited, the needle can be repositioned or, if necessary, the C-arm can be repositioned a few degrees in all directions. For the **S1** nerve root, the needle is advanced into the center of the sacral foramen until radicular pain is elicited (Fig. 4-8).

Regardless of the level injected, depth of needle penetration should be evaluated periodically with lateral fluoroscopy. For the S1 nerve root injection, the needle is placed until it contacts one of the bone margins of the sacral foramen. The needle is then advanced into the foramen a few millimeters until radicular pain is elicited.

When the needle tip touches the nerve root, the patient generally reports intense pain in a specific distribution. If this pain is concordant with the patient's typical pain distribution, 0.5 to 1.0 mL of nonionic myelographic contrast medium may be injected to confirm the needle position in the nerve root sheath (this step is optional) (Fig. 4-9).

Intermittent gentle negative aspiration should be performed during the injection to make sure that the needle tip has not entered a vascular structure. Injection of contrast agent is performed for several reasons. First, it will indicate whether the needle is properly in the nerve root sleeve and not within the nerve root itself. Injection of the nerve root directly can cause severe, sustained radicular pain, which should be avoided if possible. Second, contrast agent injection will also confirm that the needle is not positioned within a vascular structure, a situation that would remove the injectate from the injection site and negate any diagnostic or

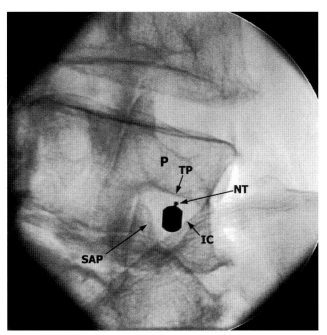

Figure 4-7 ■ LAO radiograph depicting proper needle position for right L5 SNRB. The triangular target site is bordered by the right L5 transverse process (TP) superiorly, the right S1 superior articular process (SAP) posteromedially, and the right iliac crest (IC) anterolaterally. The needle tip (NT) is seen a few millimeters inferior and lateral to the right L5 pedicle (P).

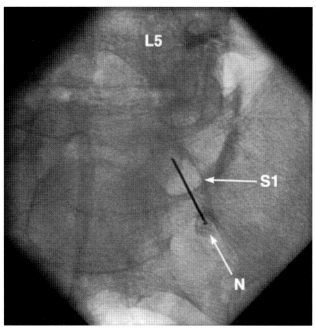

Figure 4-8 ■ Shallow LAO radiograph (5 to 10 degrees) showing proper needle position for right S1 SNRB. The S1 sacral foramen (S1) is seen as a rounded lucency inferior to the lumbosacral junction. The needle (N) is seen entering the center of the S1 neural foramen at an oblique orientation from lateral to medial. L5 = L5 vertebra.

therapeutic benefit. Also, if the needle was placed within a vascular structure, a therapeutic injection with a particulate steroid could result in vascular occlusion or thrombosis. In the case of the artery of Adamkiewicz, this could lead to spinal cord infarction. The argument against contrast agent injection is that the patient experiences continuous radicular symptoms while the contrast agent is being injected. In practice, the time between contrast agent injection and nerve block is relatively short.

Once proper needle position has been established, the injectate (diagnostic or therapeutic) is instilled into the nerve root sleeve. This is done slowly to minimize the amount that might flow retrograde into the epidural space, which would make the injection less specific. The needle is then removed. The patient's skin is then cleansed, and an adhesive bandage is applied to the puncture site.

Thoracic

Selective thoracic nerve root blocks are rarely performed, but there are occasional instances when thoracic SNRBs are necessary for diagnostic purposes. A thoracic SNRB is no more difficult to perform than lumbar or cervical SNRBs, and it is performed in similar fashion. Thoracic SNRBs carry the additional risk of a pneumothorax from inadvertent puncture of the pleura.

With fluoroscopic guidance, the thoracic SNRB is performed in a fashion identical to the previously described lumbar SNRB. One must remember to keep the needle tip just inferior and lateral to the pedicle (with the exception of T9 to T12 as described in the lumbar section), while remaining lateral to the medial border of the pedicle to avoid entering the spinal canal and medial to the ipsilateral head of

the rib and the posteromedial lung margin (Fig. 4-10). It is important to visualize the three-line configuration consisting of, from lateral to medial, the anteromedial lung, the posterolateral margin of the vertebral body, and the posteromedial lung. This will ensure that the needle does not pass

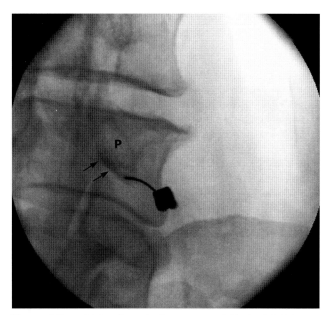

Figure 4-9 ■ LAO radiograph of contrast material in the right L4 nerve root sleeve. The needle tip is seen a few millimeters inferior to the right L4 pedicle (*P*). Curvilinear region of contrast (*arrows*) extends from the needle tip along the inferomedial aspect of the pedicle without entering the epidural space.

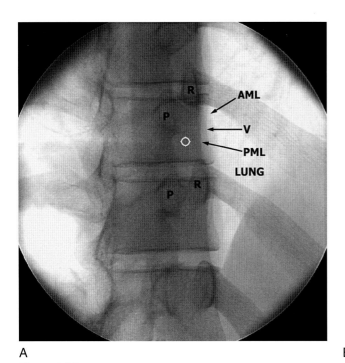

A

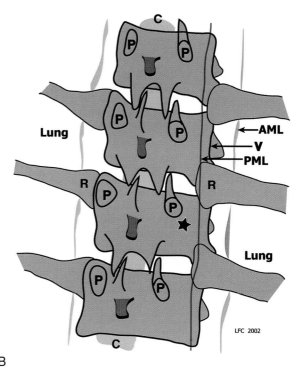

B

Figure 4-10 ■ LAO radiograph (*A*) and illustration (*B*) demonstrate positioning for thoracic nerve block. Target zone (*white target, A; star, B*) is a few millimeters inferior and lateral to the pedicle (P). One must be familiar with the three-line configuration of the anteromedial lung (AML), the vertebral margin (V), and the posteromedial lung (PML). The needle tip should remain medial to the PML and lateral to the medial border of the pedicle to avoid pneumothorax and spinal canal (C) puncture. R = head of rib.

through the pleura and potentially cause a pneumothorax. The remainder of the procedure is performed as described in the lumbosacral section. The examination can also be performed by using CT guidance in a fashion similar to that of a cervical SNRB, with the exception that the patient is placed prone (Fig. 4-11). For thoracic SNRB, we find the CT-guided method more difficult to perform than the fluoroscopic method. However, it is possible that the risk of pneumothorax and canal puncture is less when CT guidance is used. CT guidance is best used with the gantry straight so that craniocaudal angulation is fixed at 0 degrees and all one need be concerned with is the anteroposterior and mediolateral directions of the needle. Without angulation, the entire length of the needle is often not imaged on a single slice, because significant cranial or caudal angulation is often necessary to project the rib articulation and/or the transverse process out of the way to achieve the proper orientation to enter the thoracic neural foramen. Therefore, we believe that fluoroscopic guidance is best suited for a thoracic SNRB.

Cervical

Informed consent is obtained. The patient's upper extremity strength is evaluated for comparison with post-procedure strength. An intravenous line is placed in a peripheral vein. The cervical nerve roots must be approached from the anterolateral aspect of the neck because of the lateral mass obstructing a posterolateral or lateral approach. Of course, the anterolateral approach has greater risk because the ipsilateral carotid sheath, adjacent nerves, and vertebral artery are along the needle pathway. Therefore, we believe the safest approach for cervical SNRB is with CT guidance. If

there is no specific allergy or renal impairment, it may be helpful to inject 100 mL of nonionic iodinated contrast agent intravenously during the localization phase to opacify the vessels of the neck before CT localization. This will

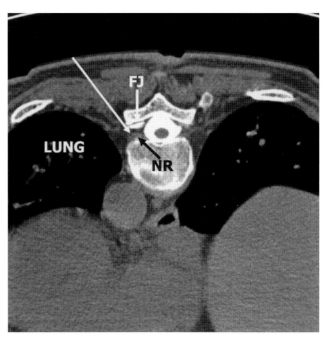

Figure 4-11 ■ Prone axial CT, thoracic disc level. *White arrow* demonstrates that the safe approach to the thoracic nerve root sheath (NR) is lateral to the facet joint (FJ) and medial to the lung.

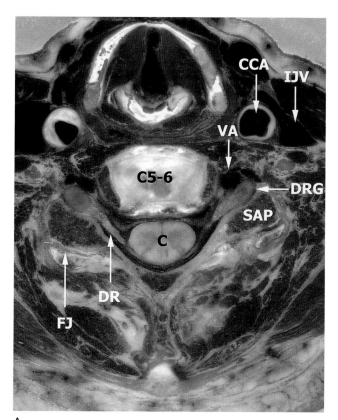

A

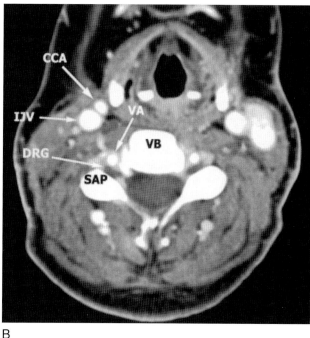

B

Figure 4-12 ■ Cryomicrotome (*A*) and contrast medium-enhanced CT scan (*B*) of the cervical spine, C5-6 disc level. DR = dorsal nerve root; SAP = C6 superior articular process; FJ = right C5-6 facet joint; C = cervical spinal cord; CCA = common carotid artery; IJV = left internal jugular vein. Note the close relationship between the vertebral artery (VA) and the dorsal root ganglion (DRG). (A from Cryomicrotome image collection compiled from work by Peter Pech, MD, and Victor M. Haughton, MD, included here with permission of Victor M. Haughton.)

demonstrate the location of the carotid sheath structures and vertebral artery (Fig. 4-12). Although contrast medium will have equilibrated with the body by the time the nerve injection procedure has begun, the initial enhanced images can be useful to identify the location of the vascular anatomy. It is still possible to perform the procedure without intravenous contrast medium enhancement, but it is more difficult. A thorough understanding of neck anatomy is a minimum requirement for CT-guided soft tissue neck procedures.

The patient is placed on the CT table in the lateral decubitus position with the side to be injected up. A cushion is placed under the head and/or neck to make the patient more comfortable and also to keep the patient's neck in neutral position without any significant lateral flexion. Most importantly, the neck should not be flexed toward the side to be injected, because this narrows the ipsilateral neural foramen. Slight lateral flexion contralateral to the side of puncture may further facilitate needle placement into the target foramen. Many patients have their neck flexed anteriorly when placed in the lateral decubitus position. The patient's neck is optimally positioned in neutral position by slight "hyperextension" relative to the beginning position. Another obstacle may be visualizing the upper cervical nerve roots in a patient who has metallic dental work. This may cause significant streak artifact and suboptimal visualization of the nerve root. If it is anticipated that streak artifact will significantly alter the CT image quality, we position the patient's head in mild hyperextension to raise the jaw out of the scanning

plane. If this does not work, asking the patient to open his or her mouth during the procedure may reduce the streak artifact.

Because there is only a very narrow window in which to safely access the cervical nerve root, it is extremely important that the site of skin puncture be as close as possible to the preplanned trajectory. We have used two different methods for puncture site localization.

First, before the skin is cleansed, a radiopaque grid is taped to the side of the patient's neck with the center placed where the target neural foramen is believed to be (Fig. 4-13). Scout CT views of the neck are obtained, and the grid can be adjusted appropriately so that it overlies the target neural foramen (Fig. 4-14). It is sometimes useful to inject 100 mL of nonionic iodinated contrast material into a peripheral intravenous line 20 to 25 seconds before scanning. Then 1-mm axial CT scans are obtained from the top of the vertebral body above the foramen to the bottom of the vertebral body below the foramen. The images are evaluated to determine the optimal approach to the nerve root (Fig. 4-15). The table position is noted, as is the portion of the grid that will yield the optimal skin puncture site. The CT table is then placed at the noted table position, and the laser light is turned on. This will project a thin linear beam of light onto the grid and neck (Fig. 4-16). An indelible marker is used to mark a point on the patient's neck where the laser light intersects with the portion of the grid, decided on earlier, that allows the best trajectory to the nerve root (Fig. 4-17). The

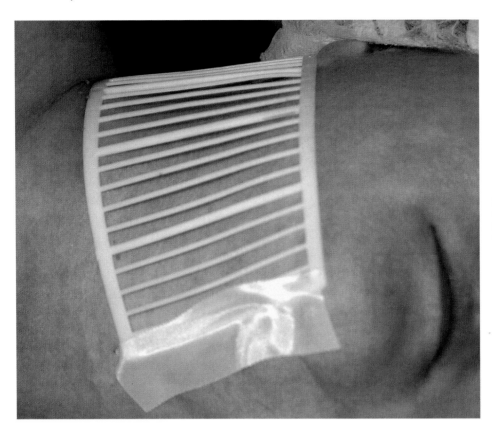

Figure 4-13 ■ Patient in left lateral decubitus position with grid affixed to the right side of the neck over the target foramen.

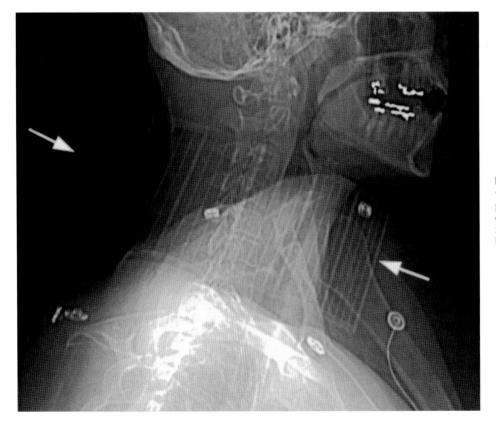

Figure 4-14 ■ Scout CT image with patient in left lateral decubitus position. The radiopaque grid (*arrows*) overlies the soft tissues of the neck from C2-3 to the mid-C7 vertebral body.

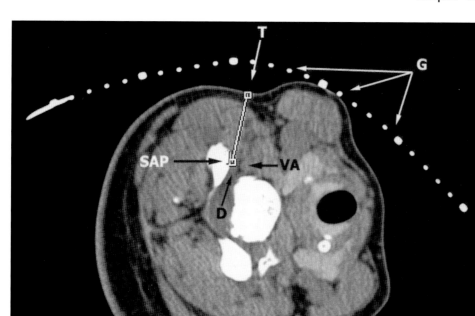

Figure 4-15 ■ Axial CT image at the level of the neural foramen. The radiopaque grid (G) is seen as multiple radiodense foci that target the optimal skin entrance. The needle trajectory (T) is plotted from the skin to the dorsal root ganglion (D) and remains posterior to the vertebral artery (VA). The number of grid points should be counted from either end of the grid, and the table position is noted before skin marking. SAP = superior articular process.

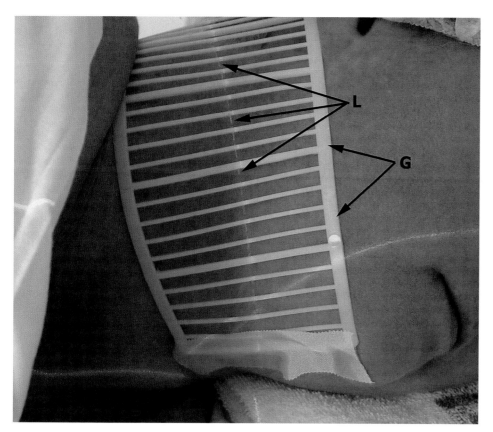

Figure 4-16 ■ Patient in left lateral decubitus position with grid affixed to the right side of the neck. The laser light (L), which corresponds to the table position for optimal skin puncture, is displayed over the grid (G).

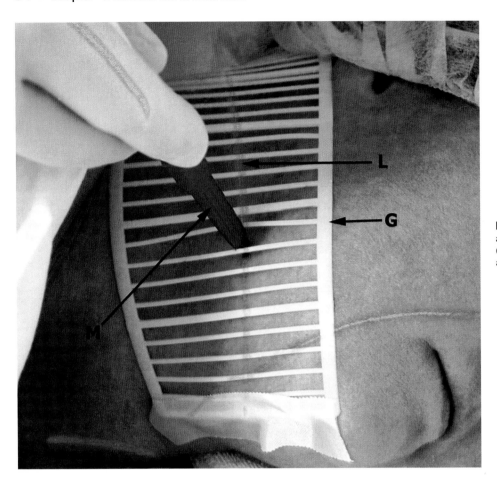

Figure 4-17 ■ With the grid (G) affixed to the neck and the laser light (L) on, the entry point is marked with an indelible marker (M).

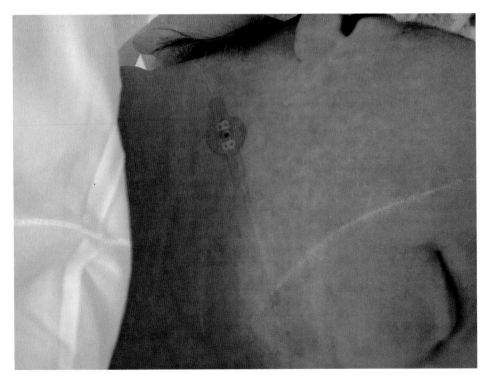

Figure 4-18 ■ Patient in left lateral decubitus position. A metallic BB has been affixed to the right side of the neck along the path of the CT laser light.

grid is then removed, and the patient is prepared and draped in a sterile fashion.

The second method uses a small metallic BB pellet marker to localize the puncture site instead of the grid. A series of localizer CT scans are first obtained. Next, the BB pellet marker is placed on the skin demarcated by the laser light (Fig. 4-18). A single CT image is then obtained to see how close the estimate is to the optimal skin puncture site. The metallic marker can be moved and additional imaging can be obtained, or one can estimate how far the skin puncture must be made in relation to the metallic marker along the laser light line. This point is then marked with indelible marker and the patient is prepared and draped in a sterile fashion.

ASSESSING PROPER NEEDLE POSITION: CERVICAL

Once the optimal entrance point has been established, superficial local anesthesia can be delivered. A 25-gauge, 3.5-inch styleted spinal needle is passed through the skin and advanced approximately 2 cm toward the target. Unless CT fluoroscopy is being used, the needle must be advanced in small increments to avoid the vital structures. Although some physicians praise CT fluoroscopy, we find it difficult to follow the needle in real time and to obtain a 3- to 5-mm window. With CT fluoroscopy, forceps should be used on the needle to keep the hands out of the primary CT beam and thereby minimize operator exposure to radiation. However, when forceps are used, it is difficult to make subtle changes in direction with a small-gauge needle. It is better to use hand-directed needle guidance and to apply those methods of steering a beveled-edge needle that are discussed in Chapter 1 on the techniques of needle manipulation. After each needle adjustment, the patient is repositioned within the CT gantry and images are obtained to evaluate the location of the needle tip. Readjustments of the needle are then made as necessary. The needle tip is advanced slightly posterior to the target toward the superior facet to avoid the vertebral artery (Fig. 4-19). Once contact has been made with the superior facet, the needle can be withdrawn a few millimeters and redirected by advancing slowly and in small increments into the posterior aspect of the neural foramen (Fig. 4-20). Again, the needle position is confirmed by CT images. The needle is then slowly advanced and adjusted until the patient experiences radicular symptoms.

When the needle tip touches the nerve root, the patient generally reports intense pain in a specific distribution. If this pain is concordant with the patient's typical pain distribution, the needle position may be confirmed (this step is optional) by injecting 0.2 to 0.5 mL of nonionic myelographic contrast material, after gentle negative aspiration to ensure that the needle is not within a vascular structure (Fig. 4-21).

Once the needle has been properly positioned, the injectate (diagnostic or therapeutic) is instilled into the nerve root sleeve. This is done slowly to minimize the amount of injectate that may flow retrograde into the epidural space, which could elicit a patient response that is difficult to interpret. One should remember always to use intermittent negative aspiration during any injection to verify that the needle has not entered a vascular structure. The needle is then removed. The patient's skin is cleansed, and an adhesive bandage is applied to the puncture site.

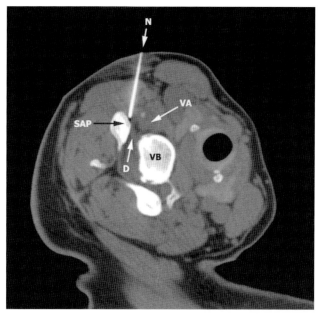

Figure 4-19 ▪ Axial CT left lateral decubitus position. The needle (N) is initially advanced posterior to the target dorsal root ganglion (*D*) to strike the superior articular process (SAP). This path is chosen to avoid vital structures, such as the vertebral artery (VA), on the initial pass. VB = vertebral body.

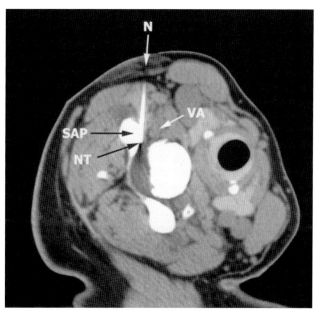

Figure 4-20 ▪ Axial CT left lateral decubitus position. The needle tip (NT) has been repositioned anteriorly into the posterior neural foramen but remains posterior to the vertebral artery (VA). SAP = superior articular process; N = needle.

Pain Response Assessment in Nerve Root Blocks

When radicular pain is elicited, it is essential to question the patient about the pain distribution. Often, the patient describes the procedurally induced pain as much more severe and often in a larger distribution than expected. This response may still be considered concordant if the patient's

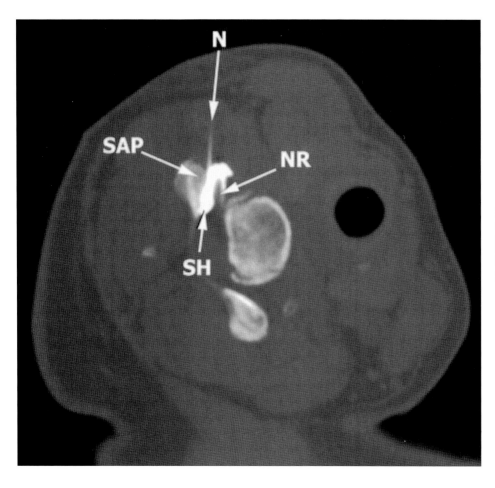

Figure 4-21 ■ Axial CT left lateral decubitus position. Contrast material in the nerve root sheath (SH) is seen outlining the nerve root (NR). N = needle; SAP = superior articular process.

typical radicular pain is a subset of this larger distribution. If the procedural pain is entirely discordant with the patient's typical pain, the SNRB for this nerve root should be abandoned and either another nerve root level should be selected or the procedure should be aborted. If the patient is uncertain whether the procedural pain is concordant or discordant, that level can be injected and the patient can be reassessed before discharge. If, at the time, the patient's symptoms have resolved, there is nothing further to do. If the patient remains symptomatic, either another level can be injected at that time or the patient can be brought back in a few days after any available imaging has been reassessed.

It is common for a patient to experience numbness in the distribution of the nerve injected. This typically lasts less than 3 hours, although it can persist for up to 24 hours. Mild, persistent pain may linger, but severe pain after injection is unusual. For a lumbar injection, it is important to observe the patient's stability on standing immediately after the procedure because motor nerve fibers can also be affected. The response should be compared with the pre-procedure evaluation. Weakness is more often seen when 0.5%, as opposed to 0.25%, bupivacaine is used. Patients are often not aware that they are weak until they try to walk, and so it is important to assist them when they stand and walk initially as they get up from the table. Weakness may last 1 to 3 hours, and the patient's post-procedure stay should be extended if weakness is observed after SNRB. For a cervical injection, the patient's upper extremity strength should be tested and compared with the pre-procedure evaluation. **For any**

SNRB, the patient should refrain from performing tasks that require the strength and dexterity of the affected muscles, at least for the remainder of the day and until pre-procedure strength and dexterity have returned.

Rarely, bilateral epidural spread may occur after SNRB that may affect sensation or cause weakness bilaterally. SNRB may rarely be associated with vasovagal reactions.

POTENTIAL COMPLICATIONS

- Bleeding
- Infection
- Thecal sac puncture and headache
- Allergic reactions pertaining to the medications
- Risk of pneumothorax for thoracic nerve block
- Vasovagal reactions and ataxia, especially for cervical nerve block
- Paraplegia caused by damage to the artery of Adamkiewicz[4]

POST-PROCEDURE CARE/FOLLOW-UP

After the procedure, the patient is placed first in a sitting position and then in a standing position with the assistance of one or more persons. If the patient has no appreciable loss of motor strength or coordination, he or she can be observed for 30 minutes, reevaluated, and then discharged. If there is some loss of motor strength or coordination, the patient is placed in a bed or lounge chair and is reevaluated every 30 minutes until he or she returns to normal levels of strength. Until that time, the patient is allowed to ambulate only with assistance. All patients having SNRB are discharged into the care of a responsible person. The patient is asked not to drive or perform any heavy tasks that would require the use of the affected musculature until at least the next morning, at which time strength should be reevaluated.

Immediate[5]

1. The patient should be observed for at least 30 minutes after SNRB or longer if there is a motor deficit.
2. The patient may sit in a reclining lounge chair; however, if there is significant post-procedure pain, or if the patient received intravenous sedation, he or she should be placed at bed rest.
3. Blood pressure, pulse, heart rate, and respiration are evaluated every 30 minutes.

Discharge[5]

1. The patient is discharged into the care of a responsible person.
2. The patient is instructed not to drive or perform any other tasks that require quick reaction time for the remainder of the day, especially if sedation was given.
3. A 2- to 3-day nonrenewable prescription for a narcotic pain reliever and/or a muscle relaxant is given to the patient.
4. Multiple adhesive bandages may be on the patient's back or neck. These should remain dry for at least 24 hours, at which point they can be removed.
5. Patients are instructed to continue to take their prescription medication, although pain medication may be tapered as indicated.
6. A discharge sheet should be given to the patient outlining the following:
   a. Which procedure was performed and at what levels
   b. Procedurally related symptoms that typically resolve in 7 to 10 days
      • Pain at the needle puncture site(s)
      • Mild increased back or neck stiffness
      • Deep back or neck pain
   c. Treatment for mild post-procedure symptoms
      • Rest the affected area for 3 to 4 days.
      • Avoid movements that aggravate the pain.
      • Use cold compresses to the painful area.
   d. Signs and symptoms of infection
      • Fever
      • Chills
      • Swelling or drainage from the puncture sites
      • New back or neck pain that is different from the usual pain
   e. Signs and symptoms of possibly more serious problems
      • Stiff neck
      • Increasing pain
      • Motor dysfunction such as difficulty walking or lifting
      • Bowel or bladder dysfunction

   f. Physician name and contact number if the patient has any concerns or if any problems were to arise as a result of the procedure
   g. Patients are then asked to follow up by phone with their referring physician approximately 3 days after the injection to report on their condition and on how they responded to the injection.

SAMPLE DICTATIONS

Lumbar Spine

Procedure: Fluoroscopically guided selective nerve root block
Date of Procedure: Month/day/year
Facility: Name of facility
Level Treated: Left L4

The procedure and potential complications were explained to the patient, and voluntary informed, signed consent was obtained. The patient was a candidate for conscious sedation. The patient was placed prone on the table. The patient's back was prepped and draped in usual sterile fashion. Subcutaneous lidocaine was instilled into the superficial soft tissues of the patient's back for local anesthesia. Under fluoroscopic guidance, a 22-gauge, 6-inch spinal needle was advanced just inferior and lateral to the left L4 pedicle. This elicited radicular pain in the distribution of L4 that the patient stated was quite typical of the usual pain. Then, 1.0 mL of myelographic contrast (Iohexol, 300 mg I/mL) was slowly instilled through the needle. It demonstrated filling of the nerve root sleeve without significant retrograde epidural spread. A single radiograph was obtained in the AP plane for documentation. Subsequently, a mixture of 0.5 mL lidocaine-MPF (1%), 1.0 mL bupivacaine-MPF (0.25%), and 0.5 mL betamethasone (6 mg/mL) was instilled slowly through the needle. The needle was removed. The patient's skin was cleansed, and an adhesive bandage was placed on the puncture site. The patient was then allowed to ambulate and demonstrated no evidence of subjective or objective motor loss. No complications were observed during the procedure or immediately afterward. The patient described being free of the usual left lower extremity pain.

Cervical Spine

Procedure: CT-guided selective nerve root block
Date of Procedure: Month/day/year
Facility: Name of facility
Level Treated: Left C5

The procedure and potential complications were explained to the patient, and voluntary informed, signed consent was obtained. The patient was a candidate for conscious sedation. The patient was placed in the right lateral decubitus position on the table. Initial CT of the neck was performed for localization of the left C4-5 neural foramen. The left lateral neck was prepped and draped in usual sterile fashion. Subcutaneous lidocaine was instilled into the superficial soft tissues of the patient's left lateral neck for local anesthesia. With CT guidance and confirmation after each manipulation, a 22-gauge, 3.5-inch spinal needle was advanced, using an anterolateral approach, until it made contact with the superior articulating process of C5. The needle was then withdrawn a few millimeters, walked anterior to the superior articulating process, and advanced a few millimeters into the posterior C4-5 foramen. This elicited radicular pain in the distribution of C5, which the patient stated was quite typical of the usual pain. Then, 0.2 mL of myelographic contrast (Iohexol, 300 mg I/mL) was slowly instilled through the needle. It demonstrated filling of the nerve root sleeve with-out significant retrograde epidural spread. Subsequently, a mixture of 1.0 mL bupivacaine-MPF (0.25%) and 0.5 mL betamethasone (6 mg/mL) was instilled slowly through the needle. The needle was removed. The patient's skin was cleansed, and an adhesive bandage was placed on the puncture site. The patient was then evaluated for any loss of motor strength and coordination. No complications were observed during the procedure or immediately afterward. The patient reported relief of the usual left upper extremity pain.

CASE REPORTS

CASE 1

Clinical Presentation

The patient is a 63-year-old woman with right lower extremity pain. She had a right L4-5 laminectomy 1 year ago for similar pain. Her pain has never gone away and has steadily increased over the past few months. It is situated low in the back and wraps around the right hip in a narrow band along the right anterolateral thigh, across the knee, and along the inside of the leg (Fig. 4-22A and B). She occasionally has pain that travels into the right great toe; even less

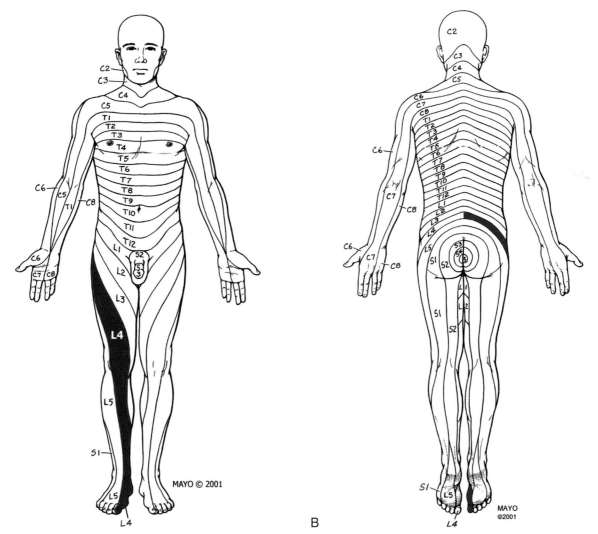

Figure 4-22 ■ Anterior (*A*) and posterior (*B*) illustrations of the distribution of the patient's pain along the right L4 dermatome.

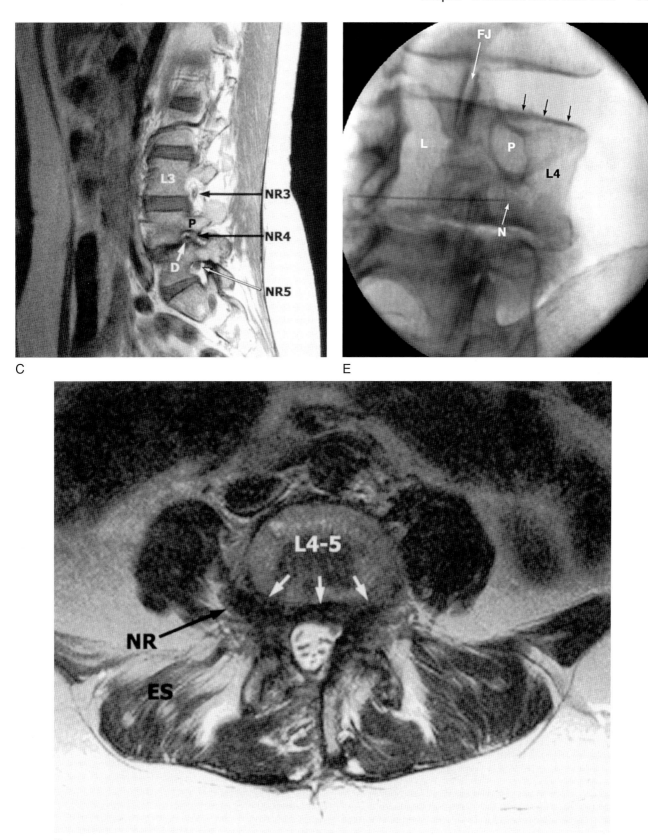

Figure 4-22 *(Cont'd)* ■ *C*, Right parasagittal T1-weighted MR image showing normal appearance of the right L3 (NR3) and L5 (NR5) roots in their foramina. The L4 nerve root (NR4) is compressed between the L4 pedicle (P) and the bulging disc (D). L3 = L3 vertebral body. *D*, Axial T2-weighted fast spin echo MR image at L4-5 disc level. The right L4 nerve root (NR) is being compressed by a bulging disc (*white arrows*). Note atrophy of the right erector spinae muscle (ES). *E*, Before administration of lidocaine, the needle tip (N) is used to localize the target site below right L4 pedicle (P). Note the superimposed anterior and posterior portions of the superior end plate of L4 (*arrows*). FJ = right L3-4 facet joint; L = laminectomy defect.

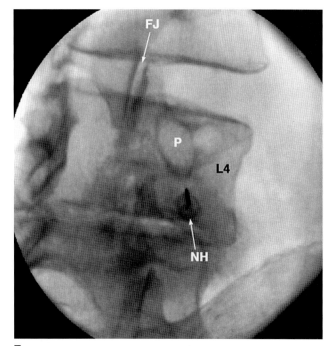

F

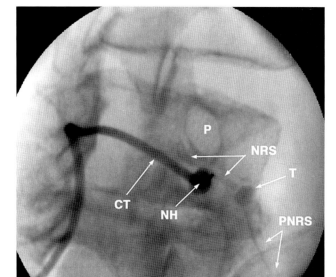

G

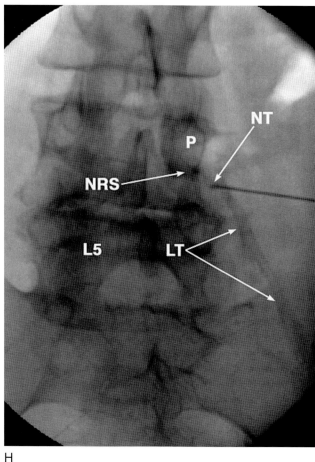

H

Figure 4-22 *(Cont'd)* ▪ *F*, Needle hub (NH) is superimposed over the needle with the tip directed slightly cephalad but below the right L4 pedicle (P). FJ = right L3-4 facet joint. *G*, Contrast agent–filled connecting tube (CT) joins the needle hub (NH). Contrast agent has been injected into the right L4 nerve root sheath (NRS) below the right L4 pedicle (P). Note filling of a Tarlov cyst (T) and peripheral nerve root sheath (PNRS). *H*, AP radiography after right L4 root block. The needle tip (NT) is at the injection site below the L4 pedicle (P). The nerve root sheath (NRS) and the sheath for the lumbosacral trunk (LT) are opacified with contrast agent. L5 = L5 vertebra.

frequently, there is left leg pain. Straight-leg raising is positive at 45 degrees on the right and negative to 90 degrees on the left. Pulses in both feet are satisfactory.

Imaging and Therapy

Pre-SNRB MR imaging demonstrated foraminal narrowing caused by a diffusely bulging disc with compression of the right L4 nerve root (see Fig. 4-22C and D). Atrophic right erector spinae muscle bundles were noted (see Fig. 4-22D), a common associated

finding with long-standing neurogenic pain. For needle placement, the right superior articular process of L4 was positioned midway between the anterior and posterior margins of the superior end plate of L4, and the superior end plates were positioned parallel to the x-ray beam until they superimposed (see Fig. 4-22E). The target zone for local anesthetic placement was localized with a needle placed on the overlying skin surface. A 22-gauge needle was then placed, under fluoroscopic guidance, with its tip inferior to the right L4 pedicle (see Fig. 4-22F). With a connecting tube attached to the needle hub (see Fig. 4-22G), myelographic contrast medium was injected into the right L4 nerve sheath, opacifying not only the sheath but also a small Tarlov cyst. After proper needle tip placement was confirmed, the SNRB was performed by injecting a mixture of 0.5 mL lidocaine (1%), 1.0 mL bupivacaine (0.25%), and 0.5 mL betamethasone (6 mg/mL) into the nerve sheath (see Fig. 4-22H).

Results

When the needle contacted the right L4 nerve root, the patient felt immediate, intense pain that she stated matched the distribution of her usual pain. Two hours after the procedure, the patient stated that she was relieved of her typical right lower extremity pain and that she had no numbness or loss of strength.

CASE 2

Clinical Presentation

The patient is a 75-year-old woman with intractable left lower extremity pain. The pain radiates from the lateral left hip into the lateral thigh, across the anterior leg, and into the top of the foot (Fig. 4-23A and B). Her strength and reflexes are normal. Straight-leg raising is negative.

Imaging and Therapy

Pre-SNRB MR imaging demonstrated a left posterolateral disc herniation at the level of the L4-5 disc, causing posterior displacement of the traversing left L5 nerve root (see Fig. 4-23C). For needle placement, the left superior articular process of L5 was positioned midway between the anterior and posterior margins of the superimposed superior end plates of L5 (see Fig. 4-23D). The 22-gauge needle was advanced inferior to the pedicle. Myelographic contrast medium was injected, and it opacified the left L5 nerve sheath, with the negative defect within the sheath representing the nerve root (see Fig. 4-23D). After confirmation of proper needle placement, the sheath was injected with a mixture of 0.5 mL lidocaine-MPF (1%), 1.0 mL bupivacaine (0.25%), and 0.5 mL betamethasone (6 mg/mL).

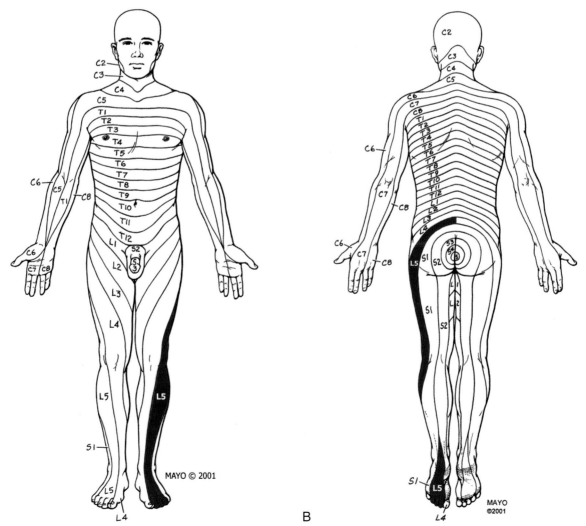

A   B

Figure 4-23 ■ Anterior (*A*) and posterior (*B*) illustrations of the distribution of the patient's pain along the left L5 dermatome.

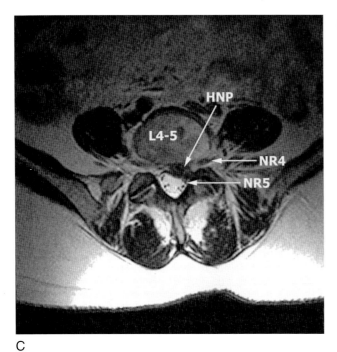

C

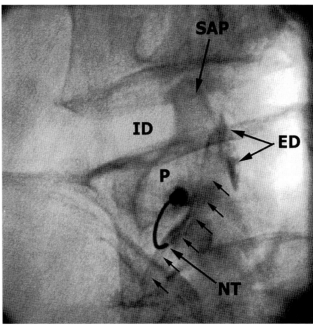

D

Figure 4-23 *(Cont'd)* ■ *C*, Axial T2-weighted fast spin echo MR image at L4-5 disc level. The traversing left L5 nerve root (NR5) is being displaced by the left paramidline herniated nucleus pulposus (HNP). The exiting left L4 nerve root (NR4) is not involved. *D*, Needle tip (NT) is positioned under left L5 pedicle (P). Contrast agent is within the left L5 nerve sheath with a negative defect of the left L5 nerve root. Note a small amount of epidural spread of contrast agent (ED). SAP = left superior articular process L5; ID = L4-5 intervertebral disc.

Results

When the needle contacted the left L5 nerve root, the patient felt sudden, intense pain in the distribution of her typical pain. Two hours after the procedure, the patient was relieved of her typical left lower extremity pain and had retained her pre-procedure strength.

CASE 3

Clinical Presentation

The patient is a 31-year-old man with right lower extremity pain. He dates the onset of symptoms to a marathon he ran 5 months ago. Approximately 1 mile into the run, numbness developed in the bottom of his right foot. This quickly progressed to a stabbing pain in the posterior thigh, knee, and leg (Fig. 4-24A and B). There were no bowel or bladder symptoms and no loss of strength. Straight-leg raising was negative to 90 degrees bilaterally, as was reverse straight-leg raising.

Imaging and Therapy

Pre-SNRB MR imaging demonstrated a moderate-sized right posterolateral disc herniation at the L5-S1 level, causing posterior displacement of the intrathecal right S1 nerve root (see Fig. 4-24C and D). For needle placement, the patient was placed prone. A 22-gauge needle was advanced superomedially into the dorsal right S1 sacral foramen (see Fig. 4-24E). Myelographic contrast medium was seen opacifying the right S1 nerve sheath (see Fig. 4-24E). After confirmation of proper needle tip placement, SNRB was performed by injecting a mixture of 0.5 mL lidocaine-MPF (1%), 1.0 mL bupivacaine (0.25%), and 0.5 mL betamethasone (6 mg/mL).

Results

When the needle contacted the right S1 nerve root, the patient experienced sudden, intense pain posteriorly in the right lower extremity into the bottom of his foot. He stated that this pain was in the usual distribution, although the procedural pain was more intense. Two hours after the procedure, the patient was free of his usual pain without loss of strength.

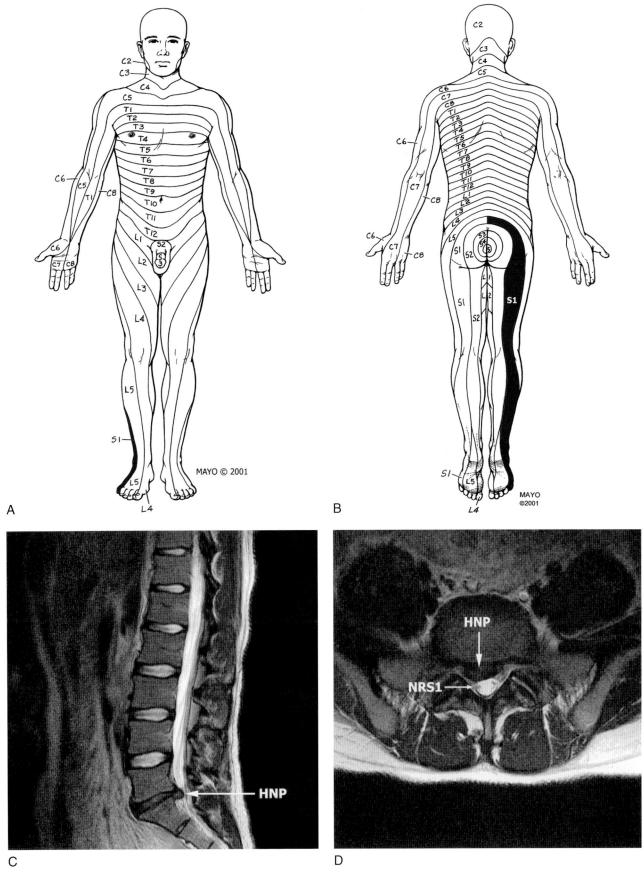

A

B

C

D

Figure 4-24 ▪ Anterior (*A*) and posterior (*B*) illustrations of the distribution of the patient's pain along the right S1 dermatome. Sagittal T2-weighted fast spin echo MR image (*C*) and axial T2-weighted fast spin echo MR image (*D*) demonstrate a moderate-sized right paramidline herniated nucleus pulposus (*HNP*) at L5-S1, causing posterior displacement of the intrathecal right S1 nerve root (*NRS1*).

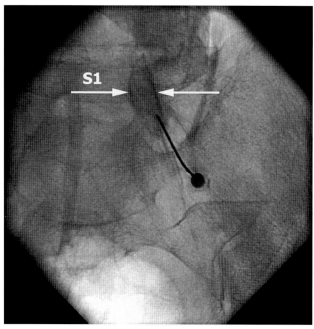

E

Figure 4-24 (*Cont'd*) ▪ *E,* Needle tip within right S1 neural foramen. Contrast material is seen outlining the right S1 nerve root sleeve (*arrows*). *S1* = S1 vertebra.

CASE 4

Clinical Presentation

The patient is an 83-year-old man with right lower extremity pain who had a right L4-5 laminectomy 45 years earlier. He has been having increasing right lower extremity pain over the past 9 months. The pain is in the right lateral thigh and courses over the anterior leg and into the great toe (Fig. 4-25A and B). Motor strength is symmetric. Straight-leg raising is negative to 90 degrees.

Imaging and Therapy

Pre-SNRB MR imaging demonstrated a large calcified facet spur projecting from the medial right L4-5 facet joint and a smaller synovial cyst along the posterior margin of the spur (see Fig. 4-25C). The intrathecal right L5 nerve root was displaced ventromedially (see Fig. 4-25C). For needle placement, the right superior

articular process of L5 was positioned midway between the anterior and posterior margins of the superimposed superior end plates of L5. A 22-gauge needle was advanced inferior and lateral to the right L5 pedicle (see Fig. 4-25D). Curvilinear myelographic contrast medium was seen opacifying the right L5 nerve sheath (see Fig. 4-25D). After confirmation of proper needle tip position, a mixture of 0.5 mL lidocaine-MPF (1%), 1.0 mL bupivacaine (0.25%), and 0.5 mL betamethasone (6 mg/mL) was instilled into the nerve sheath.

Results

When the needle contacted the right L5 nerve root, the patient had intense, concordant right lower extremity pain. Two hours after the procedure, he stated that his typical pain was alleviated without loss of motor strength.

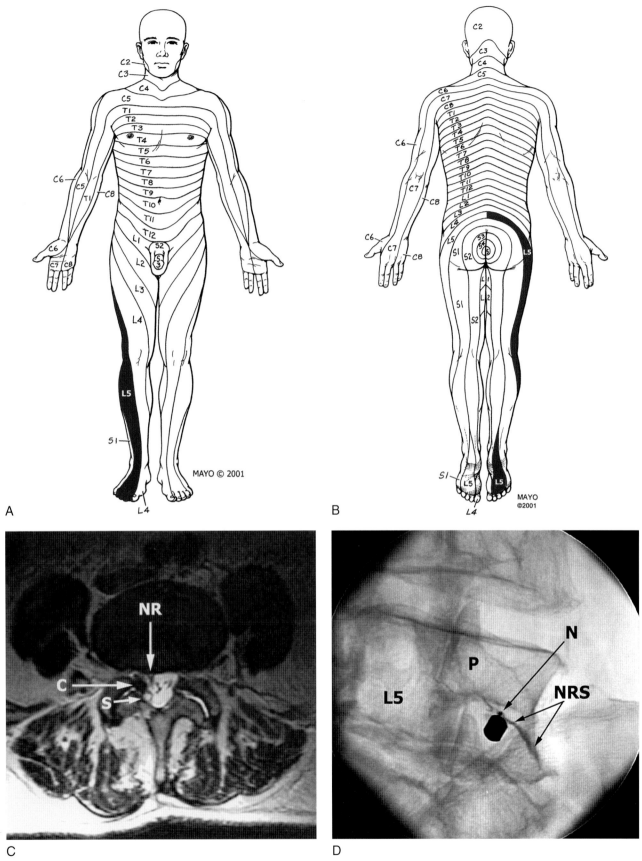

A

B

C

D

Figure 4-25 ■ Anterior (*A*) and posterior (*B*) illustrations of the distribution of the patient's pain along the right L5 dermatome. *C*, Axial T2-weighted fast spin echo MR image at L4-5 disc level. A calcified facet spur (*C*) displaces the traversing right L5 nerve root (NR). S = synovial cyst. *D*, LAO radiograph during right L5 SNRB. The needle tip (N) is inferior and lateral to the right L5 pedicle (P), with curvilinear contrast agent within the nerve root sheath (NRS).

CASE 5

Clinical Presentation

The patient is a 66-year-old woman with a 6- to 7-year history of right neck and arm pain that began without a precipitating event. The pain begins in the suboccipital region to the right of midline and courses over the anterior shoulder and into the biceps (Fig. 4-26A and B). She has significant limitation of cervical motion, particularly right lateral rotation and extension. There is -1 right deltoid and biceps paresis but otherwise normal upper extremity strength.

Imaging and Therapy

Pre-SNRB MR imaging demonstrated a prominent uncovertebral spur causing significant narrowing of the right C4-5 neural foramen (see Fig. 4-26C). With CT

guidance and with the patient in the left lateral decubitus position, a 25-gauge needle was advanced using a right anterolateral approach toward the right C4-5 neural foramen (see Fig. 4-26D). This elicited severe, sharp pain in the patient's right neck and biceps that the patient described as concordant with her usual pain. The SNRB was performed by injecting a mixture of 0.5 mL lidocaine-MPF (1%) and 0.5 mL bupivacaine (0.25%).

Results

Two hours after the procedure, the patient stated she was relieved of her usual right neck, shoulder, and biceps pain.

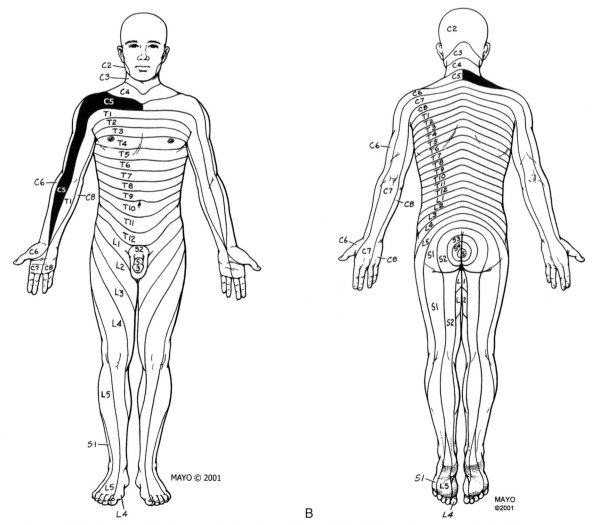

A   B

Figure 4-26 ■ Anterior (*A*) and posterior (*B*) illustrations of the distribution of the patient's pain along the right C5 dermatome.

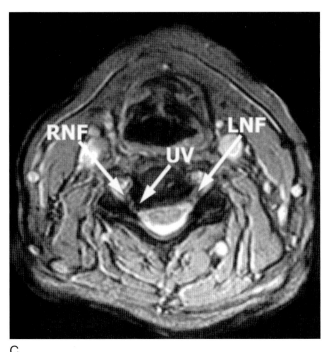

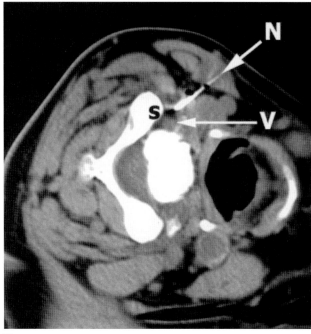

C

D

Figure 4-26 (*Cont'd*) ■ *C*, Axial T2-weighted fast spin echo MR image of cervical spine. Uncovertebral spur (UV) causes moderate narrowing of the right C4-5 neural foramen (RNF). LNF = left neural foramen. *D*, Axial CT image in left lateral decubitus position. The needle (N) is seen with the tip just lateral to the right C4-5 neural foramen. The path of the needle is posterior to the vertebral artery (V). S = superior articular process of C5.

CURRENT PROCEDURAL TERMINOLOGY (CPT) CODES

CPT codes change often and may vary from state to state. Consultation with someone experienced in CPT coding procedures is recommended to ensure that the CPT coding is appropriate for a given region or state. Below is a sample of CPT codes that are being used for the nerve block procedure at this writing.[6]

Diagnostic Radiology (Diagnostic Imaging)-Other Procedures

76005 Fluoroscopic guidance and localization of needle or catheter tip for spine or paraspinous diagnostic or therapeutic injection procedures (epidural, transforaminal epidural, subarachnoid, paravertebral facet joint, paravertebral facet joint nerve or sacroiliac joint), including neurolytic agent destruction

Introduction/Injection of Anesthetic Agent (Nerve Block), Diagnostic or Therapeutic

64479 Injection, anesthetic agent and/or steroid, transforaminal epidural; cervical or thoracic, single level

64480 cervical or thoracic, each additional level

(List separately in addition to code for primary procedure)

(Use code 64480 in conjunction with code 64479)

64483 lumbar or sacral, single level

64484 lumbar or sacral, each additional level

(List separately in addition to code for primary procedure)

(Use code 64484 in conjunction with code 64483)

XXXXX-50 Use modifier if bilateral

99141 Sedation with or without analgesia (conscious sedation); intravenous, intramuscular, or inhalation

References

1. Derby R, Kine G, Saal J, et al. Response to steroid and duration of radicular pain as predictors of surgical outcome. Spine 1992; 17(6S):S176-S183.
2. Physicians' Desk Reference, 56th ed. Montvale, NJ: Medical Economics Company, 2002.
3. Alleyne CH Jr, Cawley CM, Shengelaia GG, et al. Microsurgical anatomy of the artery of Adamkiewicz and its segmental artery. J Neurosurg 1998; 89:791-795.
4. Windsor RE, Falco FJE. Paraplegia following selective nerve root blocks. Int Spinal Inject Soc Sci Newsletter 2001; 4(1):53.
5. Fenton DS, Czervionke LF. Discography. In Williams LA, Murtagh FR (eds). Handbook of Diagnostic and Therapeutic Spine Procedures. St. Louis: CV Mosby, 2002, pp 187-188.
6. CPT 2002, CPT Intellectual Property Services. Chicago: American Medical Association, 2002.

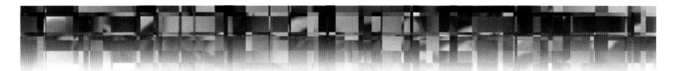

A Spine Surgeon's Perspective

Selective Nerve Root Block

Joseph T. Alexander, MD

Widespread degenerative changes in the thoracic and lumbar spine are ubiquitous with the aging process. Disc degeneration and bulging, as well as facet joint and ligamentum flavum hypertrophy, resulting in neural foraminal and lateral recess stenosis are often seen at multiple spinal levels, even in asymptomatic patients. In my clinical practice, I commonly find that the symptomatic spinal segment is not the most impressive radiographically. The reason for this is probably that in advanced spinal degeneration the affected segment becomes effectively fused, and motion, and therefore further nerve irritation and pain, are thereby prevented.

As the number of spinal segments treated surgically increases, the rates of immediate and delayed complications increase, the recovery process slows, and the overall success rate declines. Minimally invasive surgical techniques can also decrease postoperative pain and speed recovery, but they must be directed at a specific target, because overall visualization of the spine is decreased.

When faced with a patient who has intractable radicular symptoms that are non-localizing clinically and with multilevel degenerative changes on imaging studies, I have found selective nerve root blocks to be useful diagnostically and for surgical planning. I am careful to tell the patient that I do not expect any long-term relief of symptoms, although I have actually seen this occur in several cases. Because I am using this procedure for localization, I never request more than one nerve root level to be injected at one session, and I advise the patient that multiple sessions may be necessary if we do not localize the correct level during the initial evaluation. It is very important to question the patient carefully a few days after the procedure. Most will initially say, "It did not work," because their pain has already recurred. However, I consider the test to have been positive if the patient had appreciable relief of symptoms for the duration of action of the local anesthetic agent used in the procedure, whether or not any steroid was also injected. In addition, it is not unusual to produce "concordant" pain during the procedure.

Using this technique, I have succeeded in limiting some decompression and fusion procedures to a single level despite widespread degenerative changes. I have also found that a positive response seems to be a favorable prognostic sign for surgery.

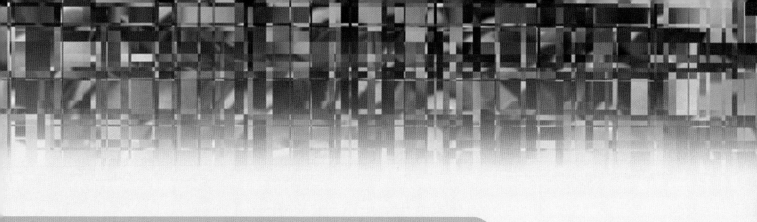

Chapter 5

Epidural Injections

- B. Todd Sitzman, MD, MPH

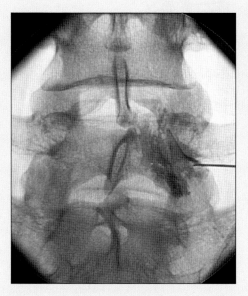

BACKGROUND

Back pain affects nearly everyone at some point in his or her adult life, with most episodes resolving spontaneously. In approximately 10% of persons, the pain persists despite conservative management and results in significant individual disability and societal cost.[1-4] Those with persistent, chronic back pain are often referred to medical specialists for evaluation and frequently receive invasive pain therapies.

Historically, the "epidural steroid injection" has been the first-line invasive therapeutic procedure of choice. First described in 1953, epidural steroids have since been administered to millions of patients for treatment of axial and radicular back pain.[5] Despite the widespread use of therapeutic epidural steroid injections, controversy remains over the efficacy of this procedure. There have been only six prospective, blinded, randomized, controlled trials reporting the efficacy of epidural steroid injections. Of these, two reported significant improvement of symptoms[6,7] and four did not.[8-11] A meta-analysis of the epidural steroid injection literature from 1966 to 1993 revealed a 14% positive treatment effect over placebo.[12]

Many less rigorously designed studies have supported the beneficial role of epidural steroid injections, although it is difficult to draw conclusions from these studies because of limitations, such as small sample size, variations in inclusion criteria, lack of diagnostic test standardization, lack of control group, variations in injection technique, and differences in duration of follow-up. Furthermore, the earlier studies were performed with "blind" techniques (i.e., without fluoroscopic guidance), a major limitation that will be discussed later in this chapter.

Thus, there is evidence that epidural steroid injections are more effective than placebo, local anesthetic alone, or bed rest for nerve root irritation or inflammation, regardless of the cause. Additionally, favorable outcomes are more common with acute pain conditions rather than chronic pain states.[13] Of those patients who do respond favorably, the majority (more than 90%) do so within 6 days of injection.

Proposed Mechanisms of Benefit

Significant controversy remains regarding the mechanism of therapeutic benefit from steroids placed in the epidural space. Several mechanisms have been proposed, including anti-inflammatory effects, direct neural membrane stabilization effects, and modulation of peripheral nociceptor input.

Axial and radicular pain symptoms may arise from any anatomic structure capable of transmitting pain (i.e., the pain generator), including the disc, spinal nerve, dura, muscle, fascia, ligament, and facet joint. Injury to any of these structures results in the release of inflammatory mediators. For example, any acute or chronic disc injury (e.g., disc herniation, annular tear, degenerative disc disease) results in the release of phospholipase A_2 from the nucleus pulposus into the epidural space.[14] Phospholipase A_2, an enzyme found in high concentration in disc material, is responsible for initiating the arachidonic acid cascade, which results in the production of prostaglandins, leukotrienes, and other mediators of inflammation.[15] The end result is further inflammation of the intervertebral disc itself, the dura, the posterior longitudinal ligament, and the nerve roots. Steroids inhibit the activity of phospholipase A_2 and thereby inhibit the inflammatory process.[16] Another possible mechanism involves the dilution of inflammatory mediators by the volume of injection material (injectate) around the affected nerve root. This may account for the beneficial effects of epidural normal saline or local anesthetics alone, although these are short lived in comparison with the effects of steroid injections. Additionally, the superior effectiveness of epidural steroid injections in acute injury, in contrast to chronic pain conditions, is purported to result from inhibition of the inflammatory process before it progresses to fibrosis and scarring.

Although evidence supporting the anti-inflammatory effects of epidural steroids is convincing, other mechanisms of action have been proposed. Steroids placed into the epidural space have been shown to inhibit normal nociceptive C fiber transmission but not A-B fiber transmission.[17] Because this effect was reversed when the corticosteroid was removed, a direct membrane effect was suggested. Also, glucocorticoid receptor sites have been located on norepinephrine and 5-hydroxytryptamine neurons within the dorsal horn substantia gelatinosa, which are known pathways of pain transmission.[18, 19] This suggests that epidural steroids may modulate nociceptive input from peripheral nociceptors by direct action on the spinal cord.

ANATOMIC CONSIDERATIONS

Knowledge of the epidural space anatomy is of great importance to the interventional pain physician. The epidural space lies between the osseoligamentous structures lining the vertebral canal and the dural membrane surrounding the spinal cord and the nerve roots. In the adult, the thecal sac extends from the foramen magnum to approximately the S2 level; however, the epidural space continues inferiorly within the bony sacral canal, terminating at the sacral hiatus at the S4 or S5 level (Fig. 5-1).

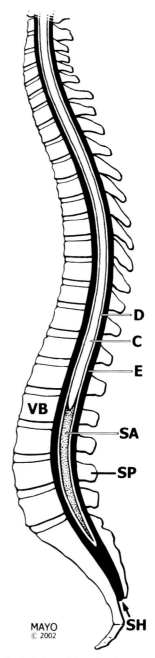

Figure 5-1 ■ Sagittal view of the spine demonstrating the osseous vertebral bodies (VB) and spinous processes (SP), the epidural space (E), the subarachnoid space (SA), the dura mater (D), and the spinal cord (C). Note that the epidural space extends from the foramen magnum to the sacral hiatus (SH).

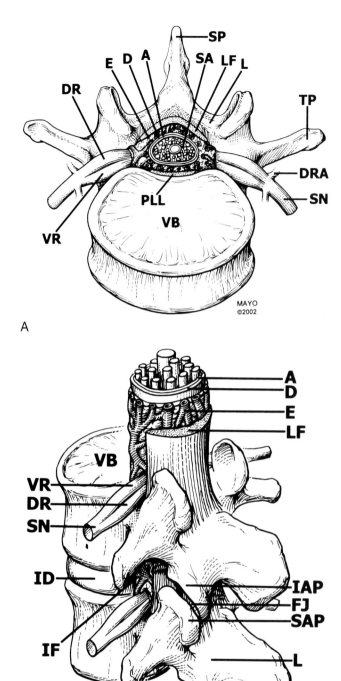

A

B

Figure 5-2 ■ Cross-sectional view of the lower lumbar spine (*A*) and oblique view of the lower lumbar spine (*B*). SP = spinous process; L = lamina; LF = ligamentum flavum; E = epidural space (containing epidural veins, lymphatics, and adipose); D = dura mater; A = arachnoid mater; SA = subarachnoid space (containing cerebrospinal fluid, cauda equina, filum terminale); PLL = posterior longitudinal ligament; VB = vertebral body; TP = transverse process; DR = dorsal root; VR = ventral root; SN = spinal nerve (continuation of the ventral ramus); DRA = dorsal ramus; FJ = facet joint (superior articular process [SAP] and inferior articular process [IAP]); IF = intervertebral foramen; ID = intervertebral disc.

The epidural space is subdivided into anterior and posterior compartments.[20, 21] The anterior epidural space is bordered anteriorly by the vertebral body, intervertebral disc, and posterior longitudinal ligament and posteriorly by the thecal sac. The posterior epidural space is bordered anteriorly by the thecal sac and posteriorly by the ligamentum flavum and the laminae. The posterior epidural space is somewhat triangular and varies in its anteroposterior diameter throughout the length of the spine: 1.5 to 2 mm at C7, 4 mm at T2, 5 to 6 mm at L2, and 2 mm at S1. The contents of the epidural space include adipose tissue, loose areolar tissue, arteries, lymphatics, and an abundant venous plexus (Fig. 5-2).

Each spinal nerve exists within an intervertebral foramen, bordered anteriorly by the vertebral body and disc, posteriorly by the facet joint, and superiorly and inferiorly by the pedicles of the adjacent vertebrae. A dural sleeve composed of dura mater and arachnoid mater, along with the epidural space, accompanies the exiting nerve roots as far as the intervertebral foramen. At this site, the dura thins to form the epineurium of the proximal spinal nerve. It is important to note that within the intervertebral foramen, the dorsal and ventral nerve roots coalesce to form the exiting spinal nerve. If there is significant narrowing of the intervertebral foramen, the spread of epidural injectate (e.g., contrast material, local anesthetic, steroid) may be limited and hence the substance may not reach its intended site of action.

CONTROVERSIES

Before proceeding to epidural techniques, it is important to clarify terminology involved with epidural injections. Foremost, not all epidural injections are alike, especially with regard to the approach used to gain access to the epidural space. The ***interlaminar*** approach (both midline and paramedian) involves insertion of an epidural needle midway between the laminae of adjacent vertebrae, whereas the ***transforaminal*** approach involves insertion of a spinal needle into the superior portion of an intervertebral foramen just inferior to the pedicle (Fig. 5-3).

Historically, the epidural space was accessed inferiorly through the caudal approach (i.e., sacral hiatus) or posteriorly through the interlaminar approach, often without the use of fluoroscopy. A major criticism of most of the early studies on epidural steroid efficacy is their use of "blind" approaches (i.e., without fluoroscopy) and therefore their lack of target specificity. Even when performed by experienced clinicians, blind epidural injections result in incorrect placement of the injectate more than 25% of the time.[22, 23] Additionally, earlier studies did not involve administration of contrast agent before the injection of local anesthetic and/or steroid. Injection of contrast medium is now strongly recommended to confirm correct needle placement within the epidural space. For these reasons, most pain specialists have abandoned "blind" epidural injections in favor of a fluoroscopically guided approach.

Interlaminar and caudal epidural injections, compared with transforaminal injections, have fallen out of favor with pain interventionalists for several reasons. Both require relatively large volumes of injectate to deliver steroids, with

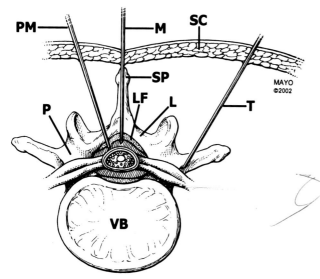

Figure 5-3 ■ ■ Percutaneous approaches to the epidural space: interlaminar approaches (paramedian [PM] and midline [M]) and transforaminal approach (T). SP = spinous process; L = lamina; P = pedicle; SC = subcutaneous tissue; LF = ligamentum flavum; and VB = vertebral body.

or without local anesthetic, to the presumed pathologic site (i.e., the pain generator); the result is minimal, if any, diagnostic benefit. For example, in back pain of discogenic etiology, only the transforaminal approach reliably delivers injectate into the anterior epidural space and thereby reaches the potential pain generators.[24]

Caudal and interlaminar approaches also involve increased risk of extraepidural and intravascular needle placement.[25, 26] Additionally, because of the presence of epidural fibrosis or adhesions (idiopathic or postsurgical), the injectate may never reach its intended target site (e.g., a compressed spinal nerve) and in this way hinder the physician's ability to appropriately interpret the effects of the injection. Any combination of these factors may increase the risk of false-positive and false-negative results. For these reasons, the transforaminal epidural injection under fluoroscopic guidance has emerged as the preferred approach to the epidural space.

Another controversy involves the terminology used to describe epidural injections. Medical journals and texts often incorrectly refer to transforaminal epidural injections as "selective epidural injections," "selective nerve root blocks," or "nerve root sleeve injections." Interlaminar epidural injections are often referred to as "translaminar" epidural injections. However, the International Spinal Injection Society (ISIS), promoting the utilization of nomenclature based on precise anatomic descriptors, recommends "transforaminal" and "interlaminar" when describing epidural injections.[27]

One should keep in mind that a transforaminal epidural injection, although more "selective" than an interlaminar epidural injection, has diagnostic specificity for radicular pain only–not for axial back pain. The local anesthetic/steroid injectate not only affects the spinal nerve at the level injected but may also affect several of its proximal branches, including the sinuvertebral nerve and the medial branch of

the dorsal primary ramus. For this reason, a transforaminal epidural injection using a small volume of local anesthetic will anesthetize the spinal nerve (relieving the radicular component) and partially anesthetize the dura, the posterior longitudinal ligament, the intervertebral disc, and the zygapophysial (facet) joint (axial components) at the level of injection.

PATIENT SELECTION

Experienced clinicians often face challenges when determining the cause of acute or chronic back pain. In the absence of clear-cut disc herniation with neurologic deficit, the accurate diagnosis of spinal pain involves a thorough physical examination, imaging studies, and neurophysiologic studies, and it may involve diagnostic injections. Blind interlaminar and caudal epidural injections have little diagnostic role. However, transforaminal epidural injections may assist in the diagnosis of radicular pain conditions resulting from nerve root compression, and they may have a prognostic role in planning for decompressive surgery.[28–30]

The therapeutic role of epidural injections with steroid is less controversial and can be divided into five main indications:

1. Disc degeneration or herniation
2. Spinal nerve root compression
3. Spinal nerve root inflammation–traumatic
4. Spinal nerve root inflammation–infectious (e.g., acute or subacute herpes zoster, postherpetic neuralgia)
5. Spinal stenosis

CONTRAINDICATIONS

Contraindications to epidural injection may be absolute or relative, as follows:

- Patient unwilling to consent to the procedure
- True allergy to the local anesthetic, corticosteroid, or contrast agent
- Infection at the site of injection
- Coagulopathy (International Normalized Ratio [INR] >1.5 or platelets <100,000/mm³)
- Pregnancy (because of the teratogenic effect of radiation)

PROCEDURE

Equipment/Supplies

Tuohy epidural needles, 18- and 20-gauge, 3.5-inch (for interlaminar or caudal approaches) (Tuohy epidural needle, Becton Dickinson & Co., Franklin Lakes, NJ)

Spinal needle, 22-gauge, 3.5-inch (for transforaminal approach) (Quinke type point, Becton Dickinson & Co., Franklin Lakes, NJ)

Epidural catheter (Perifix, B. Braun Medical, Inc., Bethlehem, PA)

Needle, 25-gauge, 1.5-inch (for subcutaneous local anesthetic and cervical transforaminal injections)

Syringe, 5 mL (for subcutaneous local anesthetic)

Syringe, 10 mL, glass (for interlaminar approach)–glass provides smooth plunger movement and improved tactile feel for the "loss of resistance" technique

Syringe, 10 mL (for caudal or interlaminar epidural injectate)

Syringe, 3 mL (for transforaminal epidural injectate)

Syringe, 3 mL (for contrast agent)

Sterile gloves, drapes, towels, gauze, gown

Povidone-iodine (Betadine)/chlorhexidine prep

Adhesive bandage

Lead apron, hat, mask

Fluoroscopy, C-arm or biplane

Medications

Sterile saline, preservative free (as diluent and as injectate during interlaminar epidural approach–"loss of resistance" technique)

Lidocaine hydrochloride, 1%, 2 to 5 mL (for subcutaneous local infiltration)

Nonionic iodinated myelographic contrast agent, 300 mg I/mL (Omnipaque [Iohexol] Injection, Nycomed, Inc., Princeton, NJ) (2+ mL for caudal and interlaminar; 0.5 to 1 mL for transforaminal)

Lidocaine hydrochloride, 1% preservative free (Xylocaine-MPF 1%, AstraZenca LP, Wilmington, DE) (5 to 10 mL for caudal and interlaminar; 1 mL for transforaminal)

Bupivacaine, 0.25%, preservative free (Sensorcaine-MPF Injection 0.25%, AstraZeneca LP, Wilmington, DE) (5+ mL for caudal and interlaminar; 1 mL for transforaminal)

Betamethasone sodium phosphate and betamethasone acetate injectable suspension, 6 mg/mL (Celestone Soluspan, Schering Corporation, Kenilworth, NJ)

Triamcinolone diacetate, 25 mg/mL (Aristocort, Fujisawa Healthcare, Inc., Deerfield, IL)

Methylprednisolone acetate injectable suspension, 40 mg/mL (Depo-Medrol, Pharmacia, Peapack, NJ)

Injection Mixtures

Caudal Approach

(10 to 15 mL total volume)

Combine:

2 mL of either betamethasone 6 mg/mL or triamcinolone 25 mg/mL

5 mL of either 0.25% bupivacaine or 1% lidocaine

3 to 8 mL sterile normal saline

Interlaminar Approach

Lumbar or Thoracic (6 to 8 mL Total Volume)

Combine:

2 mL of either betamethasone 6 mg/mL or triamcinolone 25 mg/mL

4 to 6 mL of either 0.25% bupivacaine or 1% lidocaine

Cervical (4 to 6 mL Total Volume)

Combine:

1 to 2 mL of either betamethasone 6 mg/mL or triamcinolone 25 mg/mL

2 mL 1% lidocaine

1 to 2 mL preservative-free normal saline

Transforaminal Approach

Lumbar or Thoracic (2 mL Total Volume)

Combine:

1 mL of either betamethasone 6 mg/mL or triamcinolone 25 mg/mL

1 mL of either 0.25% bupivacaine or 1% lidocaine

Cervical (1 to 2 mL Total Volume)

0.5 to 1 mL of either betamethasone 6 mg/mL or triamcinolone 25 mg/mL

0.5 to 1 mL 1% lidocaine

Local anesthetics should be from single-use vials and be preservative free to prevent flocculation of the steroid.[31] Local anesthetics should also be epinephrine free to reduce the potential risks associated with neuraxial vasospasm, especially in the cervical region.

Caudal Technique

After informed consent, the patient is positioned prone on the fluoroscopic table. It may help to straighten the lumbar curve by placing a small pillow or roll under the patient's lower abdomen/upper pelvis. A wide area of the patient's lower back and buttocks, specifically the gluteal cleft, is prepped with povidone-iodine (Betadine) and draped in sterile fashion. Sterile gauze should be placed in the midgluteal cleft below the expected needle entry point for increased sterility. The caudal epidural space is approached via the sacral hiatus; even with the use of fluoroscopy, this procedure may require manual identification of the sacral cornua. The sacral cornua are located on either side of the sacral hiatus. Rotating the patient's feet inward will often help relax the patient's gluteal muscles and make palpation of the sacral cornua easier. Fluoroscopic imaging will often reveal an opaque "∩" (inverted "U"-shaped) landmark as the entry to the sacral hiatus (Fig. 5-4).

After the sacral hiatus has been located, 1% lidocaine is used to infiltrate the skin and subcutaneous tissues. A 20-gauge Tuohy epidural needle is advanced cephalad toward the sacral hiatus at a 45-degree angle. It is common for the needle tip to contact the periosteum of the sacral canal. If this occurs, the needle is withdrawn slightly and advanced at a different and often more shallow angle. Initially, resistance is felt as the needle enters the sacrococcygeal ligament, followed by a loss of resistance as the needle enters the caudal epidural space. At this point, the angle of the needle is lowered and the needle is advanced 0.5 to 1 cm into the epidural space. It is mandatory to gently aspirate for the presence of blood or cerebrospinal fluid before injecting any medication into the epidural space. One should remember that the dural sac extends to the S2 level in adults. It is advisable to use a shorter needle (2-inch rather than 3.5-inch) and

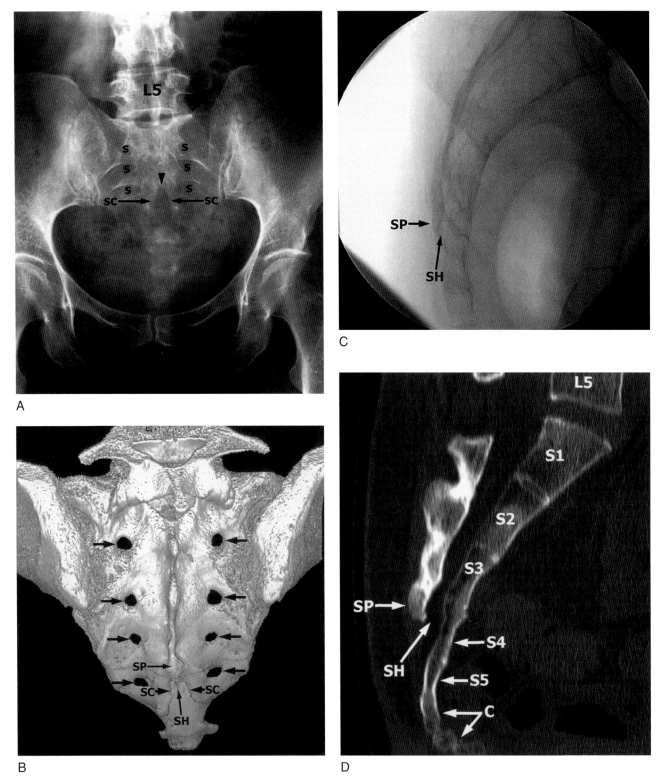

Figure 5-4 ■ *A*, Plain radiograph revealing sacral anatomy. L5 = 5th lumbar vertebra; S = sacral formina; SC = sacral cornua; *arrowhead* = sacral hiatus. *B*, Three-dimensional CT surface rendering of sacral landmarks. *Black arrows* = sacral foramina; SP = spinous process/median sacral crest; SC = sacral cornu, SH = sacral hiatus. *C*, Lateral fluoroscopic image of sacrum. SP = sacral spinous process/median sacral crest; SH = sacral hiatus at the entry to the caudal epidural space. *D*, Lateral CT image revealing the sacral spinal canal. L5 = fifth lumbar vertebra; S1-S5 = first through fifth sacral vertebrae; SP = sacral spinous process/median sacral crest; SH = sacral hiatus; C = coccygeal vertebrae.

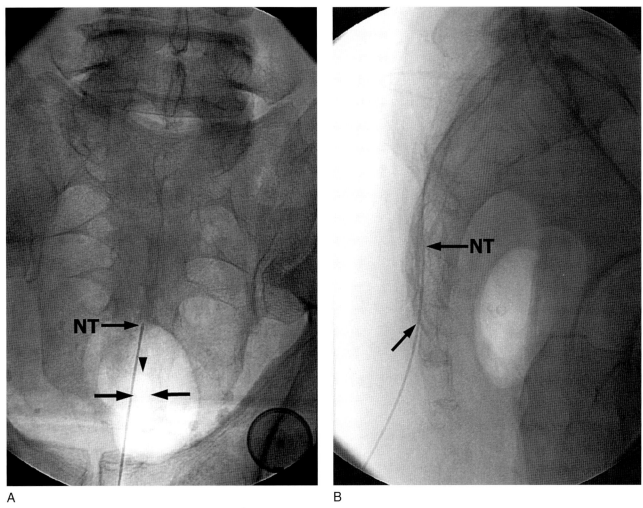

A   B

Figure 5-5 ■ *A,* AP fluoroscopic image revealing distal needle tip (NT) within the caudal epidural space. *Arrowhead* = sacral hiatus; *arrows* = sacral cornua. *B,* Lateral fluoroscopic image. NT = distal needle tip within the caudal epidural space; *arrow* = sacral hiatus.

to advance the needle tip no more than 1 cm into the sacral hiatus to decrease the risk of inadvertent dural puncture (Fig. 5-5).

Confirmation of proper position within the caudal epidural space requires the use of 1 to 3 mL of nonionic contrast agent. Ease of injection (i.e., low resistance) and spread of the agent in a cranial direction–it often exits 1 or more anterior sacral foramina–confirm the proper location of the needle tip in the caudal epidural space (Fig. 5-6).

Caudal epidural injections require larger volumes than lumbar, thoracic, and cervical epidural injections. Depending on the proposed pathologic site (i.e., the pain generator), 10 to 15 mL of injectate is recommended. This will often require dilution of the steroid with sterile saline and bupivacaine or lidocaine.

The use of a local anesthetic often results in pain relief within 15 minutes, which provides clinical confirmation that the steroid injectate has reached its intended site of action.

Lumbar Techniques

Interlaminar Approach

After informed consent, the patient is positioned prone on the fluoroscopic table. A small pillow is placed under the patient's lower abdomen/upper pelvis to increase the lumbar interlaminar space. With the use of fluoroscopic guidance, the interlaminar target site to be injected is identified and the skin over this site is marked with indelible ink. The intended target is the interlaminar space itself (Fig. 5-7). The skin over this site is prepped with povidone-iodine three or more times and draped in sterile fashion. The skin and overlying subcutaneous tissue are anesthetized with 1% lidocaine. With intermittent fluoroscopy, an 18-gauge Tuohy epidural needle is then advanced toward the interlaminar space (Fig. 5-8). The needle is slowly advanced by means of the "*loss-of-resistance*" technique, as follows:

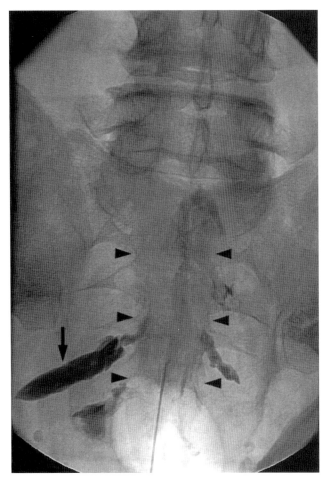

Figure 5-6 ▪ AP fluoroscopic image of caudal epidural contrast agent injection. *Arrowheads* = outline and lateral borders of caudal epidural space; *arrow* = extravasation and pooling of contrast agent through the left-sided S4 neural foramen.

1. A 10-mL glass syringe, filled with air or sterile saline, is used.
2. The clinician's nondominant thumb and index finger firmly grasp the base of the needle at the skin surface (Fig. 5-9).
3. The thumb of the clinician's dominant hand applies continuous pressure against the plunger of the syringe (see Fig. 5-9).
4. Using either constant pressure or gentle ballottement applied to the plunger of the syringe, one advances the needle and syringe toward the epidural space in a slow and deliberate fashion.
5. Once the tip of the epidural needle has passed through the ligamentum flavum and entered the epidural space, there is a sudden "loss of resistance," as if the contents of the syringe were being sucked into the epidural space.

Alternatively, one can advance the Tuohy needle toward the superior border of the lower lamina or inferior border of the superior lamina (Fig. 5-10*A* and *B*) until contact is made with the posterior laminar border (see Fig. 5-10*C*). This will allow accurate initial needle positioning without inadvertent entry into the spinal canal. It should be remembered that the epidural space is ventral to the lamina. The Tuohy needle is

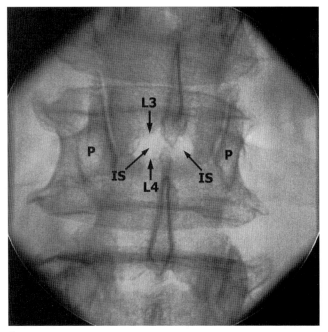

A

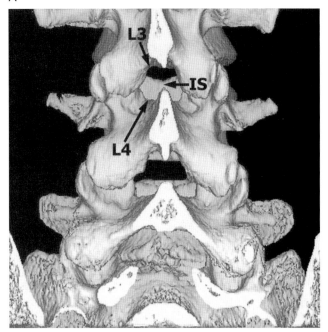

B

Figure 5-7 ▪ Image-intensified AP (*A*) and three-dimensional (*B*) views of the L3-4 interlaminar space. L3 = inferior margin of L3 lamina; L4 = superior margin of L4 lamina; IS = interlaminar space; P = pedicle of L4.

then turned so that the curved bevel is adjacent to the laminar border, which will facilitate ventral advancement of the needle. The needle can then be slowly advanced, with use of the "*loss-of-resistance*" technique, into the epidural space.

At this point, the glass syringe is removed and anteroposterior (AP) fluoroscopic imaging is performed to verify that the epidural needle is between the laminae. With a 3-mL syringe containing 2 mL of nonionic contrast agent, gentle aspiration is performed to evaluate for the presence of blood

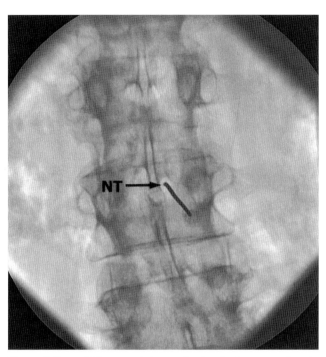

Figure 5-8 ▪ AP fluoroscopic image of an interlaminar approach to the L3-4 epidural space. NT = 18-gauge Tuohy epidural needle tip.

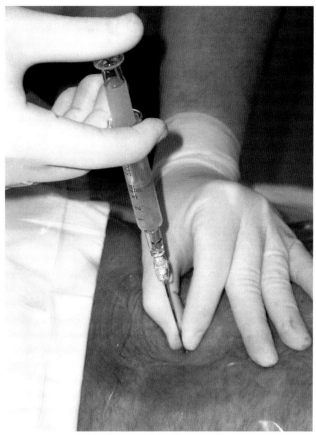

Figure 5-9 ▪ Proper hand position for the "loss-of-resistance" technique used for interlaminar epidural steroid injections. Note that the nondominant thumb and index finger secure the base of the Tuohy epidural needle while either continuous pressure or gentle ballottement is applied to the syringe plunger by the clinician's dominant thumb.

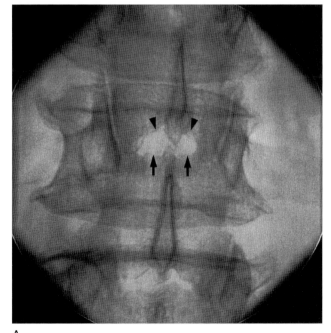

A

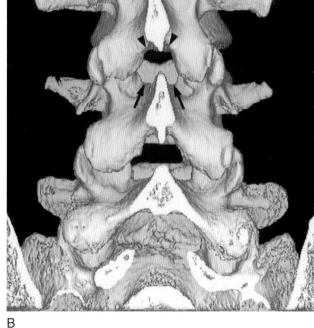

B

Figure 5-10 ▪ *A*, Image-intensified AP fluoroscopic image of the interlaminar approach to an L3-4 lumbar epidural steroid injection. *Arrowheads* = inferior margin of L3 lamina; *arrows* = superior margin of L4 lamina. *B*, Three-dimensional rendering of the L3-4 interlaminar space. *Arrowheads* = inferior lamina of L3; *arrows* = superior lamina of L4.

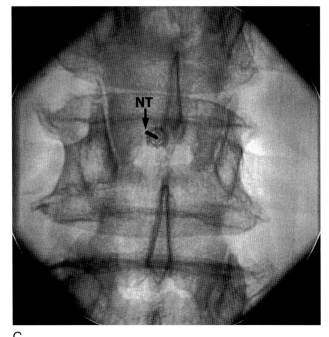

C

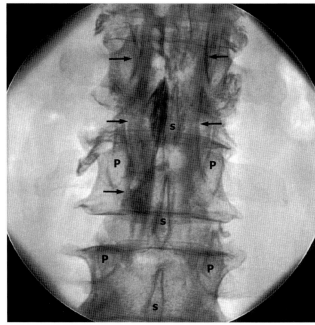

D

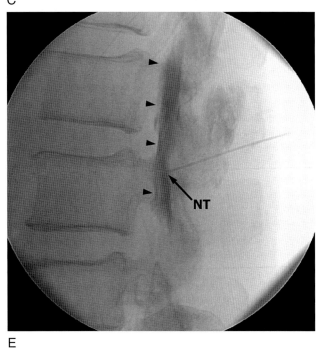

E

Figure 5-10 *(Cont'd)* ■ *C*, An 18-gauge Tuohy epidural needle tip (NT) contacting the inferior laminar border of L3 en route to the lumbar epidural space. *D*, AP fluoroscopic image of contrast outlining the lumbar epidural space. *Arrows* = lateral epidural border; P = pedicle; S = spinous process. *E*, Lateral fluoroscopic image revealing contrast agent within the lumbar epidural space. *Arrowheads* = anterior epidural border; NT = needle tip confirmed within the posterior epidural space.

or cerebrospinal fluid. If none is present, 1 mL of nonionic contrast agent is injected under continuous fluoroscopic imaging. This will reveal an even spread of agent within the epidural space (see Fig. 5-10*D* and *E*). It is advisable to obtain a lateral-view fluoroscopic image to confirm that the needle tip and contrast agent are indeed within the posterior epidural space.

A paramedian modification to the midline interlaminar approach utilizes the same technique as just described, the only exception being that the epidural needle tip is directed laterally and enters the epidural space on the patient's symptomatic side. Thus, there will be preferential spread of contrast medium within the ipsilateral epidural space,

depending on the direction of the opening of the Tuohy needle tip.

Transforaminal Approach

After informed consent, the patient is positioned prone on the fluoroscopic table. With fluoroscopic imaging, an oblique view is obtained, with the final position of the pedicle of the superior vertebra aligned with the superior articular process of the inferior vertebra (Fig. 5-11). The intended target is the 6 o'clock position of the pedicle. The skin over this site is marked, prepped with povidone-iodine, and draped in sterile fashion. The skin and subcutaneous tissues

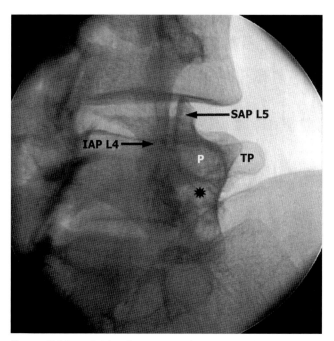

Figure 5-11 ■ LAO radiograph revealing landmarks for a right-sided L5 lumbar transforaminal epidural steroid injection. SAP L5 = superior articular process of the L5 vertebra; IAP L4 = inferior articular process of the L4 vertebra, P = pedicle of L5; TP = transverse process of L5; *star* = needle tip target site.

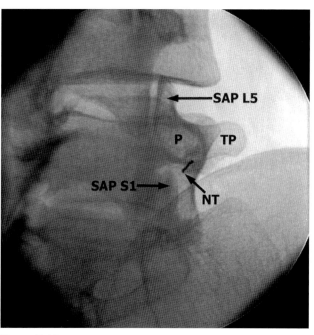

Figure 5-12 ■ LAO radiograph revealing proper needle tip location for a right-sided L5 lumbar transforaminal epidural steroid injection. SAP L5 = superior articular process of the L5 vertebra; SAP S1 = superior articular process of the sacrum; P = pedicle of L5; TP = transverse process of L5; NT = needle tip.

are anesthetized with 1% lidocaine. The tip of a 22-gauge, 3.5-inch spinal needle is slowly advanced toward the 6 o'clock position of the pedicle under intermittent fluoroscopic guidance (Fig. 5-12). It is not necessary to advance the needle until bony contact is made; however, fluoroscopic imaging in multiple planes will ensure that the needle tip is within the "safe triangle," as described by Bogduk and colleagues.[32] The corresponding sides of this inverted triangle are (1) base = inferior border of the pedicle; (2) medial side = exiting spinal nerve; and (3) lateral side = lateral border of the vertebral body (Fig. 5-13). On the AP view, the needle tip should be just below the midpoint of the pedicle and should not be medial to the mid-zygapophysial joint line.

After negative aspiration for blood and cerebrospinal fluid, injection of 1 mL of contrast agent under continuous fluoroscopic imaging should reveal contrast material spreading medially through the neural foramen and into the epidural space (Fig. 5-14). Once epidural spread has been confirmed in AP and lateral views, the steroid/anesthetic preparation is injected.

Thoracic Techniques

Interlaminar Approach

Thoracic-level epidural injections, although similar to lumbar epidural injections, require an appreciation of the anatomic

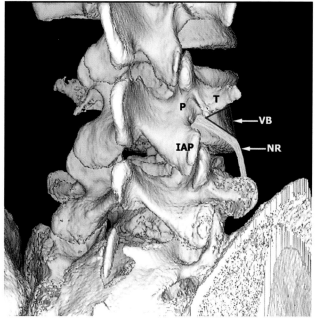

Figure 5-13 ■ Three-dimensional CT demonstrating the "safe triangle" location for lumbar transforaminal epidural steroid injection. NR = spinal nerve; VB = vertebral body; T = transverse process; P = pars interarticularis; IAP = inferior articular process. The pedicle cannot be demonstrated on a surface-rendered image.

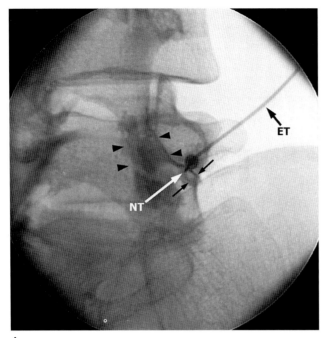

A

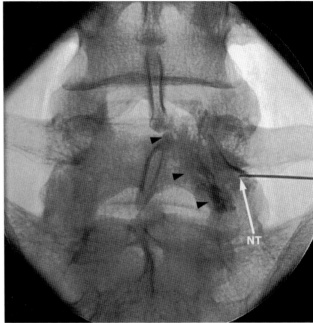

B

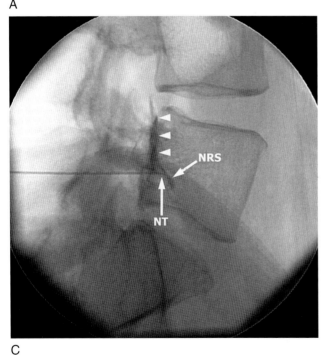

C

Figure 5-14 ▪ *A,* LAO radiograph revealing contrast agent within the right-sided L5 transforaminal epidural space. *Arrowheads* = medial spread of contrast agent into the epidural space inferior to the L5 pedicle, NT = needle tip; *arrows* = L5 spinal nerve; ET = extension tubing containing contrast agent. *B,* AP fluoroscopic image of right-sided L5 transforaminal epidural steroid injection. *Arrowheads* = medial spread of contrast agent into the epidural space; NT = needle tip. *C,* Lateral fluoroscopic image of right-sided transforaminal epidural steroid injection. *Arrowheads* = outline of contrast agent within the anterior epidural space; NT = needle tip; NRS = contrast outlining the L5 nerve root sheath.

differences between the two. The slope or inclination of the spinous processes differs throughout the thoracic spine. T1 through T4 and T10 through T12 spinous processes have little slope, and therefore a midline interlaminar approach is possible. However, the spinous processes of T5 through T9 have a significant downward slope and a midline interlaminar approach is extremely difficult, if not impossible. A paramedian midline approach must be utilized at the T5 through T9 levels. Another anatomic difference between the thoracic and lumbar epidural levels is a thinner ligamentum flavum at the thoracic level. This makes identification of the epidural space potentially more difficult and therefore

increases the risk of inadvertent dural puncture. Lastly, the thoracic epidural space is only 3 to 4 mm wide, compared with 5 to 6 mm in the lumbar region.

After informed consent, the patient is positioned prone on the fluoroscopic table. A small pillow is placed under the patient's chest to enhance the thoracic curvature and increase the interlaminar space. The technique used for T1 through T4 and T10 through T12 is similar to the lumbar interlaminar approach. However, for T5 through T9, a paramedian midline approach is used. The Tuohy epidural needle is inserted just lateral to the tip of the spinous process located below the desired interlaminar space. Note that

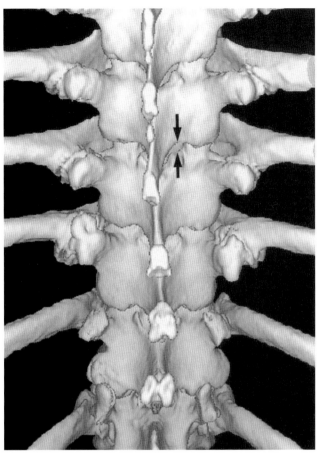

Figure 5-15 ■ Three-dimensional CT, AP rendering of the thoracic vertebral column. Note that because of its acute downward slope, the spinous process of the superior vertebra is actually inferior to the target thoracic-level interlaminar space. *Arrows* = laminae of adjacent vertebrae.

because of its acute slope, the spinous process visualized in the AP view actually corresponds to the spinous process of the superior vertebra at the target interlaminar space (Fig. 5-15). The skin over this site is prepped with povidone-iodine and draped in sterile fashion. The skin and overlying subcutaneous tissue are anesthetized with 1% lidocaine. An 18-gauge Tuohy epidural needle is then advanced toward the epidural space with the use of intermittent fluoroscopic imaging (Fig. 5-16). The needle is slowly advanced by means of the "loss-of-resistance" technique. Because of thoracic biomechanics, especially during inspiration, the epidural space pressure is significantly more negative than that in the lumbar region and the result is a more pronounced "loss of resistance."

The remainder of the thoracic interlaminar epidural injection is similar to that for the lumbar region. Once again, a lateral-view fluoroscopic image is advised to confirm that the needle tip and contrast agent are indeed within the posterior epidural space. Once confirmed, and after a negative aspiration for blood and cerebrospinal fluid, the steroid/anesthetic preparation is injected.

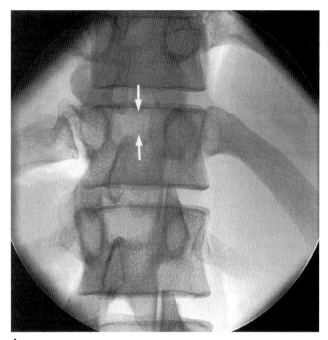

A

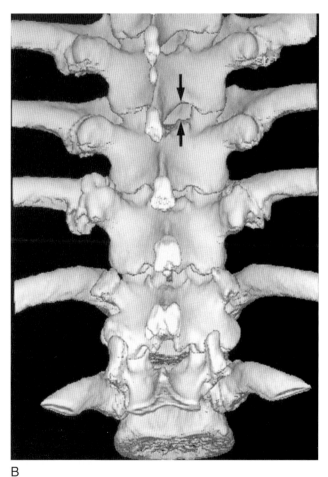

B

Figure 5-16 ■ Shallow LAO radiograph (*A*) and shallow LAO three-dimensional CT image (*B*) demonstrates target site of a thoracic interlaminar epidural steroid injection using a right-sided paramedian approach. Target between *white arrows* on *A* and *black arrows* on *B*.

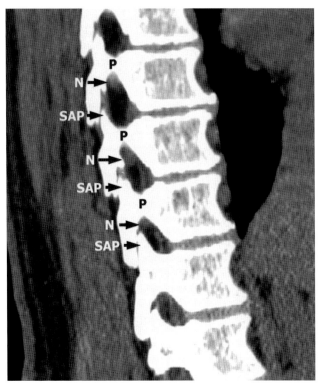

Figure 5-17 ■ Lateral CT image of the thoracic spine revealing relatively large intervertebral foramina through which thoracic spinal nerves exit. P = pedicle of vertebra; N = nerve; SAP = superior articular process of a thoracic-level facet joint.

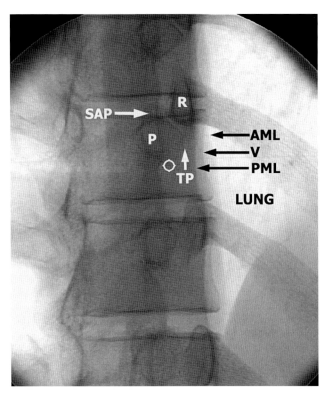

Figure 5-18 ■ Oblique fluoroscopic image of a transforaminal approach to the thoracic epidural space. *Circle* = target site of needle tip; P = pedicle; SAP = superior articular process; TP = transverse process; R = rib articulating with the superior costal facet located on the posterolateral aspect of the vertebral body; V = vertebral body margin; AML = anteromedial lung margin; PML = posteromedial lung margin.

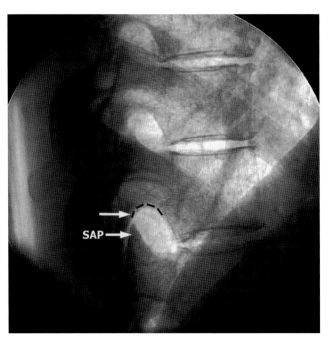

Figure 5-19 ■ Lateral fluoroscopic image of thoracic spine. *Arrow* = final distal needle tip location dorsal to the neural foramen when performing a thoracic-level transforaminal epidural steroid injection. *Dashed black lines* = undersurface of pedicle; SAP = superior articular process.

Transforaminal Approach

The transforaminal approach to the thoracic epidural space is similar, in theory, to that of the lumbar level. Again, the spinal injectionist must be aware of the anatomic differences. The pedicles of thoracic vertebrae are directed postero superiorly from the transverse process. In addition to the intervertebral articulations (zygapophysial joints), there are several costal articulations and supporting ligamentous structures that are not found at the lumbar level. The head of each rib articulates with the superior costal facet located at the posterolateral aspect of the vertebral body, just lateral to the base of the pedicle. A second costal articulation, the transverse costal facet, is located at the lateral border of the transverse process. Thoracic spinal nerves exit through relatively large intervertebral foramina bounded superiorly by the inferior vertebral notch (undersurface of the pedicle) and inferiorly by the superior articular process of the adjacent (more caudad) vertebra (Fig. 5-17).

After informed consent, the patient is positioned prone on the fluoroscopic table. With the use of fluoroscopic imaging, an AP view is obtained. The C-arm is rotated 15 to 20 degrees ipsilateral oblique. The intended target is just lateral to the 6 o'clock position of the pedicle (Fig. 5-18). The skin over this site is marked, prepped with povidone-iodine, and draped in sterile fashion. The skin and subcutaneous tissues are anesthetized with 1% lidocaine. The tip of a 22-gauge, 3.5-inch spinal needle is slowly advanced toward this target site under intermittent fluoroscopic guidance. Often the needle tip will contact periosteum and is most likely on the inferior border of the lamina. A lateral fluoroscopic image will reveal that the needle tip is dorsal to the neural foramen (Fig. 5-19). When this occurs, one simply walks off the inferolateral border of the lamina into the neural foramen.

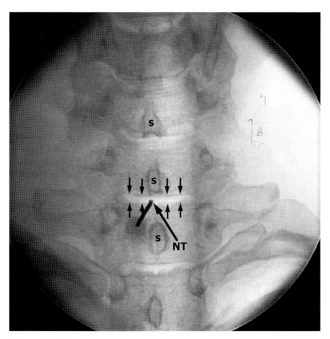

Figure 5-20 ■ AP fluoroscopic image of an interlaminar approach to the C7-T1 epidural space. *Arrows* = outline of cervical interlaminar space; NT = Tuohy epidural needle tip; s = spinous process.

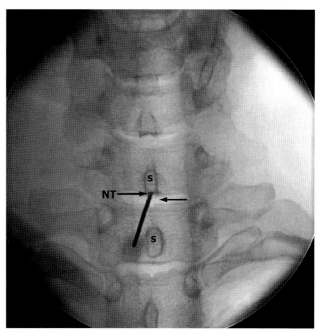

Figure 5-21 ■ AP fluoroscopic image of the final needle position of a C7-T1 interlaminar epidural injection. s = spinous process; NT = Tuohy epidural needle tip; *arrow* = C7-T1 intervertebral space.

Note that it is not necessary to advance until bony contact is made; however, fluoroscopic imaging in multiple planes is mandatory to ensure proper needle tip position.

After negative aspiration of blood and cerebrospinal fluid, injection of 1 mL of contrast agent under continuous fluoroscopic imaging should reveal spread of the contrast agent medially through the neural foramen and into the epidural space. Once epidural spread has been confirmed in AP and lateral views, the steroid/anesthetic preparation is injected.

Vigilance during aspiration for blood and direct visualization of contrast flow under fluoroscopic imaging are mandatory. The artery of Adamkiewicz is the largest of the radicular arteries supplying the anterior spinal artery of the spinal cord. It usually enters the spinal canal through the superior portion of a single intervertebral foramen between T7 and L4, usually on the left from T9 to L1.[33] Injury to this artery, either through direct needle trauma or through injection of local anesthetic/steroid, may result in anterior spinal artery ischemia and possible permanent lower extremity motor deficit. Therefore, at these levels, the needle is positioned more inferolateral in relation to the pedicle (in the inferior neural foramen) so as to decrease the risk of injury to the artery of Adamkiewicz.

Cervical Techniques

Interlaminar Approach

NEEDLE-ONLY TECHNIQUE

The cervical epidural space is extremely narrow, ranging from 1.5 to 2 mm at the C7 level to less than 1 mm at higher cervical levels. Accordingly, any pathologic process resulting in further narrowing of the spinal canal (e.g., spinal stenosis, disc herniation) would significantly limit the capacity of the cervical epidural space for injectate. For this reason, diagnostic imaging such as magnetic resonance (MR) imaging or computed tomography (CT) myelography is recommended before a cervical epidural injection is attempted via an interlaminar approach. If less than 1 mm of epidural space is identified at the C6-C7 level, a transforaminal approach is recommended instead. Also, even with adequate epidural space, patients often complain of transient axial and radicular discomfort on slow injection, attributable to the decreased capacity of the cervical epidural space.

After informed consent, the patient is positioned prone on the fluoroscopic table. A pillow is placed under the patient's chest to increase the cervical interlaminar space. With use of an AP fluoroscopic image, the spinous process of C7 and the interlaminar target site to be injected (usually the C6-C7 or C7-T1 interspace) are identified. The skin over this site is marked with indelible ink. The intended target is the superior border of the lower lamina at the desired intervertebral level. The skin over this site is prepped with povidone-iodine and draped in sterile fashion. The skin and overlying subcutaneous tissues are anesthetized with 1% lidocaine. An 18- or 20-gauge Tuohy epidural needle is then advanced toward the epidural space with the use of intermittent fluoroscopic imaging (Fig. 5-20). The needle is slowly advanced by means of the *"loss-of-resistance"* technique with normal saline (see lumbar section for details). Once the tip of the epidural needle passes through the ligamentum flavum and enters the epidural space there is a sudden "loss of resistance," as if the contents of the syringe were being sucked into the epidural space.

An AP fluoroscopic image verifies that the epidural needle is between the laminae (Fig. 5-21). With a 3-mL syringe containing 1 mL of nonionic contrast agent, one gently aspirates for the presence of blood or cerebrospinal fluid. If none is present, 1 mL of nonionic contrast agent is injected under

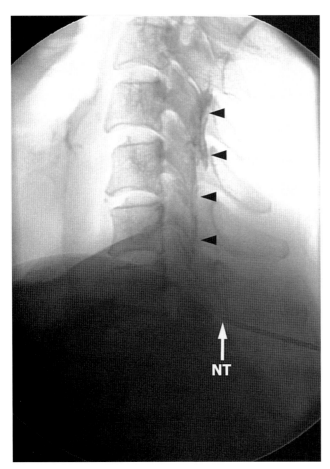

Figure 5-22 ■ Lateral fluoroscopic image of contrast medium spread within the posterior epidural space (*arrowheads*) after a C7-T1 interlaminar epidural injection. NT = Tuohy epidural needle tip.

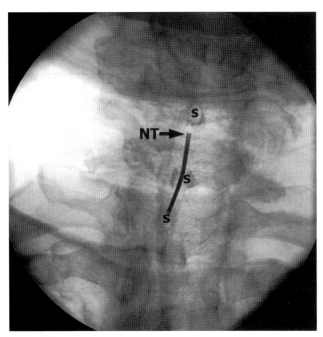

Figure 5-23 ■ AP fluoroscopic image of an 18-gauge Tuohy epidural needle within the epidural space at the C6-C7 level. s = spinous process; NT = needle tip.

continuous fluoroscopic imaging. This will reveal an even spread of contrast agent within the epidural space. A lateral fluoroscopic image will confirm contrast agent within the posterior epidural space (Fig. 5-22). The steroid/anesthetic preparation is then injected.

Because the cervical epidural space is extremely vascular, there is an increased risk of unrecognized intravascular injection. Accidental injection of even a small volume of local anesthetic into a cervical epidural vein could result in local anesthetic toxicity (i.e., seizure). Also, trauma to the epidural vasculature with subsequent bleeding could lead to spinal cord compression, especially in someone with preexisting diminished capacity of the cervical spinal canal. For this reason, all patients undergoing interlaminar cervical epidural injections are monitored for at least 45 minutes after the procedure for the development of any acute pain or neurologic deficit.

NEEDLE AND CATHETER TECHNIQUE

A variant of the interlaminar approach involves insertion of an epidural catheter through an 18-gauge epidural needle placed at C6-C7 or C7-T1. Once correct placement of the epidural needle tip within the posterior epidural space has been confirmed (Fig. 5-23), a radiopaque 20-gauge catheter is threaded cephalad within the epidural space to a specific target level (Fig. 5-24A). For example, in a patient with a right-sided C3 radiculopathy, the tip of the radiopaque epidural catheter would be threaded into the right lateral C3 epidural space under fluoroscopic guidance. After careful negative aspiration for blood and cerebrospinal fluid, 0.5 to 1 mL of nonionic contrast agent is injected (see Fig. 5-24B). Confirmation of contrast agent within the epidural space at this level precedes any injection of steroid with or without local anesthetic.

This technique has several advantages over interlaminar placement of the epidural needle at levels higher than the C6-C7 interspace:

- The interlaminar space is more accessible at lower cervical levels.
- There is a greater posterior epidural space diameter at lower cervical levels.
- There is theoretically a decreased risk of a compressive neurologic process in the event that trauma to the cervical vasculature occurs (i.e., greater epidural space capacity in the lower cervical levels).

Transforaminal Approach

After informed consent, the patient is placed in a supine oblique position on the fluoroscopic table, with the affected side up. A small pillow or wedge is often placed under the patient's shoulder to maintain this position. With the use of fluoroscopic imaging, an oblique view is obtained so that there is a clearly visible neural foramen at the intended target level. The intended target is the posteromedial aspect of the superior articular process at the waist of the foramen in the oblique view (Fig. 5-25). The skin over this site is marked, prepped with povidone-iodine, and draped in sterile fashion. The skin and subcutaneous tissues are anesthetized with 1% lidocaine. The tip of a 25-gauge needle is slowly advanced until it contacts the superior articular process (Fig. 5-26). Keeping the needle tip over the superior articular process

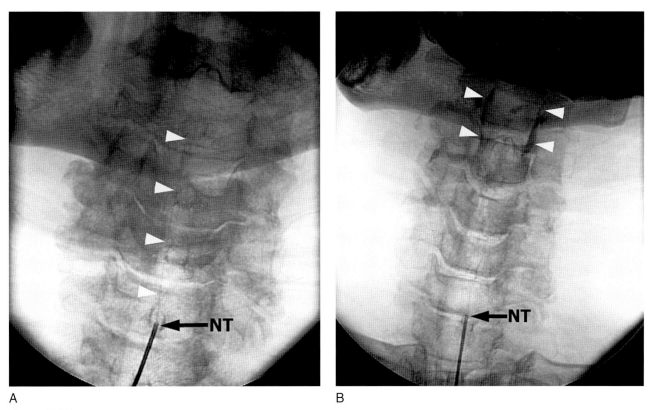

A

B

Figure 5-24 ■ *A*, AP fluoroscopic image revealing a 20-gauge radiopaque catheter (*arrowheads*) within the posterior cervical epidural space. NT = needle tip of 18-gauge Tuohy epidural needle. *B*, AP fluoroscopic image revealing localized spread of contrast medium (*arrowheads*) within the upper cervical epidural space after catheter injection. NT = needle tip.

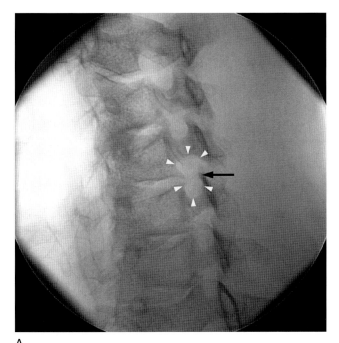

A

Figure 5-25 ■ *A*, Left-sided oblique fluoroscopic image revealing the C4 neural foramen (*arrowheads*). *Arrow* = posteromedial border of the superior articular process. *B*, Three-dimensional CT rendering of the approach to a cervical transforaminal epidural injection. *Black arrows* = contact site of needle at the posteromedial border of the superior articular process; *white arrows* = midline, posterior neural foramen where needle is "walked" into.

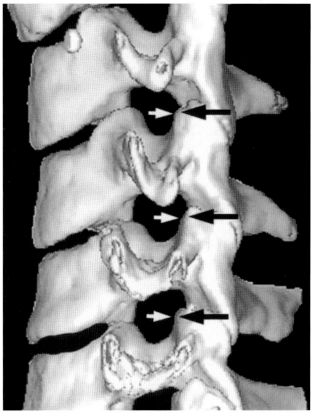

B

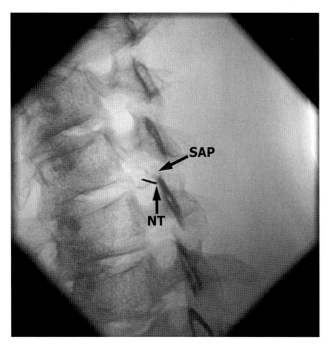

Figure 5-26 ■ Oblique fluoroscopic view revealing contact of needle tip (NT) with the superior articular process (SAP) in the approach to a cervical transforaminal epidural steroid injection.

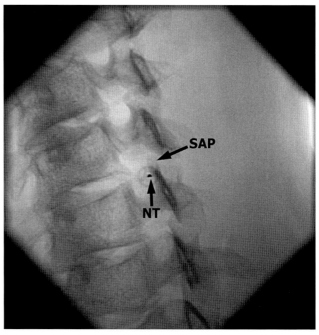

Figure 5-27 ■ Oblique fluoroscopic image revealing the final location of the needle tip (NT) location within the posterior neural foramen for a cervical transforaminal epidural steroid injection. SAP = superior articular process.

decreases the risk of traversing the foramen into the subarachnoid space and even into the cervical spinal cord. The needle is gently walked ventromedially into the posterior portion of the foramen (Fig. 5-27). Entering at this point will avoid the increased vasculature located within the superior aspect of the foramen and the anteriorly positioned vertebral artery.

After negative aspiration of blood and cerebrospinal fluid, 0.5 mL of nonionic contrast agent is injected under continuous fluoroscopic imaging. This should reveal an outline of the proximal cervical spinal nerve in the oblique view, and an AP view should reveal contrast agent spread medially through the neural foramen and into the lateral epidural space (Fig. 5-28*A*). Once epidural spread of the contrast medium has been confirmed in AP and lateral views (see Fig. 5-28*B*), the steroid/anesthetic preparation is injected.

POTENTIAL COMPLICATIONS

Complications of epidural injections are rare and are usually attributable to the needle placement or the side effects of the administered drugs.[34-46] The potential adverse effects include the following.

Needle Placement

- Pain at the injection site
- Nerve root injury
- Spinal cord injury
- Epidural hematoma
- Epidural abscess
- Meningitis

- Osteomyelitis
- Postdural puncture headache

Local Anesthetic Effect

- Weakness from motor block
- Hypotension
- Cardiac arrhythmia
- Seizure
- Allergic reaction

Steroid Effect

- Fluid retention
- Elevated blood pressure
- Hyperglycemia
- Hypothalamic-pituitary-adrenal axis suppression
- Cushing syndrome
- Steroid myopathy
- Generalized erythema/facial flushing
- Allergic reaction

POST-PROCEDURE CARE/FOLLOW-UP

Immediate

1. Have patient remain for 30 minutes after the procedure.
2. Observe for new motor/sensory deficits.
3. Observe for allergic reactions.
4. Observe for increased pain (a potential early sign of epidural hematoma).

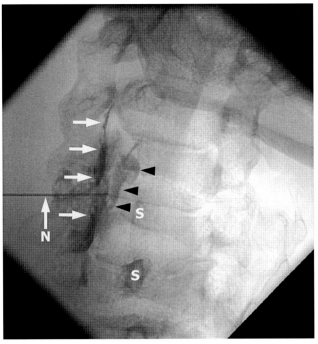

A

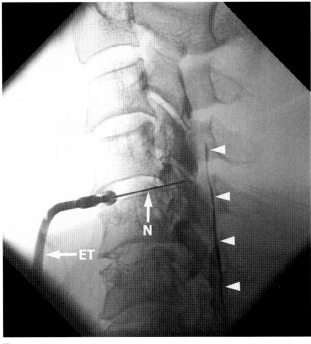

B

Figure 5-28 ■ *A*, AP fluoroscopic image of spread of contrast agent within the left-sided anterolateral epidural space (*white arrows*) during a C4 transforaminal epidural injection. *Black arrowheads* = medial spread of contrast within the posterior epidural space. S = spinous process; N = 25-gauge needle. *B*, Lateral fluoroscopic image of contrast agent within the posterior cervical epidural space (*arrowheads*) after a C4 transforaminal epidural injection. Note the diffuse spread of contrast agent throughout the lateral and anterior epidural spaces as well. N = 25-gauge, 1.5-inch needle; ET = extension tubing.

5. Observe for respiratory compromise (especially for cervical and thoracic procedures).
6. Observe for hemodynamic compromise.

Discharge

1. The patient is discharged into the care of a responsible person.
2. No driving or operating of heavy machinery is permitted for 24 hours.
3. Explanation is given of what procedure was performed and what symptoms to expect for the next few days
   a. Soreness at the puncture site(s)
   b. Initial pain relief (local anesthetic); baseline pain returns; secondary pain relief after 18 to 36 hours (steroid effect)
4. Signs and symptoms of infection are explained.
5. A contact phone number is provided if the patient has a question or concern.
6. A period of time is specified to follow-up for results of procedure.

SAMPLE DICTATIONS

Caudal Epidural Injection

Diagnostic Impression: Postlaminectomy pain syndrome with bilateral buttock/sacral radicular pain symptoms

Procedures: Caudal epidurogram with interpretation
Caudal epidural steroid injection under fluoroscopic guidance

After fully informed written consent was obtained, the patient was escorted to the fluoroscopic suite and placed in the prone position. The sacrum and sacral cornua were visualized in an AP view. The skin over the sacral hiatus (caudal epidural entry site) was marked, prepped with povidone-iodine three times, and draped in a sterile fashion. With a 25-gauge, 1.5-inch needle, 1% lidocaine was injected subcutaneously over the caudal epidural entry site. A 22-gauge, 2-inch Quincke-type styletted needle was inserted and advanced into the sacral hiatus under fluoroscopic guidance. After the needle passed through the sacrococcygeal ligament, the needle angle was lowered and the needle was advanced 1 cm. There was no evidence of paresthesias throughout needle placement. After negative aspiration for blood and cerebrospinal fluid, 1 mL of nonionic contrast agent was slowly injected. Confirmation of spread of contrast agent within the caudal epidural space was made with fluoroscopic imaging in the AP and lateral views. An additional 6 mL of agent was slowly injected. There was a clear outline of the epidural space and visualization of the sacral nerve roots. Subsequently, 12 mL of injectate (2 mL betamethasone 6 mg/mL and 10 mL preservative-free 1% lidocaine) was slowly administered without resistance. The needle was restyletted and withdrawn. There was no evidence of procedural complications.

The patient tolerated the procedure well and was able to ambulate to the recovery area, where he remained for 45 minutes after the procedure. On reexamination, there was no evidence of lower extremity weakness or sensory changes. On standing and ambulating, he reported absence of bilateral buttock pain.

Transforaminal Epidural Injection

Diagnostic Impression: Right-sided L5 neuropathic pain (post-traumatic neuralgia)
Procedure: Right-sided L5 transforaminal epidural steroid injection under fluoroscopic guidance

After fully informed written consent was obtained, the patient was escorted to the fluoroscopic suite and placed in a prone position. A right-sided oblique fluoroscopic view was obtained, with the superior articular process of S1 aligned with the pedicle of L5. The skin over the intended target site, the 6 o'clock position of the L5 pedicle, was marked, prepped with povidone-iodine three times, and draped in sterile fashion. With sterile technique, the skin and subcutaneous tissue were anesthetized with 1% lidocaine. The tip of a 22-gauge, 3.5-inch Quincke-type spinal needle was advanced toward the 6 o'clock position of the L5 pedicle under intermittent fluoroscopic guidance. Confirmation of proper needle position was made with AP, oblique, and lateral fluoroscopic views. After negative aspiration for blood and cerebrospinal fluid, 1 mL of nonionic contrast agent was injected. Fluoroscopic imaging revealed a clear outline of the L5 spinal nerve with proximal spread of agent through the neural foramen into the anterior epidural space. Subsequently, 2 mL of injectate (1 mL betamethasone 6 mg/mL and 1 mL 0.25% bupivacaine) was administered. The spinal needle was restyletted and removed. The patient tolerated the procedure well, and there was no evidence of procedural complications.

The patient was able to ambulate to the recovery area, where she was reexamined 20 minutes later. There was no evidence of lower extremity weakness or motor deficits. A sensory examination revealed a slight decrease to light touch in the right L5 distribution. The patient's right-sided buttock and posterior thigh burning dysesthesias were absent.

Cervical Epidural Injection

Diagnostic Impression: Cervical spinal stenosis (from degenerative disc and osteoarthritis)
Procedure: Cervical epidural steroid injection under fluoroscopic guidance

After fully informed written consent was obtained, the patient was escorted to the fluoroscopic suite and placed in the prone position with the head flexed midline. A pillow was placed under the patient's chest to increase the cervical interlaminar space. The C7-T1 interspace was visualized under fluoroscopic imaging, and the skin over this site was marked. After povidone-iodine preparation three times, the site was draped in sterile fashion. With sterile technique, 1% lidocaine was injected subcutaneously at the C7-T1 interspace. An 18-gauge Tuohy epidural needle was inserted and advanced toward the epidural space by means of the "loss-of-resistance" technique with normal saline. The epidural space was identified on first pass, without evidence of blood, cerebrospinal fluid, or paresthesias throughout. Needle tip placement within the epidural space was confirmed with 0.5 mL of nonionic contrast agent, with the epidural space visualized in both the AP and the lateral fluoroscopic views. A 20-gauge radiopaque epidural catheter (Perifix) was inserted through the Tuohy epidural needle and advanced within the epidural space under fluoroscopic guidance. The final distal position of the catheter was the C4-5 interspace within the posterior epidural space. There were no paresthesias during catheter insertion. After careful negative aspiration for blood and cerebrospinal fluid, 0.5 mL of nonionic contrast agent was injected through the catheter, with confirmation of epidural localization in both AP and lateral fluoroscopic views. Next, 5 mL of injectate (1.5 mL betamethasone 6 mg/mL, 2 mL 0.25% bupivacaine, and 1.5 mL preservative-free normal saline) was administered through the catheter. The epidural catheter and the Tuohy needle were gently removed together. An intact distal catheter tip was identified. There was no evidence of procedural complications.

The patient was escorted to the recovery area, where she remained for 1 hour. There was no evidence of upper extremity motor or sensory deficits after the procedure, and she reported a significant decrease in neck discomfort with range of motion.

CASE REPORTS

CASE 1

Clinical Presentation

A 73-year-old man presented with a 2-year history of progressive bilateral buttock pain with prolonged standing and ambulation. He had undergone a lumbar laminectomy with posterior fusion 4 years previously for treatment of severe multilevel spinal stenosis. He had near-complete resolution of lower extremity neurogenic claudication symptoms after surgery, but he began experiencing his current symptoms 18 months later. Physical examination revealed equivocal right-sided L5 radicular symptoms on provocative testing. There was no evidence of lower extremity weakness or motor deficits.

Imaging and Therapy

Radiographic imaging revealed an intact fusion with no evidence of instability on flexion and extension views. On

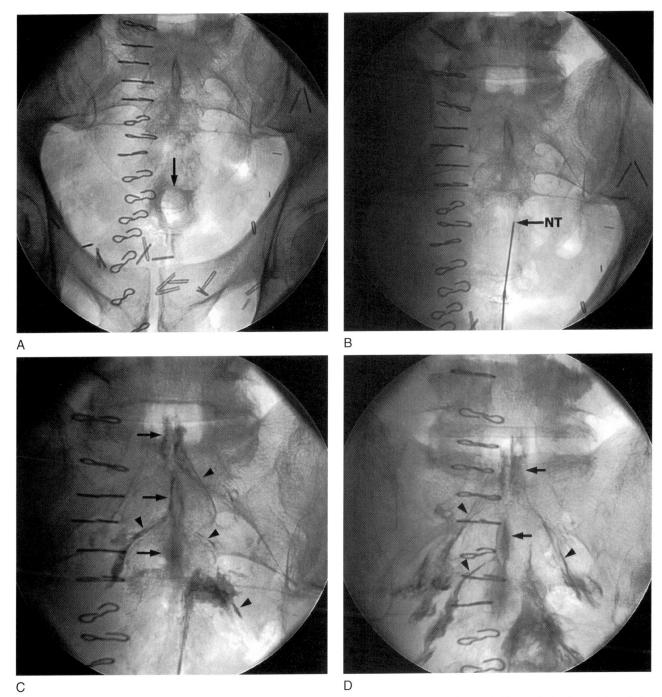

A

B

C

D

Figure 5-29 ■ *A*, AP radiograph demonstrating sacral hiatus entrance (*arrow*) to the caudal epidural space. *B*, The needle is advanced through the sacral hiatus. NT = needle tip. *C*, Contrast agent is seen outlining the caudal epidural space (*arrows*) and the exiting sacral nerves (*arrowheads*). *D*, There was significant obstruction to epidural contrast spread cephalad to L5-S1. *Arrows* = contrast agent in caudal epidural space; *arrowheads* = contrast agent outlining sacral nerves.

MR imaging, there was no evidence of disc herniation or central canal or neural foraminal stenosis.

Diagnostic Impression: Postlaminectomy pain syndrome with bilateral buttock/sacral radicular pain symptoms

Planned Procedures: Caudal epidurogram with interpretation
Caudal epidural steroid injection under fluoroscopic guidance

Procedural Report

The patient was positioned prone. An AP fluoroscopic view of the sacral hiatus revealed the entry site to the caudal epidural space (Fig. 5-29A). It was noted that the patient had had a radical retropubic prostatectomy, as evidenced by radiopaque surgical clips and sutures. With the use of sterile technique, a 22-gauge Quincke-type styletted needle was advanced through the sacral hiatus, located between the bony sacral cornua, under fluoroscopic guidance (see Fig. 5-29B). Contrast medium was injected through the needle into the caudal epidural space, revealing an outline

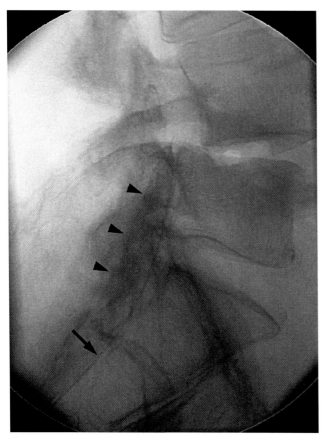

E

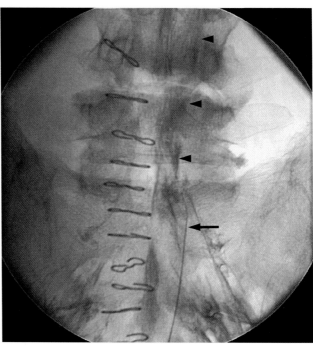

F

Figure 5-29 *(Cont'd)* ▪ *E*, An epidurolysis catheter *arrow* was inserted through the needle into the caudal epidural space to facilitate mechanical lysis of epidural adhesions. *F*, After lysis, contrast agent *(arrowheads)* flowed cephalad to L5-S1. *Arrow* = epidurolysis catheter.

of the caudal epidural space as well as the sacral nerves exiting though the sacral neural foramina (see Fig. 5-29C). Even after the injection of additional contrast agent, there was significant obstruction to spread of epidural contrast medium at the L5-S1 junction (see Fig. 5-29D), most likely representing epidural fibrosis as a result of the previous lumbar laminectomy. A radiopaque epidurolysis catheter was then inserted into the caudal epidural space to facilitate mechanical lysis of epidural adhesions (see Fig. 5-29E). A subsequent AP fluoroscopic image after epidural contrast agent and steroid injection confirmed

spread within the caudal and lumbar epidural spaces, proximal to the site of the previous obstruction (see Fig. 5-29F).

Results

The patient tolerated the procedure well and was able to ambulate to the recovery area, where he remained for 45 minutes after the procedure. On reexamination, there was no evidence of lower extremity weakness or sensory changes. On standing and ambulating, he reported absence of bilateral buttock pain.

CASE 2

Clinical Presentation

A 26-year-old woman was referred with a 6-month history of constant right-sided buttock and posterior thigh burning dysesthesias. The pain began after a traumatic fall while she was playing softball, and it had not responded to conservative treatment, including nonsteroidal anti-inflammatory medications, muscle relaxants, and physical therapy. Physical examination revealed allodynia over the right lateral buttock and posterior thigh in the L5 distribution. There was no evidence of reflex abnormalities, weakness, or lower extremity radicular pain. Also, intra-articular hip, sacroiliac, pyriformis, and lumbar facet-loading

provocative maneuvers failed to reproduce the patient's pain symptoms.

Imaging and Therapy

Plain film, MR imaging, and electromyographic studies were negative for anatomic or electrophysiologic pathology.

Diagnostic Impression: Right-sided L5 neuropathic pain (post-traumatic neuralgia)

Planned Procedure: Right-sided L5 transforaminal epidural steroid injection under fluoroscopic guidance.

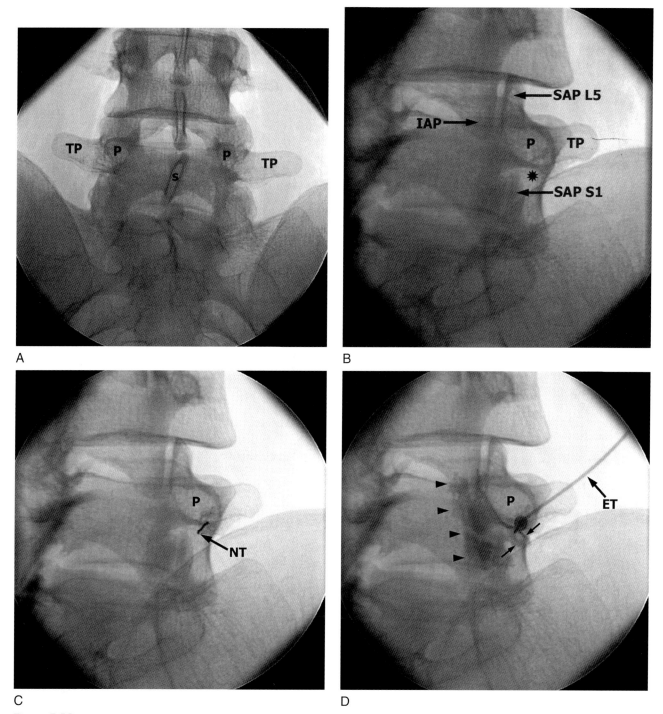

A

B

C

D

Figure 5-30 ■ *A*, AP radiograph was centered at the L5-S1 intervertebral space. TP = transverse process; P = pedicle; s = spinous process. *B*, LAO image demonstrated the target site (*asterisk*) for a right-sided L5 transforaminal epidural steroid injection at the 6 o'clock position of the L5 pedicle (P). TP = transverse process; SAP S1 = superior articular process of S1; SAP L5 = superior articular process of L5; IAP = inferior articular process of L4. *C*, Needle tip (NT) was advanced toward the target site below the L5 pedicle (P). *D*, Contrast agent injection demonstrated medial spread of contrast agent inferior to the L5 pedicle (P) into the anterolateral epidural space (*arrowheads*) and an outline of the L5 nerve root sleeve (*arrows*). ET = extension tubing containing contrast agent.

The patient was placed in the prone position with an AP image centered on the L5-S1 intervertebral space (Fig. 5-30A). A left anterior oblique position revealed the target site for a right-sided L5 transforaminal epidural steroid injection at the 6 o'clock position of the L5 pedicle (see Fig. 5-30B). With the use of sterile technique, the tip of a 22-gauge spinal needle was advanced toward the target site below the L5 pedicle (see Fig. 5-30C). Injection of contrast agent revealed medial spread of contrast medium inferior to the L5 pedicle into the anterolateral epidural space and opacification of the L5 nerve root sleeve (see Fig. 5-30D). Before injection of local anesthetic and steroid, the C-arm was returned to the AP position to confirm

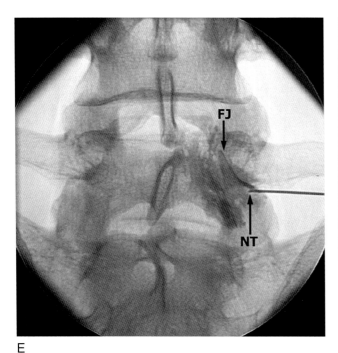
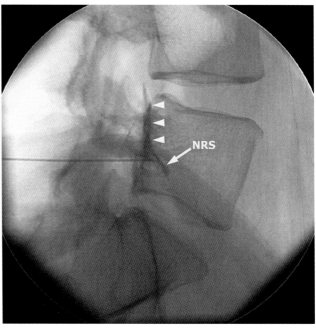

E   F

Figure 5-30 (*Cont'd*) ■ *E*, AP radiograph confirmed the position of the needle tip (NT) lateral to the facet joint (FJ). *F*, Lateral radiograph demonstrated contrast agent in the anterior epidural space (*arrowheads*) and outlining the proximal L5 nerve root sheath (NRS).

proper needle tip location lateral to the facet joint. The contrast revealed an outline of the right-sided L5 neural foramen and medial spread of contrast agent into the epidural space (see Fig. 5-30E). A lateral fluoroscopic image was also obtained to confirm correct needle tip location, with contrast agent outlining the neural foramen, the anterior L5 nerve root dural sleeve, and the anterior epidural space (see Fig. 5-30F).

Results

The patient was able to ambulate back to the recovery area, where she was reexamined 20 minutes later. There was no evidence of lower extremity weakness or motor deficits. A sensory examination revealed a slight decrease to light touch in the right L5 distribution. The patient's right-sided buttock and posterior thigh burning dysesthesias were absent.

CASE 3

A 42-year-old female medical transcriptionist presented with a 3-year history of progressive neck pain with intermittent painful radiation into the left scapular region. Conservative therapy had included nonsteroidal anti-inflammatory medications, acetaminophen, and brief physical therapy. Physical examination revealed limited cervical spine range of motion in all directional planes, without reproduction of radicular pain. Facet-loading maneuvers were negative bilaterally. Upper extremity strength, reflexes, and sensory examinations were within normal limits.

Imaging and Therapy

Cervical spine MR imaging revealed moderate degenerative disc changes from C3 through C7, with loss of disc height and osteophytic ridging. There was moderate central canal stenosis from C4 through C6, with moderate to severe foraminal narrowing at C4-5 bilaterally.

Diagnostic Impression: Cervical spinal stenosis (secondary to degenerative disc and osteoarthritic etiologies)

Planned Procedure: Cervical epidural steroid injection under fluoroscopic guidance

Procedural Report
The patient was placed in a prone position on the fluoroscopy table (Fig. 5-31A). With the use of sterile technique, the tip of an 18-gauge Tuohy epidural needle was advanced toward the posterior epidural space by means of the "loss of resistance" technique with normal saline (see Fig. 5-31B). A radiopaque catheter was inserted through the Tuohy needle into the epidural space under continuous fluoroscopic imaging. The distal catheter tip lay at the symptomatic level, C4-5. After careful negative aspiration for blood and cerebrospinal

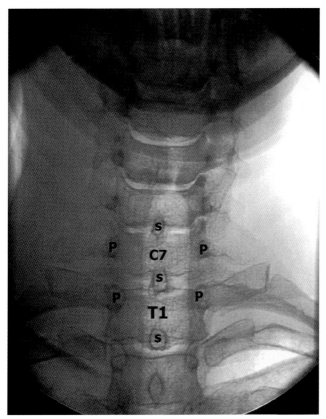

A

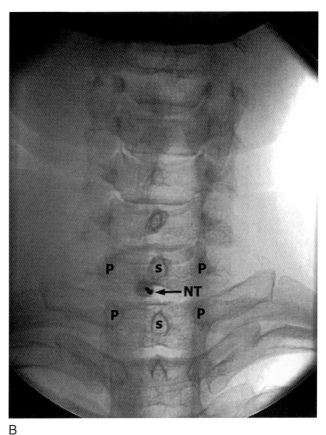

B

C

Figure 5-31 ■ *A,* AP radiograph, patient prone. C7 = seventh cervical vertebra; T1 = first thoracic vertebra; P = pedicle; s = spinous process. *B,* An 18-gauge Tuohy epidural needle was advanced toward the posterior epidural space. The needle tip (NT) was near midline. P = pedicle; s = spinous process. *C,* Radiopaque catheter (*arrows*) was inserted through the Tuohy needle (NT) into the epidural space. The distal catheter tip was at the C4-C5 level. Contrast material (*arrowheads*) was seen to outline the upper epidural space.

fluid through the catheter, contrast medium was slowly injected. It revealed an outline of the epidural space at the desired level (see Fig. 5-31C), with further spread after injection of the local anesthetic and steroid mixture (see Fig. 5-31D). A lateral fluoroscopic image confirmed spread of contrast agent within the posterior epidural space (see Fig. 5-31E).

Results

The patient was escorted to the recovery area, where she remained for 1 hour. There was no evidence of upper extremity motor or sensory deficits after the procedure, and she reported a significant decrease in neck discomfort with range of motion.

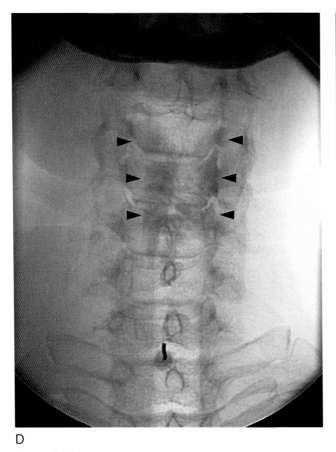

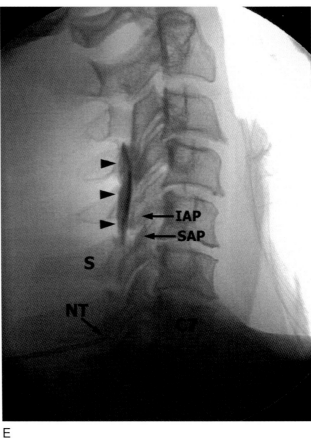

D   E

Figure 5-31 (*Cont'd*) ■ *D*, Further symmetric spread of contrast material (*arrowheads*) after injection of the local anesthetic and steroid mixture. *E*, Lateral radiograph confirmed epidural contrast agent spread within the posterior epidural space (*arrowheads*). NT = needle tip; S = spinous process; C7 = C7 vertebral body; IAP = inferior articular process of C5; SAP = superior articular process of C6.

CURRENT PROCEDURAL TERMINOLOGY (CPT) CODES

CPT codes may vary from year to year. It is recommended that one consult with someone experienced in CPT coding procedures to ensure that the CPT coding is appropriate for one's region or state. Below is a sample of CPT codes that are being used for epidural injections at this writing.[47]

Note that injection of contrast agent during fluoroscopically guided epidural injections is an inclusive component of CPT codes 62280, 62281, 62282, 62310, 62311, 62318, and 62319. Fluoroscopic guidance and localization is reported by code 76005.

Spine and Spinal Cord–Injection, Drainage, or Aspiration

62280 Injection/infusion of neurolytic substance (e.g., alcohol, phenol, iced saline solutions), with or without other therapeutic substance; subarachnoid

62281 epidural, cervical or thoracic

62282 epidural, lumbar, sacral (caudal)

62310 Injection, single (not via indwelling catheter), not including neurolytic substances, with or without contrast (for either localization or epidurography), of diagnostic or therapeutic substance(s) (including anesthetic, antispasmodic, opioid, steroid, other solution), epidural or subarachnoid; cervical or thoracic

62311 lumbar, sacral (caudal)

62318 Injection, including catheter placement, continuous infusion or intermittent bolus, not including neurolytic substances, with or without contrast (for either localization or epidurography), of diagnostic or therapeutic substance(s) (including anesthetic, antispasmodic, opioid, steroid, other solution), epidural or subarachnoid; cervical or thoracic

62319 lumbar, sacral (caudal)

76005 Fluoroscopic guidance and localization of needle or catheter tip for spine or paraspinous diagnostic or therapeutic injection procedures (epidural, transforaminal epidural, subarachnoid, paravertebral facet joint, paravertebral facet joint nerve or sacroiliac joint), including neurolytic agent destruction

99141 Sedation with or without analgesia (conscious sedation); intravenous, intramuscular or inhalation

Extracranial Nerves, Peripheral Nerves, and Autonomic Nervous System–Introduction/Injection of Anesthetic Agent (Nerve Block), Diagnostic or Therapeutic

64479   Injection, anesthetic agent and/or steroid, transforaminal epidural; cervical or thoracic, single level

64480   cervical or thoracic, each additional level (List separately in addition to code for primary procedure)

64483   lumbar or sacral, single level

64484   lumbar or sacral, each additional level (List separately in addition to code for primary procedure)

References

1. Frymoyer JW, Cats-Baril WL. An overview of the incidences and costs of low back pain. Orthop Clin North Am 1991; 22:263–271.
2. Bush K, Cowan R, Katz DE, et al. The natural history of sciatica associated with disc pathology: A prospective study with clinical and independent radiologic follow-up. Spine 1992; 17:1205–1212.
3. Cassidy JD, Carroll LJ, Cote P. The Saskatchewan health and back pain survey. Spine 1998; 17:1860–1867.
4. Guo HR, Tanaka S, Halperin WE, et al. Back pain prevalence in US industry and estimates of lost workdays. Am J Public Health 1999; 89:1029–1035.
5. Lievre JA, Bloch-Michel H, Pean G, et al. L'hydrocortisone en injection locale. Rev Rhumat Mal Osteoartic 1953; 20:310–311.
6. Dilke TFW, Burry HC, Grahame R. Extradural corticosteroid injection in management of lumbar nerve root compression. BMJ 1973; 2:635–637.
7. Carette S, Leclaire R, Marcoux S, et al. Epidural corticosteroid injections for sciatica due to herniated nucleus pulposus. N Engl J Med 1997; 336:1634–1640.
8. Snoek W, Weber H, Jorgensen B. Double blind evaluation of extradural methylprednisolone for herniated lumbar discs. Acta Orthop Scand 1977; 48:635–641.
9. Ridley MG, Kingsley GH, Gibson T, et al. Outpatient lumbar epidural corticosteroid injection in the management of sciatica. Br J Rheumatol 1988; 27:295–299.
10. Cuckler JM, Bernini PA, Wiesel SW, et al. The use of epidural steroids in the treatment of lumbar radicular pain: A prospective, randomized, double-blind study. J Bone Joint Surg Am 1985; 67:63–66.
11. Bush K, Hillier S. A controlled study of caudal epidural injections of triamcinolone plus procaine for the management of intractable sciatica. Spine 1991; 16:572–575.
12. Rapp SE, Haselkorn JK, Elam K, et al. Epidural steroid injection in the treatment of low back pain: A meta-analysis. Anesthesiology 1994; 81:A923.
13. Van Tulder MW, Waddell G. Conservative treatment of acute and subacute low back pain. In Nachemson AL, Jonsson E (eds). Neck and Back Pain: The Scientific Evidence of Causes, Diagnosis, and Treatment. Philadelphia: Lippincott Williams & Williams, 2000, pp 341–269.
14. Rydevik B, Brown MD, Lundborg G. Pathoanatomy and pathophysiology of nerve root compression. Spine 1984; 9:7–15.
15. Saal JS, Franson RC, Dobrow R, et al. High levels of inflammatory phospholipase A2 activity in lumbar disc herniations. Spine 1990; 15:674–678.
16. Delaney TJ, Rowlingson JC, Carron H, Butler A. Epidural steroid effects on the nerves and meninges. Anesth Analg 1980; 59:610–614.
17. Johansson A, Hao J, Sjolund B. Local corticosteroid blocks transmission in normal nociceptive C-fibres. Acta Anaesthesiol Scand 1990; 34:335–338.
18. Fuxe K, Harfstrand A, Agnati LF, et al. Immunocytochemical studies on the localization of glucocorticoid receptor immunoreactive nerve cells in the lower brain stem and spinal cord of the male rat using monoclonal antibody against rat liver glucocorticoid receptor. Neuroscience Lett 1985; 60:1–6.
19. Hua SY, Chen YZ. Membrane receptor-mediated electrophysiological effects of glucocorticoid on mammalian neurons. Endocrinology 1989; 124:687–691.
20. Hogan QH. Epidural anatomy examined by cryomicrotome section: Influence of age, vertebral level and disease. Reg Anesth 1996; 21:295–306.
21. Bogduk N. Clinical Anatomy of the Lumbar Spine and Sacrum, 3rd ed. New York: Churchill Livingstone, 1997.
22. White AH, Derby R, Wynne G. Epidural injections for diagnosis and treatment of low back pain. Spine 1980; 5:78–86.
23. Renfrew DL, Moore TE, Kathol MH, et al. Correct placement of epidural steroid injections: Fluoroscopic guidance and contrast administration. AJNR 1991; 12:1003–1007.
24. Lutz GE, Vad VB, Wisneski RJ. Fluoroscopic transforaminal epidural steroids: An outcome study. Arch Phys Med Rehabil 1998; 79:1362–1366.
25. White AH, Derby R, Wynne G. Epidural injections for diagnosis and treatment of low back pain. Spine 1980; 5:78–86.
26. Mehta M, Salmon N. Extradural block: Confirmation of the injection site by x-ray monitoring. Anaesthesia 1985; 40:1009–1012.
27. Pauza KJ. Nomenclature and terminology for spine specialists. ISIS Scientific Newsletter 2001; 4:24–25.
28. Derby R, Kine G, Saal JA, et al. Precision percutaneous blocking procedures for localizing spine pain: II. The lumbar neuraxial compartment. Pain Digest 1993; 3:175–188.
29. Dooley JF, McBroom RJ, Taguchi T, et al. Nerve root infiltration in the diagnosis of radicular pain. Spine 1988; 13:79–83.
30. Stanley D, McLaren MI, Euinton HA, Getty CS. A prospective study of nerve root infiltration in the diagnosis of sciatica: A comparison with radiculography, computed tomography, and operative findings. Spine 1990; 15:540–543.
31. Physicians' Desk Reference, 56th ed. Montvale, NJ: Medical Economics Company, 2002.
32. Bogduk N, Aprill C, Derby R. Epidural steroid injections. In White AH, Schofferman J (eds). Spinal Care Diagnosis and Treatment. St. Louis: CV Mosby, 1995, pp 322–344.
33. Alleyne CH Jr, Cawley CM, Shengelaia GG, et al. Microsurgical anatomy of the artery of Adamkiewicz and its segmental artery. J Neurosurg 1998; 89:791–795.
34. Abram SE, O'Connor IC. Complications associated with epidural steroid injections. Reg Anesth 1996; 21:149–162.
35. Williams KN, Jackowski A, Evans PJ. Epidural haematoma requiring surgical decompression following repeated cervical epidural steroid injections for chronic pain. Pain 1990; 42:197–199.
36. McLain RF, Fry M, Hecht SI. Transient paralysis associated with epidural steroid injection. J Spinal Disord 1997; 10:441–444.
37. Chan ST, Leung S. Spinal epidural abscess following steroid injection for sciatica: Case report. Spine 1989; 14:106–108.
38. Goucke CR, Graziotti P. Extradural abscess following local anesthetic and steroid injection for chronic low back pain. Br J Anaesth 1990; 65:427–429.
39. Cooper AB, Sharpe MD. Bacterial meningitis and cauda equina syndrome after epidural steroid injections. Can J Anaesth 1996; 43:471–474.
40. Waldman SD. Complications of cervical epidural blocks with steroids: A prospective study of 790 consecutive blocks. Reg Anesth 1989; 14:149–151.
41. Williamson JA. Inadvertent spinal subdural injection during attempted spinal epidural steroid therapy. Anaesth Intensive Care 1990; 18:406–408.
42. Kay J, Findling JW, Raff H. Epidural triamcinolone suppresses the pituitary-adrenal axis in human subjects. Anesth Analg 1994; 79:501–505.
43. Tuel SM, Meythaler JM, Cross LL. Cushing's syndrome from epidural methylprednisolone. Pain 1990; 40:81–84.
44. Boonen S, Van Distel G, Westhovens R, et al. Steroid myopathy induced by epidural triamcinolone injection. Br J Rheumatol 1995; 34:385–386.
45. DeSio JM, Kahn CH, Warfield CA. Facial flushing and/or generalized erythema after epidural steroid injection. Anesth Analg 1995; 80:617–619.
46. Simon DL, Kunz RD, German JD, et al. Allergic or pseudoallergic reaction following epidural steroid deposition and skin testing. Reg Anesth 1989; 14:253–255.
47. Derived from CPT 2002, CPT Intellectual Property Services. Chicago: American Medical Association, 2002.

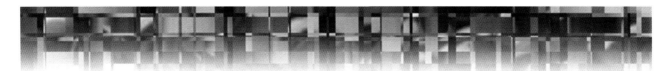

A Spine Surgeon's Perspective

Epidural Injections

Joseph T. Alexander, MD

Fortunately, it is unusual for a herniated disc to manifest as a severe neurologic deficit such as a cauda equina syndrome or a myelopathy that would require immediate surgical intervention. In the great majority of cases, even those with significant radicular findings, the symptoms will resolve without surgical decompression. Initially, however, many patients have excruciating pain that limits their activity and their ability to participate in rehabilitation activities. Another common clinical scenario is a patient who has radicular pain after a fall or accident. Radiographic evaluation reveals obviously long-standing degenerative changes with foraminal stenoses but no true disc herniation. I have found an epidural steroid injection to be quite effective for both of these types of patients, and I use it routinely. In all cases, I will evaluate the effectiveness of each injection individually rather than proceed with a series of injections on a predetermined timetable.

More controversial to me is the use of epidural steroids in the setting of severe central spinal stenosis. I do not request it in cases with cervical stenosis, out of concern for potentially increasing the myelopathic symptoms that I commonly see. In the lumbar spine, I have seen temporary relief of symptoms of claudication, but rarely have I seen a lasting benefit. For patients with significant symptoms caused by lumbar stenosis, I will sometimes recommend epidural steroids as a temporizing measure, but I will also advise these patients that recurrent symptoms are likely.

A more bothersome trend that I have observed in recent years is an increasing tendency for patients with mechanical back pain to receive a series of epidural injections as *initial* treatment, sometimes before a definitive diagnosis has been made or a referral to a spine care specialist has been completed. I recently heard as an extreme example of this practice an attempt by an insurance provider to deny authorization for a magnetic resonance examination until *after a patient had failed a series of three epidural injections!* Although epidural injections may provide temporary relief of back pain in selected situations, this treatment modality should certainly be saved until at least a provisional diagnosis has been reached and less invasive treatment modalities have been offered.

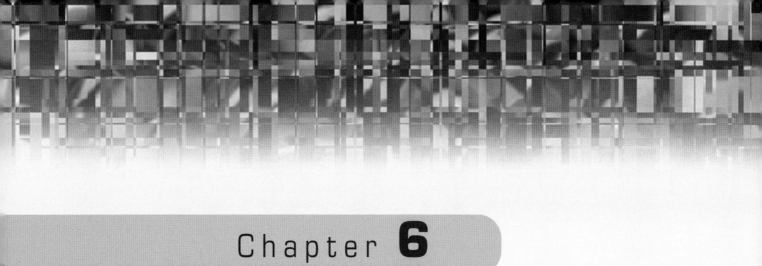

Chapter 6

Sacroiliac Joint Injection

- Mark J. Kransdorf, MD

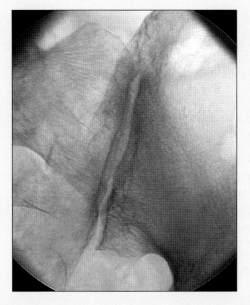

BACKGROUND

The cause of chronic low back pain is often exceedingly difficult to localize clinically, and the contribution of the sacroiliac (SI) joint to this pain is especially difficult to assess.[1] In a prospective evaluation of 85 patients, Dreyfuss and colleagues[2] evaluated the diagnostic utility of 12 of the "best" historically accepted SI joint tests used for the diagnosis of SI joint disease. They evaluated these tests against a criterion of unequivocal pain relief after an intra-articular injection of local anesthetic into the SI joint and found that none of the 12 tests demonstrated a worthwhile diagnostic value.

SI joint injection is useful in both the diagnosis and the treatment of low back pain. An SI joint injection can establish the component of pain related to the SI joint and can be used to treat inflammatory or degenerative SI joint pain.[3, 4]

Image guidance is essential for accurate intra-articular needle placement. Rosenberg and associates[5] studied 39 clinically guided SI joint injections performed in 33 patients. In a prospective, double-blind study in which contrast medium was injected along with bupivacaine and methylprednisolone, follow-up computed tomography (CT) demonstrated intra-articular injection of contrast agent in only 22% of patients. Importantly, these researchers also found epidural extension of injected contrast agent in 24% of patients and contrast agent extending within the sacral neural foramina (predominantly at

S1) in 44%. The spread of the injection material into the epidural space and along the nerve roots is believed to be responsible for the neurologic symptoms (lower extremity weakness and voiding difficulty) after SI joint injection.[5]

ANATOMIC CONSIDERATIONS

The SI joint is formed by the articulation between the sacrum and the ilium. It has two parts: (1) a true synovial-lined cartilaginous joint and (2) a fibrous articulation. The inferior one half to two thirds of the joint is the synovial portion.[6] The articular cartilage is considerably thicker on the sacral side, being 3 to 5 mm thick as compared with 1 mm on the iliac side. The posterosuperior portion of the joint is merely a cleft between the iliac wing and the superior portion of the sacral wing.[6] The obliquity of the joint varies along its course and among individuals (Fig. 6-1).

The innervation of the SI joint is predominantly from the dorsal rami of the S1 through S4 nerve roots.[7] Recent histologic analysis has revealed the presence of nerve fibers within the SI joint capsule and adjoining ligaments. The presence of these afferent fibers implies that pain originating in the SI joint could be referred to the dermatomes associated with each of the fibers found in the capsule and ligaments.[7, 8] The presence of these nerve fibers within the capsule and adjoining ligaments likely accounts for the beneficial therapeutic effects of extracapsular injections reported by some patients.

Capsular irritation of the SI joint is thought to be the underlying factor leading to lower extremity symptoms, yet the mechanism is unknown.[9] Contrast medium extravasation patterns after SI joint arthrography suggest three pathways of communication between the SI joint and nearby neural structures: (1) posterior extension of contrast agent into the dorsal sacral foramina, (2) superior recess extravasation at the sacral alar level along the fifth lumbar epiradicular sheath, and (3) ventral leakage into the lumbosacral plexus.[9]

PATIENT SELECTION

Patients who have chronic low back pain without radicular pain are candidates for SI joint injection. Routine imaging of the SI joints should be performed before injection to identify any underlying cause, such as inflammatory or crystalline arthropathy, infection, or tumor, that may alter patient management. In general, the SI joints are well visualized on radiographs, especially with the modified Ferguson view (image intensifier above the patient, central x-ray beam at L5-S1, and image intensifier angled 25 to 30 degrees toward the head).[6] CT is generally not required, but it may be a useful adjunct in patients in whom the osseous anatomy is not adequately visualized or in those with advanced degenerative disease.

SI joint injection is best used as a diagnostic or therapeutic test in patients with the following:

- SI joint–related symptoms requiring pain control, including low back pain (usually unilateral, but can be bilateral); groin pain; sitting intolerance (can sit in one place for only a short time); and possible referred numbness, burning, or tingling in the buttock and lower extremity
- No associated radiculopathy
- No underlying arthropathy

CONTRAINDICATIONS

- Coagulopathy (International Normalized Ratio [INR] >1.5 or platelets <50,000/mm^3)
- Pregnancy (because of teratogenic effects of radiation)
- Systemic infection or skin infection over the puncture site
- Severe allergy to any component of the injection mixture
- Patient has received the maximum amount of steroid, including systemic steroids, allowed for a given time period, unless the injection is to be performed without steroids

PROCEDURE

Equipment/Supplies

Procedural

Spinal needle, 22-gauge, 3.5-inch (or 6-inch) (Quincke type point, Becton Dickinson & Co., Franklin Lakes, NJ)
Luer-lock syringe, 3 mL (for injection mixture)
Control syringe, 12 mL, with 25-gauge, 1.5-inch needle for local anesthesia
Povidone-iodine (Betadine) scrub
Alcohol scrub
Sterile drapes, towels and gloves
Sterile gauze
Adhesive bandages
C-arm fluoroscopy preferred
CT guidance (not usually required but may be useful in select patients)
Lead apron

Medications

Lidocaine MPF* 1%, 9.5 mL, mixed with 0.5 mL of 8.4% sodium bicarbonate to buffer pH
Bupivacaine hydrochloride 0.5% (Sensorcaine-MPF*, AstraZeneca LP, Wilmington, DE)
Betamethasone (acetate and sodium phosphate) 6 mg/mL (Celestone Soluspan, Schering Corporation, Kenilworth, NJ)
Nonionic myelographic contrast, 300 mg I/mL
Gadolinium (magnetic resonance [MR] contrast agent) if the patient has a severe allergy to iodine

*Local anesthetics should be from single-use vials and should not contain paraben or phenol in order to prevent flocculation of the steroid.[10]

Therapeutic Injection Mixture

Combine:
Betamethasone, 1.0 mL
Bupivacaine, 1.0 mL

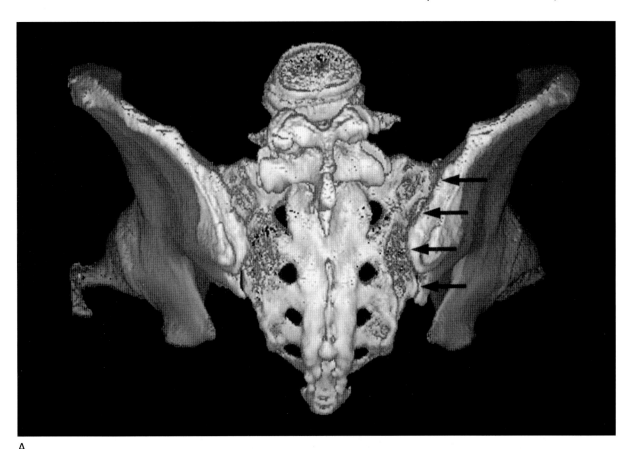

A

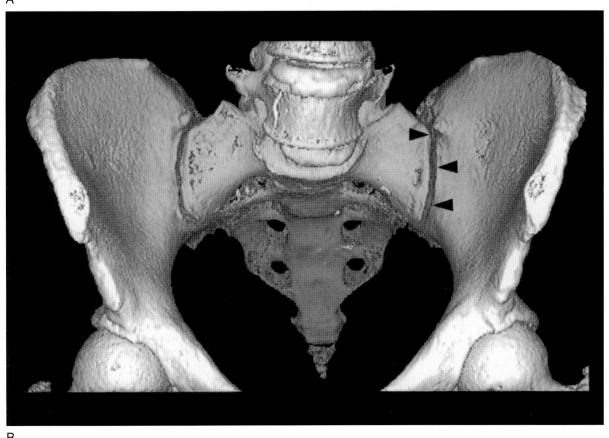

B

Figure 6-1 ■ Posterior (*A*), anterior (*B*), and RAO (*C*) three-dimensional surface-rendered CT images demonstrate the complex orientation of the SI joint (*arrows*).

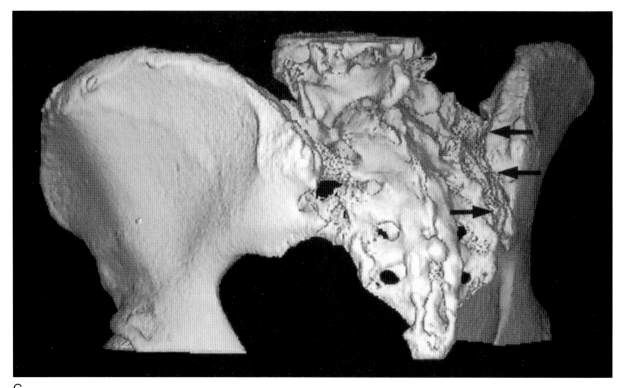

C

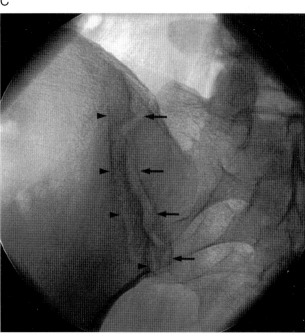

D

Figure 6-1 *(Cont'd)* ■ *C*, RAO, *D*, PA radiograph demonstrates the varying obliquity of both the anterior (*arrowheads*) and the posterior (*arrows*) joint space.

Diagnostic Injection

Bupivacaine, 2.0 mL

Therapeutic versus Diagnostic Injection

Therapeutic injections are associated with long-term symptomatic relief and are generally preferred over diagnostic studies unless there is a specific contraindication to steroid administration. Although not all patients will have a positive response, therapeutic injection obviates a second injection in

patients who experience pain relief from the initial diagnostic injection.

Methodology

Pre-procedure Guidelines

Image-guided injection of the SI joint is an outpatient procedure that can be performed with either fluoroscopic or CT guidance. Fluoroscopic guidance is generally preferred

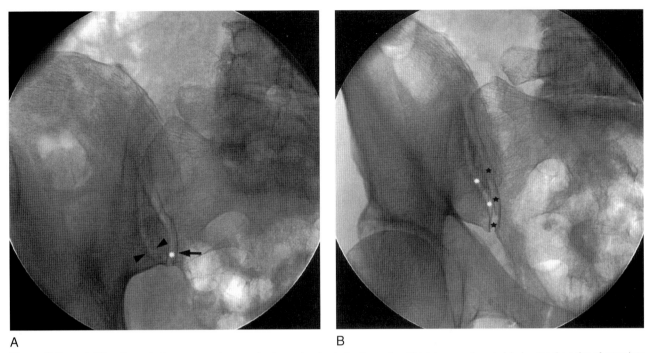

A   B

Figure 6-2 ■ *A*, PA radiograph demonstrates the posterior (*arrow*) and anterior (*arrowheads*) joint space. An asterisk denotes the point of entry into the posterior joint space. *B*, PA radiograph. Caudocranial x-ray beam angulation causes the posteroinferior joint space (*stars*) to project caudad and the anterior joint space (*asterisks*) to project cephalad.

because injection under direct visualization is faster and more cost effective. Moreover, it allows real-time evaluation of the pattern of contrast agent spread. CT may be useful in specific patients, especially those with advanced SI joint degeneration or those whose osseous anatomy and landmarks are not adequately seen under fluoroscopy. Patients are instructed to have a driver with them after the procedure as well as someone who can be responsible for their well-being for several hours after the procedure because of possible effects of the injected material.

The patient's lower extremity motor strength should be tested before the SI joint injection. This will provide a baseline for comparison with the patient's post-procedure motor strength at the time of discharge.

C-Arm Fluoroscopy

Informed consent is obtained. The patient is placed prone on the fluoroscopy table. Access to the SI joint is obtained by using a posteroinferior to anterosuperior approach. The patient is prepared and draped with sterile technique. The injection technique, described in detail by Dussault and coworkers,[11] can be easily accomplished within minutes. With the tube perpendicular to the table and the patient prone, the inferior aspect of the joint is marked. The skin entry site projects within 1 cm of the inferior margin of the joint (Fig. 6-2A). The C-arm is angled 20 to 25 degrees caudad (image intensifier above the patient and positioned obliquely toward the patient's head). This positioning projects the posteroinferior portion of the SI joint in a caudal direction, separating it from the anterior aspect of the joint, which projects cephalad (see Fig. 6-2B). A 22-gauge, 3.5-inch spinal needle is inserted at the site previously marked

and advanced perpendicular to the table until it enters the posteroinferior aspect of the joint (Fig. 6-3A). The needle should be advanced through the capsule and ligaments of the joint; the procedure may be aided by angling the needle tip laterally, along the natural course of the SI joint.[10] Intra-articular needle position should be confirmed with injection of 0.2 to 0.5 mL of nonionic contrast medium (see Fig. 6-3B). After confirmation of the needle position, the anesthetic together with the steroid preparation is injected.

Conventional Fluoroscopy

Informed consent is obtained. The patient is placed prone on the fluoroscopy table with the contralateral hip raised 20 to 30 degrees to allow the lower third of the dependent SI joint to be viewed in profile (parallel to the x-ray beam). This position uncovers the synovial portion of the joint and allows direct entry into the joint with a vertically oriented needle.[12, 13] Clearly, the varying obliquity of the joint will necessitate somewhat different degrees of patient obliquity to see the joint in profile (Fig. 6-4). The needle tip should be placed into the lower aspect of the joint, approximately 1 cm above its inferior extent (Fig. 6-5). After determination of the appropriate puncture path, the skin is prepared and draped in the usual fashion. After local anesthesia, a 22-gauge, 3.5-inch needle is advanced into the joint. Once the posterior ligaments have been traversed, there is decreased resistance to movement. Needle tip position is confirmed as intra-articular with injection of 0.2 to 0.5 mL of nonionic contrast agent (Fig. 6-6). After confirmation of needle position, the anesthetic together with the steroid preparation is injected.

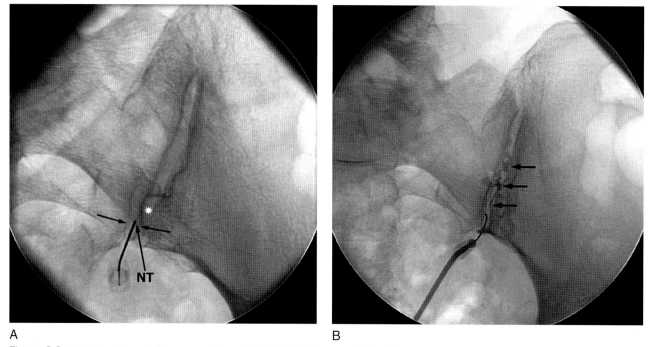

A   B

Figure 6-3 ■ *A*, PA radiograph demonstrates the needle tip (NT) in the posteroinferior joint space (*arrows*) 1 cm craniad to the inferior joint margin. *Asterisk* = anterior joint space. *B*, PA radiograph demonstrates contrast medium (*arrows*) within the joint space.

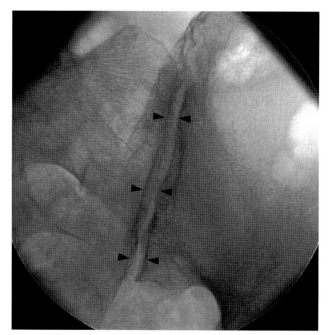

Figure 6-4 ■ RAO radiograph demonstrates a curvilinear lucency (*arrowheads*) representing overlap of the anterior and posterior SI joint space.

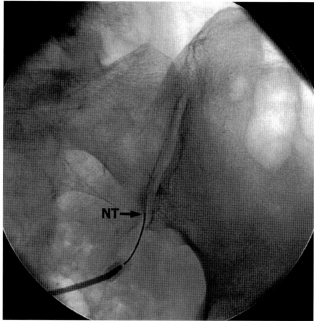

Figure 6-5 ■ RAO radiograph with the needle tip (NT) in the joint space, 1 cm craniad to the inferior joint margin.

Computed Tomography

Informed consent is obtained. The patient is placed in the prone position on the CT table. The SI joint is initially evaluated with 5-mm axial images obtained from its midportion through the inferior margin (Fig. 6-7). Needle placement is directed toward the lower third of the joint, the ideal location of the needle tip being approximately 1 cm above the inferior aspect of the joint (Fig. 6-8). After preparation of the puncture site, draping, and local anesthesia, a 22-gauge, 3.5-inch spinal needle is advanced into the joint. Access to the

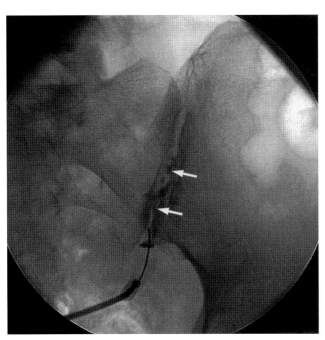

Figure 6-6 ■ RAO radiograph demonstrates contrast agent (*arrows*) within the joint space.

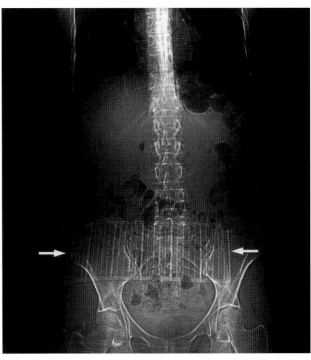

Figure 6-7 ■ Scout CT image with patient prone. Radiopaque localizer grid (*arrows*) is taped to the patient's lower back overlying the target SI joint.

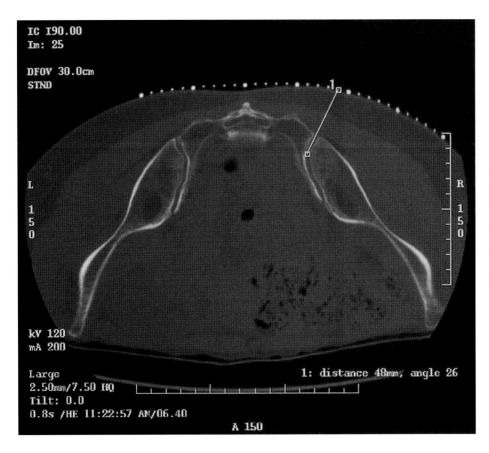

Figure 6-8 ■ Axial CT image demonstrates a radiopaque grid on the patient's posterior skin surface. A digital measurement calculates the distance from the skin surface to the posterior joint space as well as the skin entrance point and the angle necessary for joint access. The CT slice position (I90.00) gives the craniocaudad position for needle entrance.

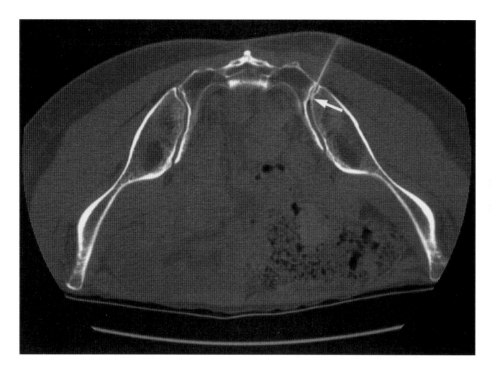

Figure 6-9 ■ Axial CT image. The needle is aligned parallel to the joint space with its tip (*arrow*) 1 cm into the posterior joint space.

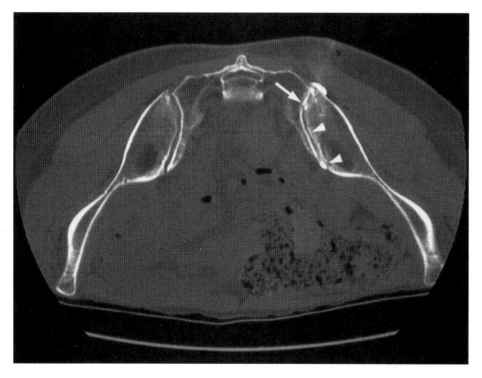

Figure 6-10 ■ Axial CT image demonstrates contrast agent (*arrowheads*) extending throughout the posterior and anterior joint space. *Arrow* = needle tip.

posterior portion of the joint is facilitated if the angle of the approach matches the orientation of the posterior aspect of the joint (Fig. 6-9). Needle tip position is confirmed as intra-articular with the injection of 0.2 to 0.5 mL of nonionic contrast medium (Fig. 6-10). After confirmation of needle position, the anesthetic together with the steroid preparation is injected.

Assessing Proper Needle Position

As noted earlier, injection of a small amount (0.2 to 0.5 mL) of contrast medium into the joint will confirm the intra-artiular position of the needle. The contrast agent will outline the margins of the joint and extend into the dependent portion of the articulation. In addition to providing a record

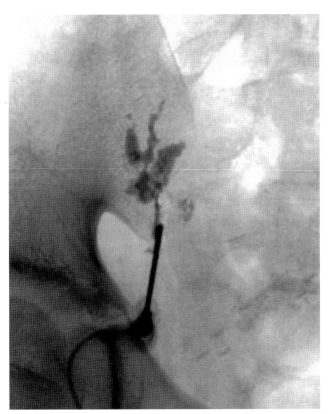

Figure 6-11 ■ PA fluoroscopic image of the SI joint after contrast injection shows nodularity with multiple small sacculations to the joint cavity, compatible with synovitis.

of correct needle placement, contrast agent injection may have diagnostic implications by identifying abnormalities in articular contour, collections of juxta-articular fluid, or synovitis (Fig. 6-11).

Pain Response Assessment in SI Joint Injections

In general, immediate pain relief is seen in 50% to 80% of patients, and 90% of patients have pain relief within 12 hours.[11, 14] The injection may function as a provocative test by distending the joint and reproducing patient symptoms. Patients with a history of previous spine surgery have definitive but less than 50% pain relief.[14] Patients will often have good pain relief for as long as 10 ± 5 months.[15]

POTENTIAL COMPLICATIONS

- Bleeding
- Infection (cellulitis, septic arthritis, or osteomyelitis)
- Drug-related allergic reactions
- Transitory lower extremity weakness
- Transitory lower extremity paresthesia
- Transitory difficulty in voiding

POST-PROCEDURE CARE/FOLLOW-UP

Immediate

1. The patient should be observed for 30 minutes after injection.
2. The patient may sit in a reclining lounge chair.
3. Blood pressure, pulse, heart rate, and respiratory rate are monitored as necessary.

Discharge[16]

1. The patient's motor strength should be evaluated and compared with pre-procedure strength. The patient should not be discharged until post-procedure strength is at or near pre-procedure strength.
2. The patient is discharged into the care of a responsible person.
3. Instructions are given for the patient not to drive for the remainder of the day.
4. An adhesive bandage may be on the puncture site. The bandage should remain dry for at least 24 hours, at which point it can be removed.
5. The patient is instructed to continue taking his or her prescription medication, although pain medication may be tapered as indicated.
6. A discharge sheet should be given to the patient outlining the following:
    a. Which procedure was performed
    b. Procedure-related symptoms that typically resolve in 7 to 10 days
        - Pain at the needle puncture site(s)
        - Mild increased back stiffness
        - Deep back pain
    c. Treatment for mild post-procedure symptoms
        - Rest the affected area for 3 to 4 days.
        - Avoid movements that aggravate the pain.
        - Use cold compresses to the area that hurts.
    d. Signs and symptoms of infection
        - Fever
        - Chills
        - Swelling or drainage from the puncture site(s)
        - New back pain that is different from the usual pain
    e. Signs and symptoms of possibly more serious problems
        - Stiff neck
        - Increasing pain
        - Motor dysfunction such as difficulty walking
        - Bowel or bladder dysfunction
    f. Physician name and contact number if the patient has any concerns or if any problems were to arise as a result of the procedure
    g. Advice to schedule a follow-up appointment with the referring physician in 7 to 10 days

SAMPLE DICTATION

With the patient's understanding and consent, a fluoroscopic-guided injection of the right SI joint was performed. The patient was placed in the prone position, and the skin was prepared in the usual fashion. A 22-gauge, 3.5-inch spinal needle was advanced into the posteroinferior aspect of the right SI joint under direct fluoroscopic visualization. After confirmation of the intra-articular position of the needle tip with injection of 0.5 mL of Omnipaque 300 contrast medium, a mixture of 1.0 mL betamethasone (6 mg/mL) and 1 mL of bupivacaine (0.5%) was injected. The patient tolerated the procedure well, without immediate complication.

Examination of the patient at the time of discharge, approximately 30 minutes after the injection, showed no motor or sensory deficit or evidence of bleeding. The patient noted marked improvement in his pain at the time of discharge. He was given a post-procedure information sheet at discharge.

CASE REPORT

CASE 1

Clinical Presentation

The patient is a 58-year-old woman with a 7-year history of right SI joint pain. She describes the pain as sharp and aching, significantly exacerbated by sitting. She has no numbness, radiculopathy, or bowel or bladder dysfunction. Previous caudal epidural provided no improvement. Clinically guided SI joint injection attempted by Pain Management was unsuccessful, and the patient was referred for image-guided SI joint injection.

Imaging and Therapy

Informed consent was obtained. The patient was placed prone on the CT table. A radiopaque grid was taped to the patient's skin overlying the right SI joint, and a scout coronal CT image was obtained (Fig. 6-12). Axial images were obtained to localize the optimal entry point and angle (Fig. 6-13). A 22-gauge, 3.5-inch spinal needle was advanced into the posterior aspect of the right SI joint (Fig. 6-14), and 0.2 mL of contrast medium was injected to confirm intra-articular needle placement (Fig. 6-15). Subsequently, a mixture of 1 mL bupivacaine (0.5%) and 1 mL betamethasone (6 mg/mL) was injected into the joint and the needle was removed.

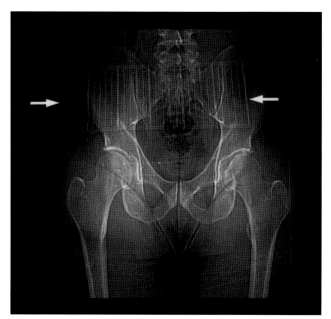

Figure 6-12 ▪ Scout CT image with patient prone. Radiopaque localizer grid (*arrows*) is taped to the patient's lower back overlying the target SI joint.

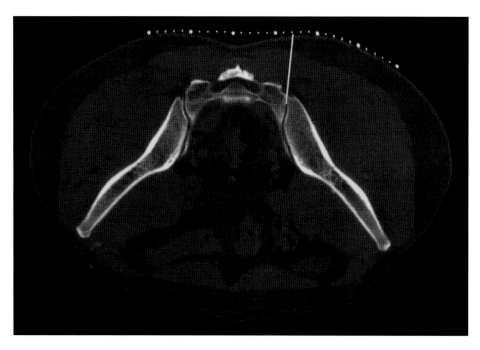

Figure 6-13 ▪ Axial CT image demonstrates a radiopaque grid on the patient's posterior skin surface. An electronic line projects the expected path of the needle into the posterior joint space.

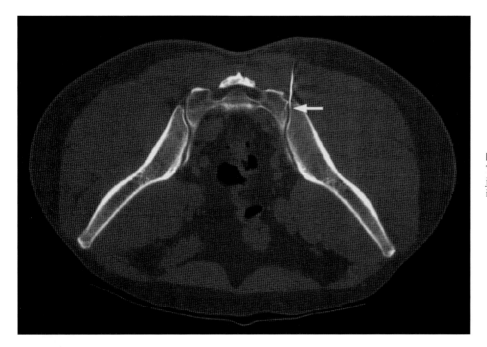

Figure 6-14 ■ Axial CT image. The needle is aligned parallel to the joint space, with its tip (*arrow*) 5 mm into the posterior joint space.

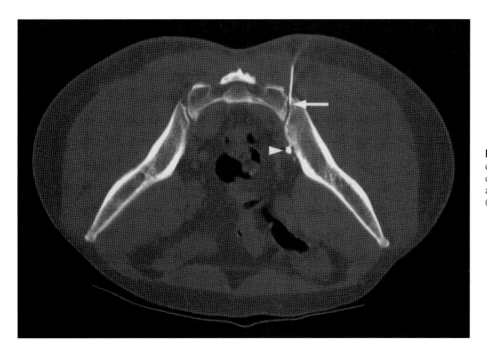

Figure 6-15 ■ Axial CT image demonstrates contrast agent that has extended through the posterior and anterior joint space into the pelvis (*arrowhead*). *Arrow* = needle tip.

Results

Follow-up evaluation showed a significant reduction in pre-procedure pain and no evidence of numbness or loss of strength.

CURRENT PROCEDURAL TERMINOLOGY (CPT) CODES

CPT codes change often and sometimes are valid only for certain states or regions. It is best to consult with coding experts to make sure that coding for one's procedures is legitimate and complete. Below is a sample of codes that are being used for SI joint injections.[17]

27096 Injection procedure for sacroiliac joint, arthrography and/or anesthetic/steroid

76005 Fluoroscopic guidance and localization of needle or catheter tip for spine or paraspinous diagnostic or therapeutic injection procedures (epidural, transforaminal epidural, subarachnoid, paravertebral facet joint, paravertebral facet joint nerve or sacroiliac joint), including neurolytic agent destruction

73542 Radiological examination, sacroiliac joint arthrography, radiological supervision and interpretation

(Do not report 76005 in addition to 73542)

99141 Sedation with or without analgesia (conscious sedation); intravenous, intramuscular or inhalation

References

1. Schwarzer AC, Aprill CN, Bogduk N. The sacroiliac joint in chronic low back pain. Spine 1995; 20:31–37.
2. Dreyfuss P, Michaelsen M, Pauza K, et al. The value of medical history and physical examination in diagnosing sacroiliac joint pain. Spine 1996; 21:2594–2602.
3. Braun J, Bollow M, Seyrekbasan F, et al. Computed tomography guided corticosteroid injection of the sacroiliac joint in patients with spondyloarthropathy with sacroiliitis: Clinical outcome and followup by dynamic magnetic resonance imaging. J Rheumatol 1996; 23:659–664.
4. Pulisetti D, Ebraheim NA. CT-guided sacroiliac joint injections. J Spinal Disord 1999; 12:310–312.
5. Rosenberg JM, Quint TJ, de Rosayro AM. Computerized tomographic localization of clinically-guided sacroiliac joint injections. Clin J Pain 2000; 16:18–21.
6. Brower AC, Flemming DJ. Arthritis in Black and White, 2nd ed. Philadelphia: WB Saunders, 1997, pp 1–32, 155–173.
7. Fortin JD, Kissling RO, O'Connor BL, Vilenesky JA. Sacroiliac joint innervation and pain. Am J Orthop 1999; 28:687–690.
8. Ikeda R. Innervation of the sacroiliac joint: Macroscopic and histological studies. Nippon Ika Daigaku Zasshi 1991; 58:587–596.
9. Fortin JD, Washington WJ, Falco FJE. Three pathways between the sacroiliac joint and neural structures. AJNR Am J Neuroradiol 1999; 20:1429–1434.
10. Physicians' Desk Reference, 56th ed. Montvale, NJ: Medical Economics Company, 2002.
11. Dussault RG, Kaplan PA, Anderson MW. Fluoroscopy-guided sacroiliac joint injection. Radiology 2000; 214:273–277.
12. Ebraheim NA, Xu R, Nadaud M, et al. Sacroiliac joint injection: A cadaveric study. Am J Orthop 1997; 26:338–341.
13. Hendrix RW, Lin PJP, Kane WJ. Simplified aspiration or injection technique for the sacro-iliac joint. J Bone Joint Surg Am 1982; 64:1249–1252.
14. Pulisetti D, Ebraheim NA. CT-guided sacroiliac joint injections. J Spinal Disord 1999; 12:310–312.
15. Bollow M, Braun J, Taupitz M, et al. CT-guided intraarticular corticosteroid injection into the sacroiliac joints in patients with spondyloarthropathy: Indication and follow-up with contrast enhanced MRI. J Comput Assist Tomogr 1996; 20:512–521.
16. Fenton DS, Czervionke LF. Discography. In Williams AL, Murtagh FR (eds). Handbook of Diagnostic and Therapeutic Spine Procedures. St. Louis: CV Mosby, 2002, pp 187–188.
17. Derived from CPT 2002, CPT Intellectual Property Services. Chicago: American Medical Association, 2002.

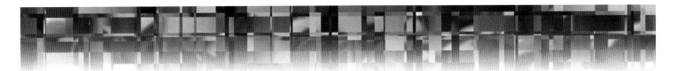

A Spine Surgeon's Perspective

Sacroiliac Joint Injection

Joseph T. Alexander, MD

Degeneration of the SI articulation is rarely treated surgically. It is troublesome to diagnose because the symptoms overlap considerably with those of other degenerative disorders of the lumbar spine and hip. Except in patients with clear-cut signs on provocative testing, it can at times be a diagnosis of exclusion when other entities have been ruled out. Symptoms can be bothersome and long lasting, and they may not respond to oral anti-inflammatory medication, pelvic stabilization exercises, gait analysis, correction of leg-length discrepancies, or other measures. In some of these cases, patients can benefit from SI joint injections, both to confirm the diagnosis and to provide relief of symptoms.

Chapter **7**

Percutaneous Spine Biopsy

- Leo F. Czervionke, MD
- Douglas S. Fenton, MD

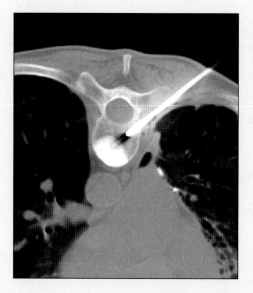

BACKGROUND

Percutaneous biopsy of the spine is not a new technique, but it has been refined over the years as new biopsy needles and imaging techniques have become more sophisticated. Percutaneous spine biopsy was first performed in the mid 1930s by Robertson and Ball using a posterolateral approach.[1, 2] In the past, needle biopsies of the spine were performed by surgeons using open surgical procedures, because early x-ray fluoroscopic images were of poor quality and computed tomography (CT) was not available. These open surgical procedures were performed with large-caliber needles and carried the risk of greater morbidity compared with the percutaneous, relatively small-caliber needle biopsy procedures commonly performed today. Fluoroscopically guided needle biopsy of the spine became popular after 1949.[3–6] CT-guided biopsy of the spine became widely accepted after 1981.[7] Before the availability of CT, percutaneous biopsy of the spine from the T2 to the T9 level was generally considered dangerous.[8] There was concern about possible inadvertent lung puncture because of the close proximity of the parietal pleura in this region, and fear of penetrating the azygous/hemiazygous system.[9, 10] As a result, an open surgical procedure for biopsy of the T2 through T9 vertebral bodies was recommended. With current image guidance methods, including real-time CT (CT fluoroscopy), percutaneous biopsy is now a safe, widely used, effective technique for biopsy of the cervical, thoracic, and lumbar vertebrae, intervertebral discs, and paraspinal soft tissues, and it is routinely performed as an outpatient procedure.[11, 12]

Percutaneous spine biopsy using modern techniques is believed to have an overall accuracy in the range of 80% to 95%.[13, 14–18] The older literature reports a lower accuracy for percutaneous biopsy.[8] Positive recovery rates are higher for osteolytic lesions and lower for sclerotic lesions of bone and for vertebral spondylodiscitis.[19, 20] The sensitivity of spine biopsy reported in the literature can be misleading because appropriate patient selection, lesion site selection, and operator experience are critical factors that can alter the accuracy. For example, if the patient has been receiving antibiotics, when a presumed infected disc is aspirated the chance of recovering viable microorganisms is lessened. Therefore, low accuracy does not necessarily indicate suboptimal technique or that the procedure is invalid.

Modern spine biopsy techniques use x-ray fluoroscopic guidance or CT guidance to assist in needle positioning. The advantage of x-ray fluoroscopy is that it provides real-time assessment of needle position. It is our preferred method for biopsy of large lesions in the spine using the transpedicular approach and for disc biopsies in the lumbar region. CT guidance is preferred when a small bone lesion is being sampled, for paraspinal masses, and for most thoracic spine biopsies, to minimize the chance of inadvertent puncture of the pleura. CT guidance is preferable for cervical spine biopsies as well. Current CT scanners have real-time CT capability. Cine magnetic resonance (MR) imaging (MR fluoroscopy) is also available as an option for image guidance. However, the stainless steel needles generate considerable artifact, and therefore precise localization of the needle tip may not be possible with MR imaging.

Complications of spine biopsy are infrequent (0.2%)[13, 14] and include hematoma, vertebral osteomyelitis, disc space infection, nerve root damage causing radiculopathy, and pneumothorax. Complications are more common with thoracic spine biopsies in general.[14] A detailed summary of potential spine biopsy complications is included later in this chapter.

PATIENT SELECTION

The indications for spine biopsy include diagnosing neoplasm (vertebral or paraspinal), disc infection, and metabolic bone disease. Most patients present with back pain and have been evaluated with CT, MR imaging, or radionuclide bone scanning before being considered for biopsy. A large-core biopsy is generally necessary to evaluate for metabolic bone disease (needle caliber diameter >3 mm); therefore, metabolic bone biopsies are usually obtained with open surgical techniques,[21] although sufficient core samples can be obtained with large-bore needles such as Craig or Jamshidi needles.[6, 22, 23] A fine-needle aspiration biopsy technique (smaller than 18- to 20-gauge) is usually sufficient for biopsy of paraspinal soft tissue masses. Such aspirates are usually insufficient for vertebral bone biopsy in which a larger core should optimally be obtained with a 16-gauge needle or larger. Fine-needle bone aspiration may be sufficient to confirm the diagnosis of multiple myeloma.[24] A large needle such as a Craig needle may actually be less optimal

for soft tissue biopsy because it can macerate soft tissue and thus make histologic assessment difficult.[25]

Major Indications

- Assess compression fracture and benign (post-traumatic or insufficiency) fracture versus pathologic (neoplastic or metabolic) fracture.
- Confirm metastatic tumor involvement of vertebrae, paraspinal soft tissue, or the epidural region in a patient with a known primary neoplasm.
- Confirm disc space infection/osteomyelitis. The diagnosis of disc space infection is usually known. The biopsy may be obtained in equivocal cases or more commonly to obtain a sample of the organism producing the infection for Gram stain, culture, and sensitivity.

Minor Indications

- Vertebral biopsy to confirm a diagnosis of multiple myeloma
- Symptomatic synovial cyst aspiration
- Facet joint aspiration to exclude septic joint

CONTRAINDICATIONS

- Coagulopathy (International Normalized Ratio [INR] >1.5, prothrombin time >1.5 times control, or platelets <50,000/mm^3)
- Pregnancy (because of teratogenic effects of radiation)
- Systemic infection or skin infection over the puncture site
- Severe allergy to any medication needed to perform the biopsy procedure
- A solid bone fusion that does not allow access to the disc for aspiration biopsy
- Patients with significant spinal cord compromise at a level to be studied, because there is a theoretical risk of causing or aggravating a myelopathy
- Epidural tumor in the spinal canal. One must exercise extreme caution in sampling an epidural tumor within the spinal canal, because the biopsy procedure may result in soft tissue swelling or bleeding in the canal, which may further compromise the spinal cord. It is always preferable to select the biopsy site in this order of decreasing preference: (1) subcutaneous soft tissue mass, (2) paraspinal soft tissue mass, (3) vertebral bone, and (4) epidural mass.

PROCEDURE

Equipment/Supplies

Control syringe, 12 mL, with 25-gauge, 1.5-inch needle containing 9.5 mL 1% lidocaine for local anesthesia and optionally adding 0.5 mL of 8.4% sodium bicarbonate injectable (1 mEq/mL) to alleviate burning pain associated with anesthetic
Povidone-iodine (Betadine) scrub
Alcohol scrub
Sterile drapes

Sterile gauze
Adhesive bandages
Lead apron (for fluoroscopic procedures) and sterile gowns
Hat, mask, and sterile gloves
Hydrogen peroxide (for cleansing the antiseptic from the skin after the biopsy)
Scalpel
Selected needle biopsy/aspiration system(s)
Radiopaque grid or marker for CT-guided procedures

Medications

For the majority of patients, intravenous sedation is usually not required for standard spine biopsy procedures that use small-caliber needles (smaller than 18- to 22-gauge). The use of large-caliber needles often requires intravenous sedation. Agents to be used include the following:

Lidocaine 1% (Xylocaine 1%, AstraZeneca LP, Wilmington, DE) for subcutaneous and periosteal local anesthesia

Midazolam (Versed, Roche Laboratories, Nutley, NJ), 1 mg, given intravenously is the routine dose for the standard patient if sedation is required for relief of anxiety during the procedure. Maximum dose is 5 mg. Caution should be exercised in older patients, who may experience respiratory depression with even small doses (0.5 to 1.0 mg) of midazolam. If sedation is required for patients older than 65 years of age, start dose at 0.5 mg intravenously.

Fentanyl, 50 to 100 μg, for intravenous use to alleviate pain during the procedure

Atropine, 0.6 to 1 mg, should be available for spine biopsy procedures in case of a vasovagal reaction.

Epinephrine should **not** be used, because of its undesirable vasoconstrictive properties, particularly in biopsy procedures of the head and neck region.

GENERAL PRINCIPLES OF SPINE BIOPSY

Pre-procedure

Percutaneous spine biopsy is performed as an outpatient or inpatient procedure. Pre-procedure laboratory studies that should be obtained include prothrombin time, partial thromboplastin time, complete blood cell count, platelet count, and International Normalized Ratio. Blood urea nitrogen and creatinine determinations are only necessary if the patient has known or suspected renal disease and will receive an intravenous contrast agent. The patient should always be questioned regarding allergies to medications.

Patients are instructed to be accompanied by a responsible adult who can drive them home and is capable of reporting any procedure-related difficulties should these occur after patients leave the department.

Patient Preparation

For all spine biopsy cases, informed consent is obtained after details of the procedure and procedural risks have been discussed. All patients, regardless of the type or location of

the spine biopsy to be performed, are prepared in a similar fashion. The patient is placed on the fluoroscopy table or within the CT gantry in a position that will most facilitate the procedure without causing undue discomfort to the patient. Monitoring of the patient's vital signs is obtained as necessary, depending on the patient's clinical situation; it is mandatory if intravenous sedation is to be used. We reserve the use of intravenous sedation for a minority of patients who are experiencing a great deal of pain or anxiety. Sedation is used more often when large-caliber bone biopsy systems are used. With the use of sterile technique, a wide area surrounding the needle entrance point is scrubbed three successive times with povidone-iodine and then with alcohol. The entry site is covered with sterile towels or an eye-hole drape. Assuming that there is no allergic contraindication, lidocaine 1% is injected into the subcutaneous tissues of the entry site and then along the expected needle path, first with a 25-gauge, 1.5-inch needle and then with a 22-gauge, 3.5-inch spinal needle (or longer if necessary). The amount of local anesthetic used varies and is often patient dependent. A skin nick is then made with a scalpel to facilitate placement of a larger-caliber needle through the superficial soft tissues. The actual technique used for spine biopsy in a given patient is tailored to that patient and is dependent on the anatomic region (cervical, thoracic, or lumbar), the location of the lesion (paraspinal, epidural, vertebral body, or posterior vertebral arch), the image-guidance method chosen for biopsy (CT vs. x-ray fluoroscopy), and the needle apparatus chosen for the biopsy.

After all procedures, the skin surface is cleansed with hydrogen peroxide to remove the povidone-iodine, and an adhesive bandage is applied to the puncture site.

Entry Site and Target Localization

Biopsies can be performed under x-ray fluoroscopic or CT guidance. Cine fluoroscopic MR guidance is a relatively new method that has recently been used for performing biopsies, but its role in performing percutaneous spine biopsy has yet to be determined. In the following sections, we discuss our preferred method of biopsy based primarily on lesion location. Before any biopsy, one should perform a thorough evaluation of all pertinent imaging studies to determine that a given biopsy is necessary and appropriate. The pre-biopsy evaluation is also essential to select the image guidance method that is optimal for biopsy, to assess the appropriate needle trajectory that would likely give the greatest diagnostic yield, and to choose the biopsy system that is most appropriate in a given situation. Patient safety is always considered in making these choices.

Fluoroscopic Guidance

The needle entry site is usually determined **after** the skin preparation. The physician performing the procedure must have a thorough knowledge of anatomy, including vertebral landmarks and adjacent soft tissues, to plan the fluoroscopically guided spine biopsy and to establish the safest and most appropriate needle trajectory.

For example, when a transpedicular approach for vertebral body biopsy is used, the target pedicle is viewed in the anteroposterior (AP) plane and is kept in the center of the

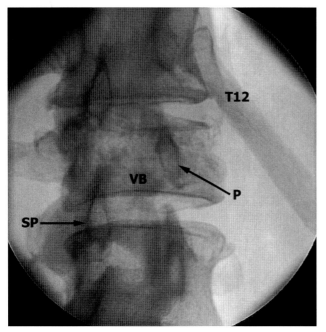

Figure 7-1 ■ Radiographic position for transpedicular biopsy. Shallow left anterior oblique (LAO) radiograph. The right pedicle (P) of L1 has an ovoid configuration when the x-ray beam is parallel to the long axis of the pedicle. SP = spinous process L1; VB = L1 vertebral body; T12 = right 12th rib. Note compression fracture of superior portion of L1 vertebral body.

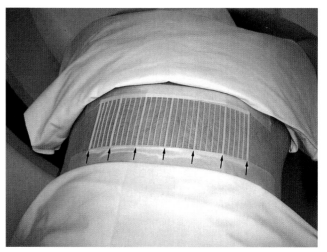

Figure 7-2 ■ Localization grid positioned on patient's back for thoracic biopsy before sterile skin preparation. Grid bars are 1 cm apart with thicker bars (*arrows*) located 5 cm apart.

field of view. A radiopaque marker such as a sterile hemostat or needle is placed on the skin surface. With continuous fluoroscopy, the C-arm is obliqued toward the side of the pedicle to view the pedicle en face. Generally, the pedicle will appear most ovoid when the x-ray beam is projecting down the long axis of the pedicle (Fig. 7-1). For a posterolateral vertebral body approach using fluoroscopy, depending on the location of the lesion within the vertebra, the

C-arm is rotated several degrees in either direction to facilitate biopsy more medially or laterally within the vertebral body.

CT Guidance

The needle entry site is determined **before** the skin preparation with a nonsterile radiopaque grid or other radiopaque marker. A radiopaque grid is optimal for CT-guided biopsy because it covers a larger area on the patient's skin and need not be repositioned to determine the desired entry site. The grid is centered over the probable needle entry site and taped to the patient's skin (Fig. 7-2).

Initial AP and lateral CT digital radiographs will demonstrate the grid in relation to the patient's vertebrae (Fig. 7-3).

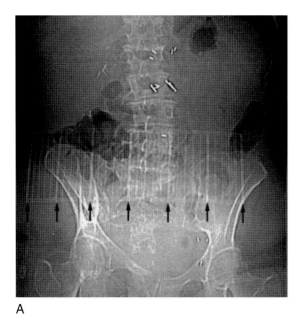

A

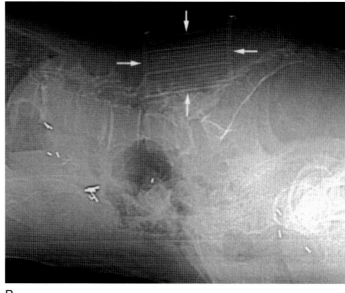

B

Figure 7-3 ■ Digital radiographs of localizer grid positioned in the lumbar region. *A*, AP digital radiograph of localization grid (*arrows*). *B*, Lateral digital radiograph of localization grid (*arrows*).

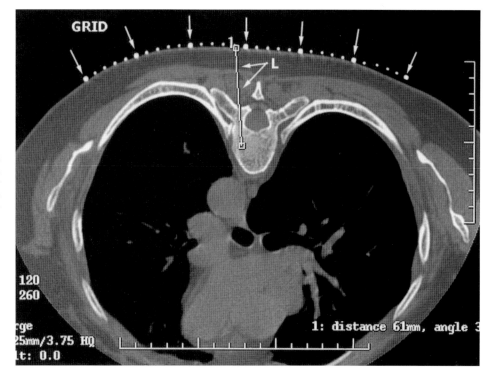

Figure 7-4 ■ Axial CT scan with localizing grid on the skin surface. The 5-cm grid bars are indicated by arrows. L = Localizer line drawn on CT image to measure the skin-to-target distance.

If the grid overlies the target vertebra, no adjustment to the grid position needs to be made. If the grid does not overly the target vertebra, the grid position is adjusted and additional scout CT digital radiographs are obtained.

It is important to choose a field of view large enough to allow visualizion not only of the pathology but also of the skin surface and the entire grid. Helical CT scans of 1- to 3-mm partitions are performed to localize the lesion. These images are then studied to determine optimal needle trajectory. A CT image is selected that optimally demonstrates the pathologic target and desired needle trajectory, and the image location number of this image is noted. A digital line is then drawn on this CT image along the desired needle trajectory to measure the distance from the skin entry site to the biopsy target location (Fig. 7-4). The point where the electronic line intersects the grid is noted. This intersection point is noted by counting from one end of the grid or the other. The CT gantry is moved to the image location number previously noted. When the CT laser light is then turned on, it will project on the grid and skin surface (Fig. 7-5). A mark is made on the skin surface with a pen where the CT laser light intersects with the grid intersection point previously noted (Fig. 7-6). The grid is then removed, and the skin is prepared and draped in sterile fashion.

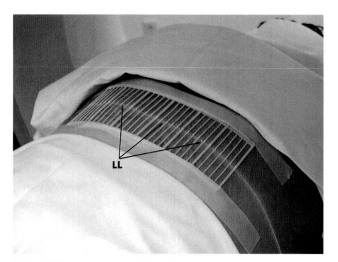

Figure 7-5 ■ After the axial CT slice location is chosen, the CT scanner table is moved until the scanner laser localizer light beam (LL) projects on the localizer grid at the desired location.

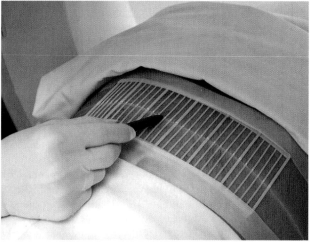

Figure 7-6 ■ Skin entry point is marked with a marking pen where the light beam intersects the grid at the desired entry point based on the axial CT scan localizer image in Figure 7-4.

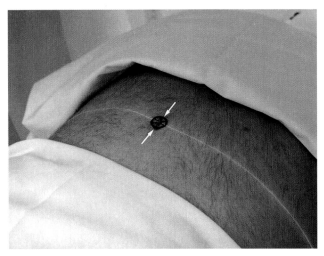

Figure 7-7 ■ Alternatively, for localization purposes a metallic BB pellet is taped to the skin over the lesion to be sampled based on preliminary axial CT scans obtained through the target lesion. After the desired axial lesion is selected and the table location is moved to the appropriate position, the skin entry point is marked where the BB pellet (*arrows*) intersects the scanner localizer light beam.

If a radiopaque grid is not available, use of a radiopaque BB pellet taped to the skin and the CT scanner laser localizer will suffice for purposes of entry site localization. This localization method usually prolongs the procedure, requiring repeated CT scan acquisitions to determine the appropriate skin entry site (Fig. 7-7).

Selecting CT versus X-ray Fluoroscopic Guidance

Either CT or x-ray fluoroscopic guidance can be used effectively to guide the percutaneous spine biopsy. The modality chosen is in part based on the experience of the physician performing the biopsy. CT is advantageous for biopsy of paraspinal soft tissue masses, when a small structure is being sampled, or when precise needle localization is critical.[15, 26] A good rule to use is to *choose the image guidance method most suitable that will visualize the target lesion being sampled and the trajectory that the needle must follow to the target to accomplish the most efficient and safe needle placement.*

For example, when performing a lumbar vertebral body transpedicular biopsy, one can visualize the pedicle with either CT or x-ray fluoroscopy. However, the fluoroscopic approach is more expeditious because the needle is directly visualized in real time passing down the long axis of the pedicle. Real-time CT fluoroscopy available on newer CT scanners provides a similar advantage, but the lumbar transpedicular biopsy is still more easily accomplished by using x-ray fluoroscopic guidance for direct visualization, especially if one is familiar with transpedicular needle placement for vertebroplasty, because the approach is identical. We also prefer x-ray fluoroscopic guidance for disc biopsy or aspiration because the disc is readily seen at fluoroscopy and the approach used is identical to that used for discography.[27]

CT is clearly advantageous for soft tissue paraspinal masses or for precise localization in small vertebral bone lesions. CT is also recommended for biopsy of posterior vertebral arch lesions because it allows direct visualization of needle depth to prevent inadvertent entry into the spinal canal or neural foramen. Posterior vertebral arch lesions are optimally sampled with the use of real-time CT fluoroscopy during needle placement. CT is the guidance method of choice for percutaneous biopsy of the cervical spine.

THREE BASIC NEEDLE BIOPSY TECHNIQUES

All spine biopsy procedures employ one of the following basic techniques for needle placement. Described below are the basic needle techniques for spine biopsy that can be used in the cervical, thoracic, or lumbar region, with CT or x-ray fluoroscopic guidance. This section is followed by a description of the specific biopsy needle systems we routinely use for spine biopsy.

Tandem Needle Technique

This technique can be used with CT or fluoroscopic guidance but is usually performed with CT.[28] A small-caliber "skinny" (22-gauge) needle is initially advanced to the margin of the bone or soft tissue mass to be sampled. This needle is used to administer local anesthetic deep to the subcutaneous tissue or to the periosteum. The skinny needle serves as a guide for a second, larger-caliber needle (e.g., 16- to 20-gauge), which is passed parallel and in close proximity to the initial needle (Fig. 7-8). Needle placement is confirmed with CT or radiographs, and the skinny needle is removed. The second, larger-caliber needle is then advanced into the vertebra or paraspinal soft tissue mass, where the biopsy specimen is collected. With available modern image guidance, we now rarely use this technique.

Coaxial Needle Technique

This is the preferred method for biopsy of deep spinal and paraspinal lesions and is used routinely at our facility, with fluoroscopic or CT guidance, for posterolateral and transpedicular approaches. The goal with a coaxial system is to minimize damage of normal tissue by using a single needle pass to obtain multiple target lesion samples. This goal is achieved with a needle system that uses a *combined large- and small-caliber needle set.* Biopsy needles used for a given biopsy may be selected from one or two different biopsy needle systems or needle sets. A large-caliber (11- to 16-gauge) spine biopsy needle with an inner stylet is placed into the structure to be sampled (i.e., vertebra or paraspinal soft tissue mass). A smaller, longer (18- to 22-gauge) biopsy needle is then inserted **through** the larger-caliber needle in coaxial fashion (Fig. 7-9) to obtain one or more aspirates or small-core biopsy specimens, according to the particular needle manufacturer's instructions. A large-core sample is finally obtained with the larger-caliber needle by advancing and withdrawing the needle using to-and-fro motion within

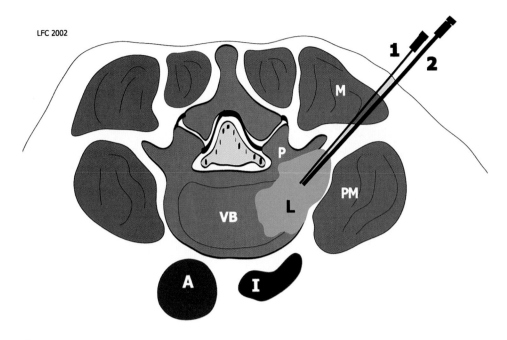

LFC 2002

A

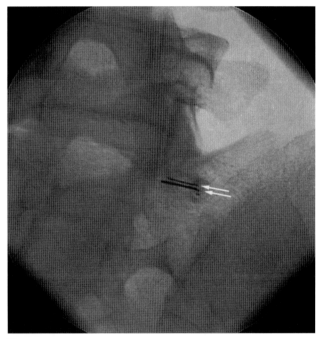

B

Figure 7-8 ■ Tandem needle biopsy approach. *A*, Illustration of tandem needle approach. Skinny needle 1 is initially advanced into the target lesion (L) using a right extrapedicular posterolateral approach. A larger-caliber biopsy needle 2 is then placed parallel to the first needle into the target lesion in vertebral body (VB). P = pedicle; M = erector spinae muscle group; PM = psoas muscle; A = aorta; I = inferior vena cava. *B*, Radiographs showing two needles placed using tandem technique. Initially a 25-gauge needle (*upper arrow*) was left in place after local anesthetic instillation. After this, a 22-gauge spinal needle (*lower arrow*) has been inserted parallel and immediately adjacent to the 25-gauge needle.

the target lesion while simultaneously applying negative suction to the needle hub by withdrawing on a syringe attached to the hub. An intervening connecting tube can be applied to the needle hub, with the aid of a gloved assistant, to apply syringe suction while the primary operator advances and twists the needle. We have found this to be an excellent method for acquiring a large vertebral body bone marrow core specimen, especially when a large-caliber needle is used for obtaining the biopsy specimen. The syringe suction is maintained while the biopsy needle containing the specimen is withdrawn slowly through the paraspinal

tissues. The syringe suction is maintained until the specimen is collected. The tissue specimen is immediately smeared onto sterile slides, and the remaining larger portion of the specimen is placed in formalin or into culture tubes (or both, depending on the situation) with the assistance of the pathology technician.

Regardless of the coaxial system, it is important to verify before the procedure that the selected inner coaxial needle will fit through the outer cannula and that the inner needle is sufficiently long to project out from the end of the outer cannula into the target lesion.

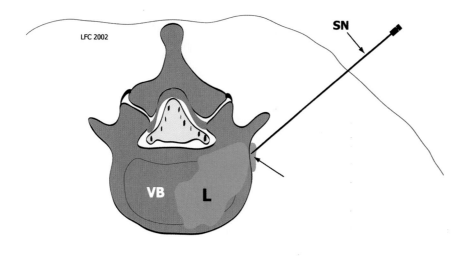

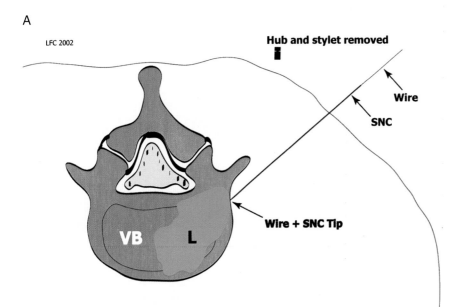

Figure 7-9 ▪ Illustration of a posterolateral approach with a coaxial needle system for biopsy of a cortically based vertebral body lesion (fashioned after the Geremia or the Elson Bone biopsy systems). *A*, After local anesthetic is administered subcutaneously, a 22-gauge skinny needle (SN) with removable inner stylet is advanced along the desired trajectory to the vertebral body periosteum where additional anesthetic agent is deposited (*arrow*). Shown is a posterolateral extrapedicular approach. VB = vertebral body; L = target lesion. *B*, The 22-gauge needle inner stylet is removed. A wire is placed coaxially into the 22-gauge skinny needle cannula (SNC), and the tip of the wire is advanced to the vertebral body periosteum within the SNC. The cannula hub is then removed. VB = vertebral body, L = target lesion. *C*, A blunt-tipped inner cannula (IC) is inserted coaxially into the outer cannula (OC) of the biopsy needle, and both are advanced over the stiffener wire (W) and skinny needle outer cannula (not visible) to the level of the periosteum. VB = vertebral body; L = target lesion; H = hub of outer cannula biopsy needle.

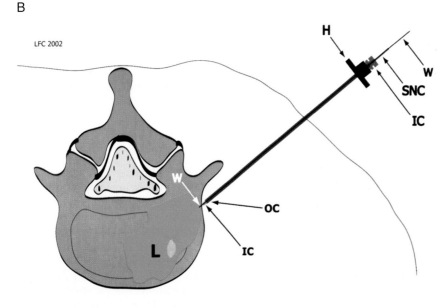

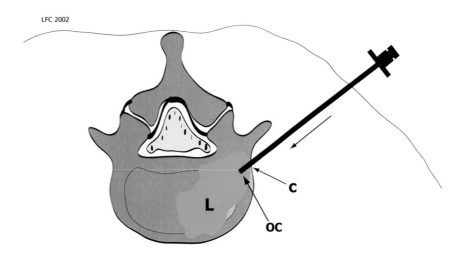

D

Figure 7-9 (*Cont'd*) ▪ *D*, After removing the blunt-tipped inner cannula, the skinny needle cannula and the wire, the outer cannula (OC) of the biopsy needle is advanced (*arrow*) through the vertebral body cortex (C) by inserting with a twisting motion. A handle (not shown) may be required for better leverage when advancing the biopsy needle through the cortex. L = target lesion. *E*, Optional step. Initial biopsy specimens may be obtained with another biopsy needle (BN1), which can be inserted coaxially through the larger outer cannula (OC) biopsy needle. To obtain the first specimen the inner biopsy needle is advanced (*arrow*) into the lesion (L) with a rotating motion while suction is applied to the needle hub of the inner biopsy needle. H = hub of outer cannula. *F*, Final biopsy specimen is obtained by advancing (*arrow*) and rotating the large outer cannula (OC) alone into the target lesion (L) while suction is applied to the needle hub to obtain a large core sample. VB = vertebral body.

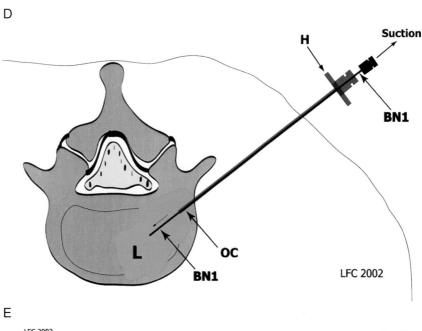

E

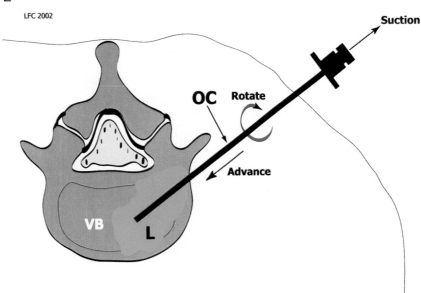

F

Single Needle Technique

A single large-caliber (11- to 16-gauge) or small-caliber (18- to 22-gauge) needle with an inner stylet can be used to biopsy a vertebra or a soft tissue mass. Care must be taken to monitor needle advancement with x-ray fluoroscopy, conventional CT, or real-time CT imaging to ensure that the needle does not puncture a vital structure such as the spinal cord, lung, or large blood vessel. In general, smaller-gauge needles produce less damage to vital structures. This technique is ideal for superficial posterior paraspinal masses, in which the tumor can be safely sampled with repeated needle passes if necessary without risk of damaging deeper structures (Fig. 7-10).

A single-needle technique can also be used to sample the vertebral body or for a posterolateral or transpedicular approach with CT or fluoroscopic guidance. To obtain a sufficient bone core sample, a 16-gauge or larger needle is

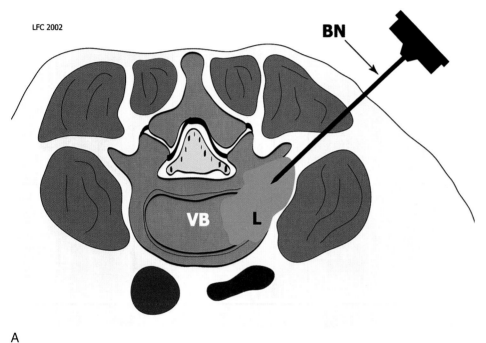

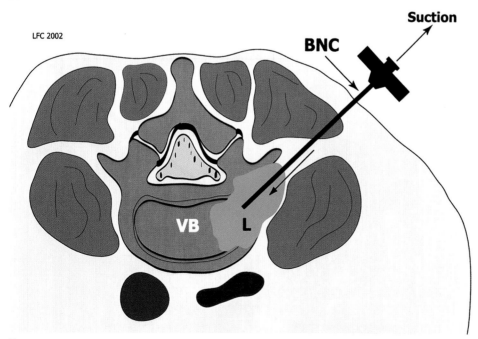

Figure 7-10 ■ Illustration of single needle biopsy approach (fashioned after Temno or Cook Bone biopsy trochar systems). *A,* After subcutaneous and deeper local anesthesia is given, the biopsy needle (BN) and inner trochar are advanced as a single unit into the target lesion (L). VB = vertebral body. *B,* The inner trochar has been removed. The biopsy needle cannula (BNC) is advanced (*arrow*) and rotated into the lesion (L) with suction applied to the biopsy needle hub by a syringe (not shown) connected to the needle hub by an intervening connecting tube (not shown).

recommended. However, only one biopsy sample can be obtained unless repeated passes are made or a coaxial modification of this technique is used.

SPINE BIOPSY TARGET CONSIDERATIONS

Five general spinal/paraspinal locations are considered for needle biopsy or aspiration:

1. Paraspinal soft tissue (anterior or posterior)
2. Vertebral body
3. Posterior vertebral arch
4. Intervertebral disc
5. Epidural space or neural foramen

Paraspinal Soft Tissue Mass

Such a mass may be located in the posterior paraspinal soft tissues or anterior paravertebral soft tissues adjacent to the vertebral body or in the posterior vertebral arch.

Most lesions in this category can be sampled with small-caliber (18- to 22-gauge) needles. Single or multiple needle passes with simple aspiration technique may be sufficient for readily accessible subcutaneous masses or large paravertebral masses. With the use of modern biopsy devices, core biopsy specimens are readily obtained with 18- or 20-gauge needles (e.g., SureCut) or semiautomatic biopsy devices (e.g., Bioptic, Temno, or Medi-tech). The samples obtained are optimally examined by a cytopathologist standing by immediately after biopsy to determine whether the sample obtained is conclusive or sufficient in quantity. If it is inconclusive, larger-core samples may be obtained with a 16-gauge needle biopsy device. For deeper paravertebral soft tissue, passing a coaxial system with a 14- or 16-gauge outer cannula is preferable, because it allows several passes into the soft tissue mass with an 18- or 20-gauge core-biopsy needle coaxially. Another advantage is that the outer cannula can usually be directed in slightly different trajectories, allowing biopsy of the mass in different locations by the selected coaxial needle biopsy system.

Vertebral Body Mass

For the vertebral body, the most commonly sampled portion of the vertebra, either a transpedicular approach or an extrapedicular posterolateral approach can be used. The vertebral body may be percutaneously sampled by means of a direct puncture, a single-needle technique, a coaxial system, or a tandem needle placement technique.

Posterior Vertebral Arch

The posterior vertebral arch is not commonly selected as a site of percutaneous biopsy. Primary tumors that arise in the vertebral arch are usually sampled by means of open surgical techniques. Care should be taken in percutaneous needle biopsy of the vertebral arch to avoid placing the needle in the spinal canal and damaging the spinal cord or nerve

rootlets within the thecal sac. CT, preferably with CT fluoroscopy, is the image guidance method of choice.

Intervertebral Disc Biopsy/Aspiration

Needle aspiration or core biopsy techniques using large- or small-caliber needles can be used to obtain disc material. An x-ray fluoroscopically guided approach is the most straightforward method for disc biopsy in the lumbar, thoracic, or cervical region. In the thoracic region, some operators feel more comfortable using CT guidance for disc aspiration to avoid inadvertent needle placement into the lung or the spinal canal.

Epidural or Foraminal Mass

The neural foramen or epidural compartments should not be sampled unless other sites are inaccessible for biopsy, because injury to the spinal cord or nerve roots is possible. Furthermore, the operator should have a clear understanding of his or her own abilities and the operation of the biopsy device being used. Unless there is a large epidural mass, a core biopsy specimen is usually not obtained. The goal in biopsy of the epidural space or foraminal soft tissues is collection of a small amount of tissue for cytologic examination using a small-caliber needle. Extra caution should be exercised in sampling epidural masses because biopsy of these lesions can produce local tissue swelling or bleeding, which could compress and compromise the nerve rootlets of the cauda equina or spinal cord.

SELECTION OF NEEDLE BIOPSY SYSTEM

The number of spine biopsy systems commercially available are too numerous to mention, and it is not our intention to do so. We mention specific needle biopsy systems only because they provide specific examples that we are familiar with in our particular practice and because they help illustrate the general instructional message of this chapter. It is important to note here that **we do not advocate or recommend a specific vendor or needle biopsy system as having an advantage over another. We receive no financial support from any of these vendors and are not shareholders in any of the companies that manufacture these needle biopsy systems.**

It is preferable that physicians performing biopsies become proficient at using two- or three-needle biopsy systems at most, based on their training and personal experience. If the operator is unfamiliar with a given needle set, it is best to seek training in the proper handling and use of the needle set for patient safety and optimal tissue sample recovery. The needle biopsy apparatus chosen is based on the location and type of mass being sampled and the familiarity of the operator with the given needle biopsy system.

A variety of bone biopsy needles are available on the market, any of which may be sufficient for recovering adequate bone biopsy specimens. All are designed to obtain a relatively large core specimen of bone (1.5 to 2.0 mm in diameter) and are therefore relatively large in caliber (i.e., 11 to 16 gauge). The Craig needle, which has traditionally been popular for CT and fluoroscopic-guided spine biopsy for many years, can provide a core sample 3 mm in diameter.[29] In general, larger biopsy needles provide better specimen samples for the pathologist to examine.[12]

Whichever needle biopsy system is chosen, the needle should always be used in accordance with the manufacturer's technical recommendations and guidelines. Careful attention must be paid to technique in placing these needle systems, because it is possible to cause damage to a blood vessel, nerve root, spinal cord, or pleura, especially with the large-caliber bone biopsy needles. **Therefore, frequent fluoroscopic or CT imaging is performed to ensure that the needle does not deviate from the intended pathway.**

EXAMPLES OF NEEDLE BIOPSY SYSTEMS

Temno™ Bone Biopsy Needle (Fig. 7-11)

- Available from Bauer Medical, Inc. (Clearwater, FL). Temno is a registered trademark of Allegiance Healthcare.
- 8-gauge, 11-, 13-, or 15-cm length (blue)
- 9-gauge, 11- or 13-cm length (green)
- 11-gauge, 11- or 13-cm length (red)
- 12-gauge, 11- or 13-cm length (orange)
- 13-gauge, 7- or 11-cm length (white)
- Diamond-shaped point inner stylet
- Oblique, sharp beveled tip of outer cannula for cutting through bone

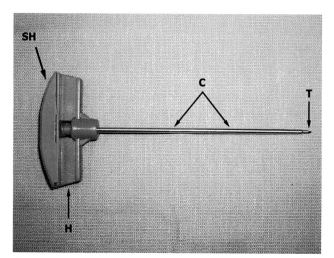

A

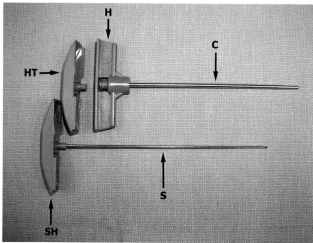

B

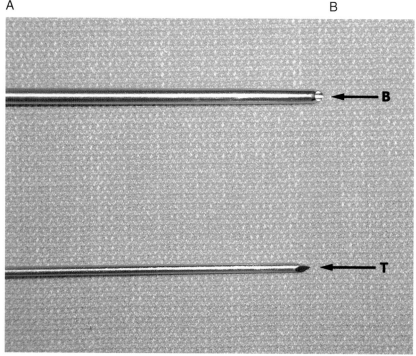

C

Figure 7-11 ■ Temno Bone Biopsy Needle System. *A*, Eleven-gauge Temno Bone biopsy nedle showing inner pointed-tip stylet (T) inserted and locked into place within outer cannula (C). H = handle component of outer cannula; SH = handle component of inner stylet. *B*, Components of the biopsy needle are separated. HT = handle top locks into handle component of cannula for better grip on handle when advancing outer cannula into bone with inner stylet (S) removed. *C*, Magnified view of oblique sharp bevel (B) of distal outer cannula and diamond point tip (T) of stylet. (*Temno™ is a registered trademark of Allegiance Healthcare. Photographed with permission from Allegiance Healthcare, McGaw Park, IL.*)

- Handle is "T" shaped with stylet portion of T-handle locking into cannula portion of the T-handle
- Metal obturator for pushing collected sample core from inside the cannula

Method

The T-handle portion of the inner stylet and T-handle portion of the outer cannula are joined together. The diamond point needle is advanced to the proximal margin of the lesion. The inner stylet is removed. The stylet handle is replaced with the plastic handle, which locks into the cannula T-handle. The handle is rotated while the outer cannula is advanced to obtain a bone sample. Alternatively, one can apply suction to the hub of the needle with a connecting tube attached to a syringe while collecting the sample. Other smaller needles can be used coaxially through the Temno cannula to collect multiple smaller tissue samples before obtaining a large-core sample with the outer cannula biopsy needle.

Geremia Needle Biopsy System
(Fig. 7-12)

- Available from Cook Incorporated (Bloomington, IN)
- 22-gauge, 25-cm introducer "skinny" needle with inner stylet (has removable plastic hub)
- 40-cm stiffener wire
- 16-gauge, 15.5-cm bone biopsy needle cannula with 1-cm markers and Franseen tip
- 16-cm, coaxial tapered introduction cannula
- Black knob (fits biopsy needle hub with or without inner cannula)
- Blunt-tipped obturator

Method

The 22-gauge, 25-cm introducer needle with stylet is placed at the periosteal margin of the vertebral body or at the disc margin at the desired location. The inner stylet is removed, and local anesthetic is given through the 22-gauge needle. The 40-cm stiffener wire is inserted through the 22-gauge cannula. This makes an exchange-length wire after the plastic hub is removed (unscrewed) from the 22-gauge introducer needle. The 16-cm tapered introduction cannula is placed through the 15.5-cm bone biopsy needle and screwed together (biopsy system). The tapered introduction cannula projects approximately 5 mm past the tip of the bone biopsy needle. The biopsy system is advanced over the exchange wire. The biopsy system is gently rotated and advanced over the wire until it contacts the bone or the disc margin. The exchange wire is removed. If the lesion is deep to the cortical margin or if a deep disc biopsy is to be performed, the inner cannula should remain attached to the biopsy needle. The black knob can be placed on the hub on the introducer needle and advanced to the proximal margin of the lesion. Once the biopsy system is at the proximal margin of the lesion, the inner cannula is removed. A 20-mL syringe is connected to the hub of the biopsy needle through a con-

necting tube to apply light continuous negative pressure to keep the specimen within the needle. The specimen is obtained by rotating the biopsy needle back and forth with mild, steady forward advancement. The biopsy needle is removed by using slow back-and-forth rotational movement while continuous gentle syringe suction is applied. The obturator is used to push the sample from the biopsy needle. One can also use smaller-caliber, longer needles through the Geremia needle for a coaxial biopsy to obtain a greater number of specimen samples.

The advantage of introducing a skinny needle initially is that it provides a safe guiding pathway for the larger coaxial needle to follow. If no radicular symptoms occur during insertion of the skinny needle, one is confident that insertion of the large-caliber needle will not cause significant injury to a nearby nerve.

Elson Bone Biopsy Needle Set
(Fig. 7-13)

- Available from Cook Incorporated (Bloomington, IN)
- 22-gauge, 25-cm introducer "skinny" needle with inner stylet (has removable plastic hub)
- 12-gauge, 14-cm blunt-tip outer cannula with tapered inner cannula
- 14-gauge, 17.1-cm bone biopsy needle cannula with 5-pointed Franseen tip and inner blunt-tipped obturator
- 14-gauge, 18.3-cm bone biopsy needle cannula with 5-pointed Franseen-type tip and inner blunt tipped obturator

Method

The 22-gauge, 25-cm introducer needle is placed at the periosteal margin of the vertebral body or at the disc margin at the desired location. The inner stylet is removed, and local anesthetic is given through the 22-gauge needle. A 40-cm stiffener wire is not packaged with the Elson system as it is in the Geremia system. However, we find that this 40-cm wire is advantageous; by allowing sufficient exchange length so that the wire is exposed when the biopsy system is coaxially placed, it permits the operator control of the wire at all times. The 40-cm wire used in the Geremia system can be purchased separately for this purpose. The 40-cm long stiffener wire is inserted through the 22-gauge introducer needle. The plastic hub is removed (unscrewed) from the 22-gauge introducer needle. The blunt inner cannula is placed through the 12-gauge blunt outer cannula (biopsy needle). These two needles **do not** connect (unlike the Geremia system); therefore, they must be held together by the operator as they are advanced through tissue and/or bone, which can be difficult at times. The exchange wire is removed. The two-piece biopsy system is advanced to the proximal margin of the target lesion. The blunt inner cannula is removed. Two 14-gauge Franseen-type tipped needles, 17.1 cm and 18.3 cm in length, are supplied for coaxial biopsy. One or both of these needles can be used to obtain specimens from different sites. In addition, other, smaller caliber, longer needles can be used in coaxial fashion through the outer cannula for biopsy and/or aspiration. Once these specimens have been obtained, a final biopsy is acquired with the 12-gauge needle.

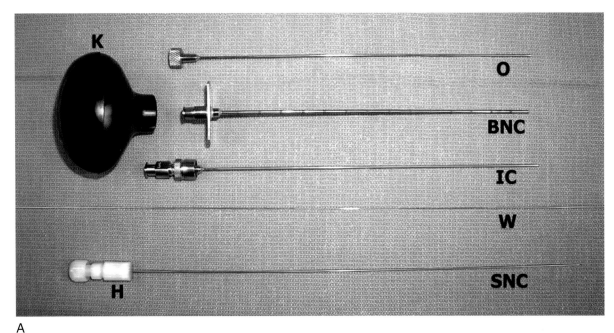

A

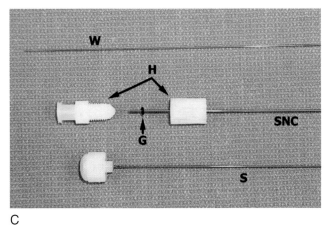

B

C

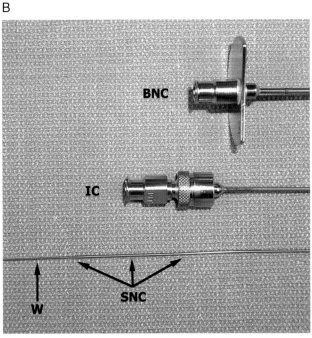

D

Figure 7-12 ■ Geremia Biopsy Needle Set (Cook Incorporated, Bloomington, IN). *A*, The biopsy set components include one 22-gauge, 25-cm introducer skinny needle cannula (SNC), with inner stylet shown inserted and removable plastic hub (H); one 40-cm stiffener wire (W); one 16-gauge, 15.5 cm bone biopsy needle cannula (BNC) with Franseen-type tip; and one 16-cm coaxial tapered introduction cannula (IC). Black knob (K) fits over biopsy needle when inner cannula is not in place for better grip when advancing biopsy needle. A blunt-tipped obturator (O) is used to push the collected specimen from the biopsy needle. *B*, The proximal end of separated skinny needle system. The skinny needle cannula (SNC) has a plastic removable hub (H). Inner stylet (S) has a plastic nonremovable hub (SH). *C*, The proximal end of the skinny needle cannula (SNC) showing components of removable plastic hub (H), rubber grommet (G), and proximal end of the skinny needle stylet. The 40-cm stiffener wire (W) can be placed coaxially through the skinny needle cannula prior to hub removal. *D*, The proximal end of Geremia coaxial system showing the hub of the biopsy needle cannula (BNC) separated from the hub of the introducing cannula (IC). The 40-cm stiffener wire (W) has been inserted coaxially into the skinny needle cannula (SNC) (with its plastic hub removed).

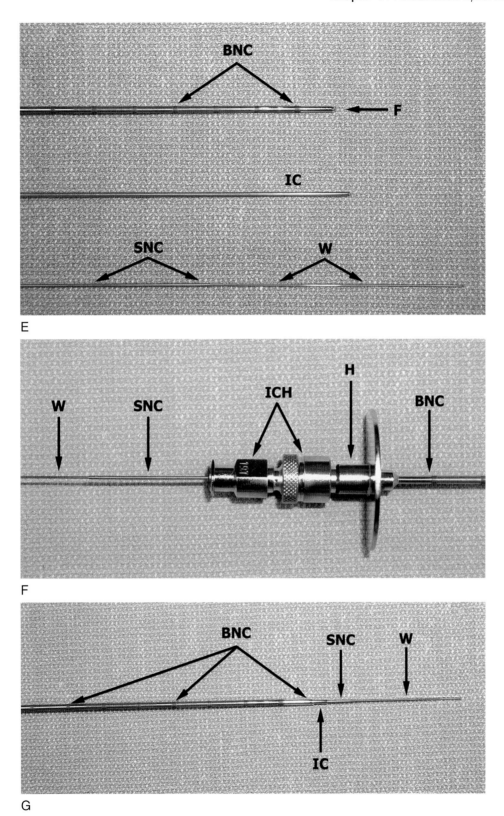

Figure 7-12 (*Cont'd*) ■ *E,* The distal end of biopsy system corresponding to D. The biopsy needle cannula (BNC) has 1-cm markers and a Franseen-type tip (F). The introducing cannula (IC) is separate from the biopsy needle. The distal end of the skinny needle cannula (SNC) is shown with the stiffener wire (W) coaxially within it. *F,* The proximal end of Geremia system is positioned coaxially. From left to right, the 40-cm stiffener wire (W) has been inserted into the skinny needle cannula (SNC), which in turn has been inserted into the introducer cannula hub (ICH), which is connected to the hub (H) of the biopsy needle cannula (BNC). *G,* The distal end of the Geremia coaxial system corresponding to F with components in place. From left to right is the biopsy needle cannula (BNC), introducer cannula (IC), skinny needle cannula (SNC), and 40-cm stiffener wire (W). (*Photographed with permission of Cook Incorporated, Bloomington, IN.*)

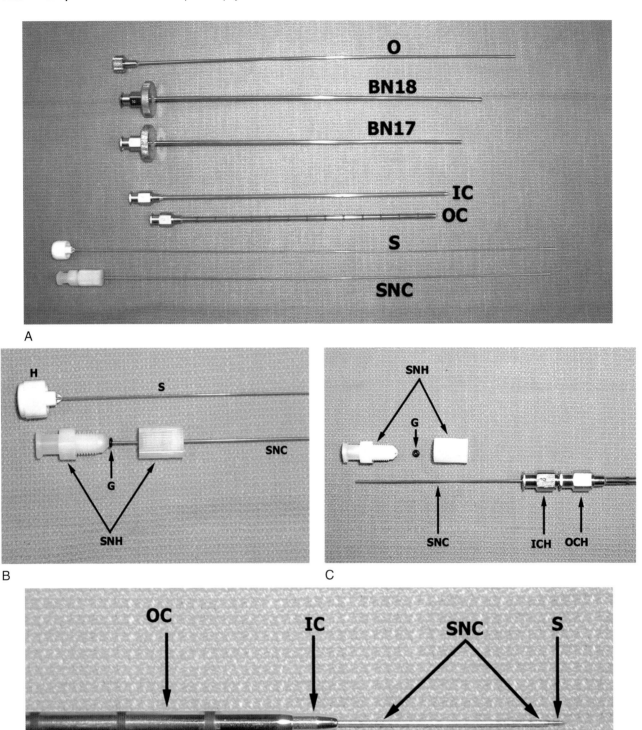

Figure 7-13 ■ Elson Bone Biopsy System (Cook Incorporated, Bloomington, IN). *A,* The biopsy system includes a 22-gauge, 25-cm skinny needle cannula (SNC) with removable plastic hub and with inner stylet (S); a 12-gauge blunt tapered-tip outer cannula (OC) and tapered-tip inner cannula (IC); a 14-gauge, 17.1-cm bone biopsy needle (BN17) with a five-pointed Franseen-type tip and inner blunt-tipped obturator; a 14-gauge, 18.3-cm bone biopsy needle (BN18) with a five-pointed Franseen-type tip; and two identical blunt-tipped obturators (O) (only one shown) for pushing the collected specimen from the biopsy needles. *B,* The skinny needle components include the inner stylet (S) and its plastic hub (H), the skinny needle cannula (SNC), its removable hub (SNH), and grommet (G). *C,* The proximal end of Elson coaxial system before biopsy needle insertion showing from left to right the skinny needle cannula (SNC); inner cannula hub (ICH); outer cannula hub (OCH) and components of the skinny needle removable plastic hub (SNH); and its grommet (G). *D,* The distal end of Elson coaxial system before biopsy needle insertion showing from left to right the outer cannula (OC); inner cannula (IC); skinny needle cannula (SNC); and stylet (S).

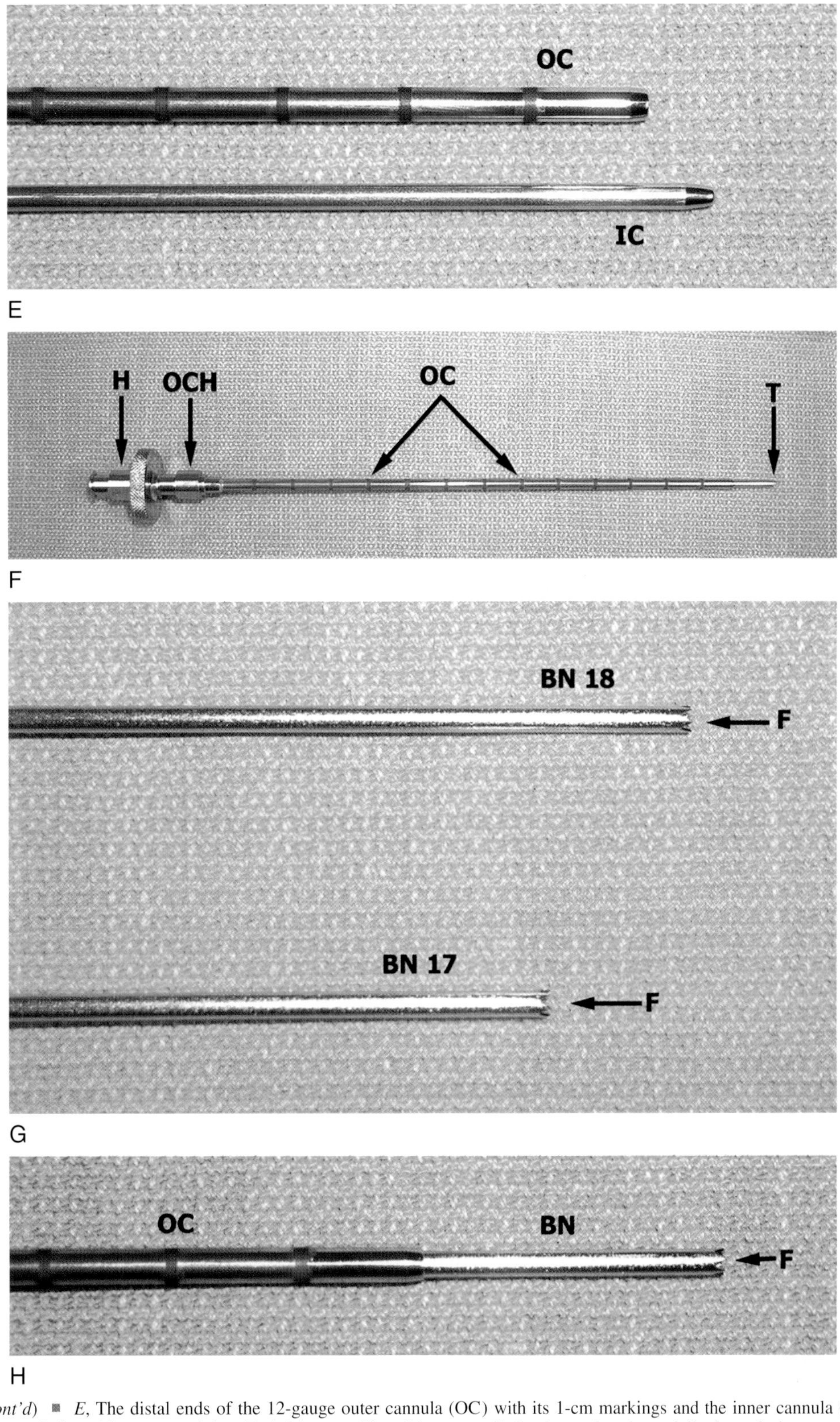

Figure 7-13 (*Cont'd*) ■ *E*, The distal ends of the 12-gauge outer cannula (OC) with its 1-cm markings and the inner cannula (IC). Both the outer cannula and inner cannula have blunt, tapered tips. *F*, A 14-gauge Elson biopsy needle has been placed coaxially through the outer cannula (OC), with 1-cm marks. OCH = outer cannula hub; T = biopsy needle tip; H = biopsy needle hub. *G*, The distal ends of the 17.1-cm and 18.3-cm Elson biopsy needles (BN17 and BN18, respectively) each with a Franseen-type tip (F). *H*, The distal end of 14-gauge Elson biopsy needle (BN) with Franseen tip (F) has been inserted coaxially through the 12-gauge outer cannula (OC). Note 1-cm markings on the outer cannula. (*Photographed with permission of Cook Incorporated, Bloomington, IN.*)

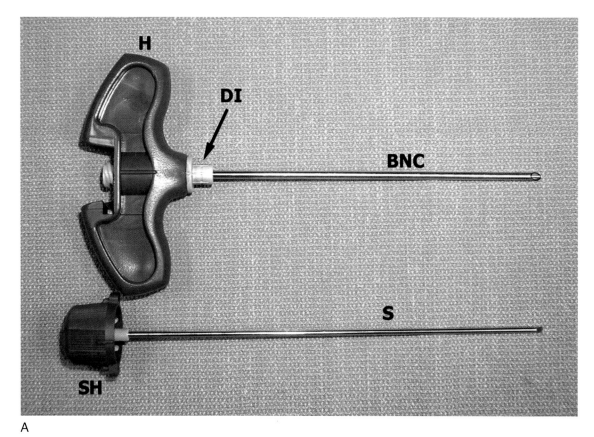

A

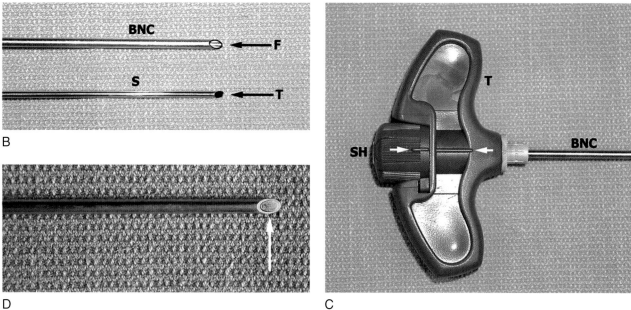

B

D

C

Figure 7-14 ■ Osteo-Site M1 Bone Biopsy Needle (Cook Incorporated, Bloomington, IN). *A*, Components include biopsy needle cannula (BNC), which has a T-shaped handle (H). Needle stylet (S) has a hub (SH) that fits into the hub on the T-handle. DI = sliding depth indicator. *B*, A close-up view of beveled tip (T) of stylet (S) and beveled face (F) of the biopsy needle cannula (BNC). *C*, A close-up view of the biopsy needle with the inner stylet locked in place. Note that the notch (*arrow*) on stylet hub (SH) aligns with notch (*arrow*) on the T-handle (H) of the biopsy needle cannula (BNC). *D*, A close-up view of the beveled needle tip with the beveled inner stylet tip inserted into the cannula, resulting in a smooth, single bevel face (*arrow*). (*Photographed with permission of Cook Incorporated, Bloomington, IN.*)

Osteo-Site Bone Biopsy Needle
(Fig. 7-14)

- Available from Cook Incorporated (Bloomington, IN)
- 11-gauge, 10-cm triple-pointed beveled outer cannula
- Diamond-tip inner stylet with small knob

Method

The inner stylet is locked into the T-handle of the outer cannula. The notch on the inner stylet knob must align with the notch on the outer cannula handle so that the diamond tip aligns properly with the triple-pointed bevel of the outer cannula. The biopsy system is advanced to the proximal margin of the lesion. The inner stylet is removed. A 20-mL syringe is attached to the hub of the needle cannula by means of a connecting tube. Gentle suction is applied to the needle while the cannula is rotated and advanced to collect the bone sample. The needle is removed while maintaining continuous gentle suction. The metal obturator is used to displace the core sample from the cannula. Again, smaller, longer biopsy needles can be placed coaxially through the bone biopsy needle to collect other smaller tissue samples before the large core is obtained with the primary biopsy needle.

TSK SureCut Modified Menghini Biopsy Needle (Fig. 7-15)

- Available from TSK Laboratory, Japan; SureCut Biopsy needle, Boston Scientific/Medi-tech
- Modified stainless steel Menghini needle with a beveled tip
- Needle calibers available: 15, 16, 17, 18, 19, 21, and 22 gauge
- Needle lengths available: 4, 5, 7, 9, 10, 12, 15, and 23 cm
- Needle removable from biopsy syringe
- Syringe plunger permanently attached to inner pencil-point stylet

Method

When the plunger is pushed into the syringe, the needle tip of the inner stylet protrudes from the needle cannula. The needle is advanced into the target biopsy tissue. The plunger of the biopsy syringe is withdrawn until the plastic clip stopper locks in place to apply negative pressure. The needle is briskly advanced a few millimeters into the target tissue while rotating 360 degrees to collect the specimen. The needle is removed from the tissue, while continuing to apply suction with the clip lock in place. When one is ready to

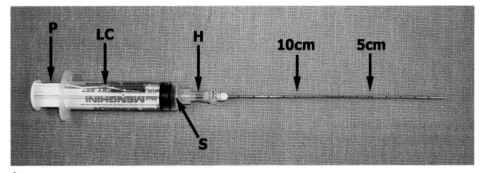

Figure 7-15 ▪ TSK SureCut Modified Menghini Biopsy Needle. *A,* The biopsy needle and inner stylet are in place. The plastic locking clip (LC) is part of the syringe plunger (P). The inner stylet (S) is attached to the black plunger piston tip. The plastic hub (H) of the biopsy needle cannula can be removed from the syringe. Note that the marks on the biopsy needle are in 1-cm increments, with double marks located 5 cm and 10 cm from the needle tip. *B,* Suction is applied to the needle tip before specimen collection by withdrawing plunger (P) until the plastic locking clip (LC) catches on the proximal margin of the syringe barrel (B), which maintains the suction. The inner stylet (S) is visible through the distal portion of the syringe. (*SureCut Biopsy needle, Boston Scientific/Medi-tech, photographed with permission.*)

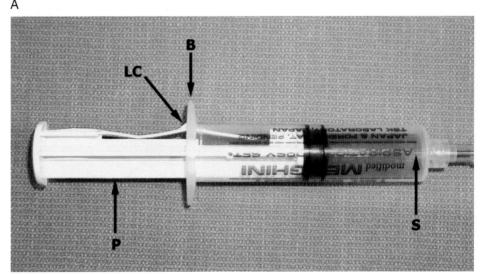

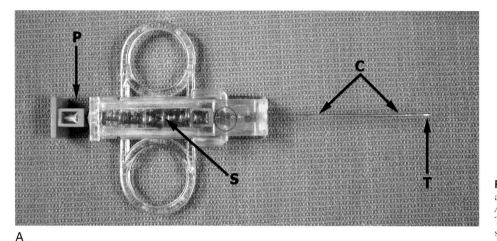

A

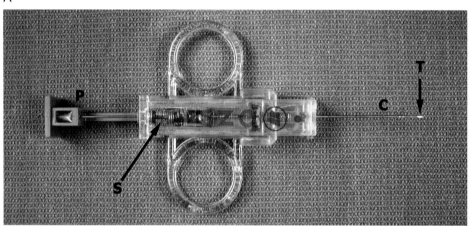

B

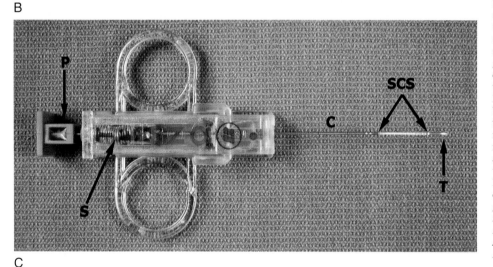

C

Figure 7-16 ■ Temno Semi-automated Throw Biopsy Needle. *A*, The pre- and post-firing positions. The appearance of the biopsy needle system is the same before the plunger (P) is cocked and after the biopsy needle is fired. Note that the spring (S) within the syringe chamber is relaxed. C = outer cannula of biopsy needle; T = tip of inner stylet. *B*, The device cocked with the inner stylet still covered by the needle cannula. The plunger (P) has been pulled back, causing retraction of both the needle cannula (C) and the inner stylet into the plastic syringe. Note that the spring (S) in the syringe is in a cocked position. Only the tip (T) of the inner stylet projects beyond the needle cannula as in A. *C*, The device is cocked, with the inner stylet exposed, and is now in position to collect the specimen. With the spring (S) still cocked, the plunger (P) has been pushed forward to allow the stylet specimen collection segment (SCS) to project from the cannula (C) Note that the stylet collection segment is seen en face in the photograph. T = stylet needle tip. *D*, The device is cocked as in C. A close-up tangential view of the specimen collection segment (SCS) of the stylet before the sample is collected. When the plunger is pushed to fire the mechanism, the needle cannula (C) moves in the direction of the long arrow toward the fixed stylet tip (T), which traps the specimen in the collection segment. After firing, the device will look identical to photograph A. (*Temno™ is a registered trademark of Allegiance Healthcare. Photographed with permission from Allegiance Healthcare, McGaw Park, IL.*)

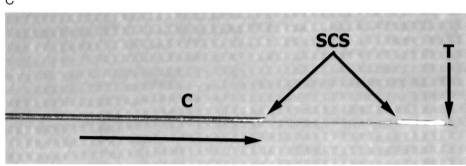

D

deposit the sample onto a slide or into a collection tube, the plastic plunger clip is released by gently pushing the plunger in until the inner stylet pushes the sample out of the needle cannula. This biopsy needle may be used alone for a single pass into a soft tissue mass or coaxially through a larger-caliber needle.

Temno Adjustable Throw Biopsy Device (Fig. 7-16)

- Available from Bauer Medical, Inc., Clearwater, FL. Temno is a registered trademark of Allegiance Healthcare.
- 18-gauge, 6-, 9-, 15-, and 20-cm length (orange)
- 20-gauge, 6-, 9-, 15,- and 20-cm length (green)
- 22-gauge, 6-, 9-, 15,- and 20-cm length (gray)
- Nonremovable notched inner stylet
- Spring-loaded mechanism, semiautomated gun mechanism

Before using this needle, the operator must be keenly aware of the tissues in and near the intended target tissue being sampled that could be within the throw length of the needle, to avoid injury to important normal anatomic structures such as blood vessels or neural tissue.

Method

The needle is advanced to the proximal margin of the lesion. The spring-loaded gun is cocked by withdrawing the plunger, which pulls the inner stylet and cannula back a short distance. The biopsy system is held by placing one's thumb on the plunger and two fingers through the loops. The plunger is advanced halfway to allow the notched portion of the distal stylet to project into the tissue to be sampled. To obtain the biopsy specimen with this needle, the plunger is pushed in the remainder of the way to activate the biopsy system. The outer cannula snaps forward over the inner stylet, and a small piece of tissue is captured in the notched portion of the stylet.

This needle system can be used coaxially through a larger caliber biopsy needle.

LUMBAR SPINE BIOPSY PROCEDURES

Vertebral Body Biopsy

Two basic approaches are used to obtain bone core samples from the vertebral body: the *transpedicular* approach and the *extrapedicular posterolateral* approach (Fig. 7-17). Either can be used for disease processes that completely replace a given lumbar vertebral body, and either can be performed with CT or x-ray fluoroscopic guidance. The posterolateral approach or the transpedicular approach using CT guidance is preferred for smaller vertebral body lesions. The extrapedicular approach is also used when the target is a paraspinal soft tissue mass. The transpedicular approach with x-ray fluoroscopic guidance is preferred when the vertebral body has been completely replaced by tumor and precise positioning of the needle in the vertebral body is not

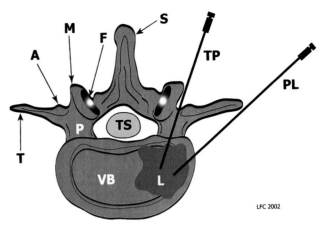

Figure 7-17 ■ Illustration of the lumbar vertebral body biopsy needle approaches. A biopsy needle inserted using the transpedicular approach (TP) enters the pedicle in a groove between the mamillary process (M) (of the superior articular process) and the accessory process (A) (of the transverse process). The needle traverses the pedicle long axis before entering the vertebral body (VB) target lesion (L). A biopsy needle, inserted using the posterolateral approach (PL), courses through the soft tissues lateral to the transverse process (T) and pedicle (P) before entering the vertebral body cortex. S = spinous process; TS = thecal sac; F = articular facet.

critical, because it can be performed more expeditiously. Some prefer a transpedicular approach for vertebral body biopsy for tumor diagnosis because of the shorter distance the needle must traverse to reach the intended target and to minimize the theoretical risk of disseminating malignant cells in paraspinal tissues, such as into the pleural cavity.[17]

Transpedicular Approach: Fluoroscopic Guidance

Depending on the location of the lesion in the vertebral body, the C-arm fluoroscope is rotated 10 to 30 degrees in oblique position on the ipsilateral side of the lesion until the eye of the "Scotty dog," representing the pedicle, is optimally seen (see Fig. 7-1). A large-caliber needle (11- to 16-gauge) with diamond-pointed stylet (e.g., Osteo-Site, Cook) is passed through the paraspinal soft tissues to the pedicle under direct fluoroscopic visualization (Fig. 7-18). After the needle tip has been centered on the pedicle, the needle handle is gripped and forward manual pressure is applied to the needle while the needle tip is rotated through the cortex. It is advantageous to hold the handle with one hand and the needle at the skin surface with the other hand as one would hold a pencil. This keeps the needle shaft straight. Special care is taken not to penetrate the medial cortex of the pedicle. When the cortex is penetrated by the diamond-pointed needle, a release in resistance is felt. The needle tip is advanced to the proximal margin of the lesion. A biopsy specimen may be obtained with the large outer needle biopsy cannula at this juncture, but it is preferable to remove the inner stylet and coaxially place a smaller-gauge needle of greater length (e.g., 14-gauge Elson, Geremia needle biopsy set,[30] or 18-gauge SureCut), through the larger needle cannula. This allows retrieval of one or more specimens before the larger core biopsy specimen is obtained with the larger biopsy needle.

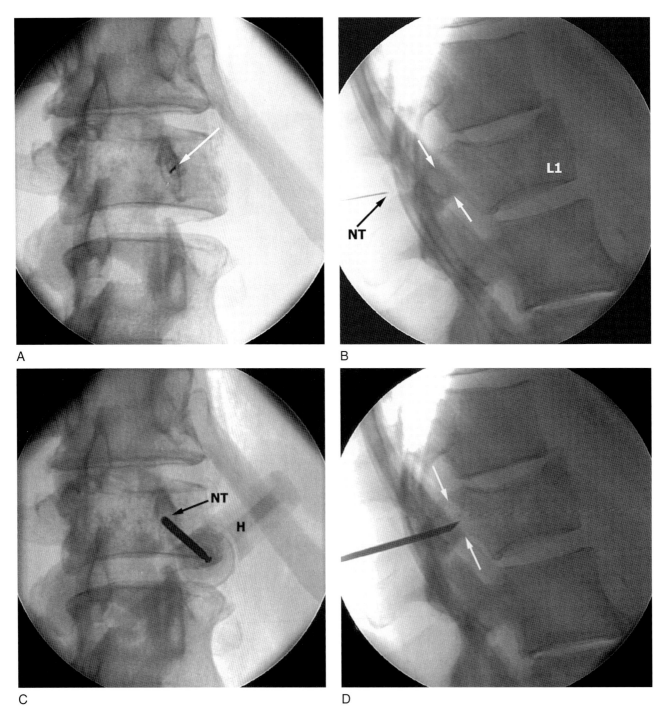

A

B

C

D

Figure 7-18 ■ Transpedicular biopsy of L1 in a patient with metastatic lung carcinoma. *A*, An LAO radiograph at the L1 level demonstrates an 18-gauge spinal needle (*arrow*) superimposed over the right pedicle of L1. *B*, Lateral radiograph. An 18-gauge spinal needle with the needle tip (NT) projecting posterior to the L1 pedicle (*arrows*). Note the compression fracture of the L1 vertebral body. *C*, In the same projection, an 11-gauge Cook M1 biopsy needle has been inserted into the pedicle. NT = needle tip; H = needle handle. *D*, Lateral radiograph. The biopsy needle tip projects over the L1 pedicle (*between arrows*).

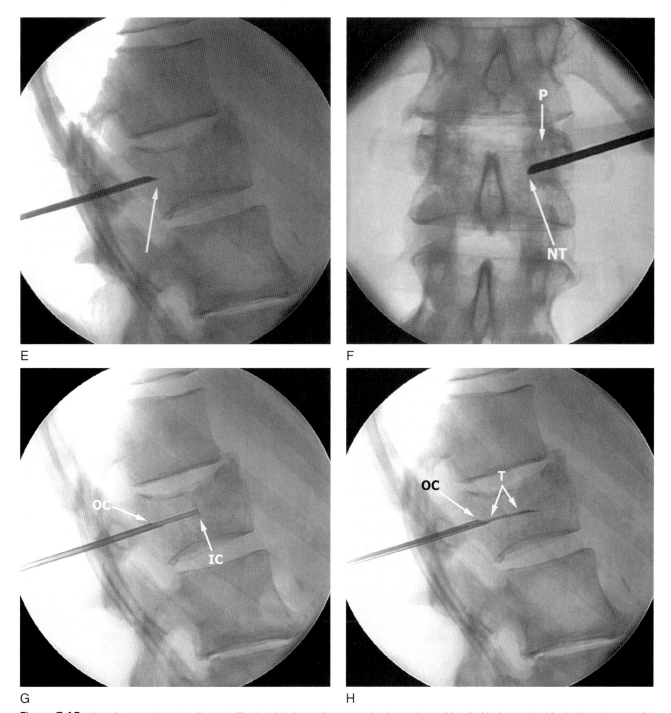

E

F

G

H

Figure 7-18 (*Cont'd*) ■ *E*, Lateral radiograph. The beveled-tip needle (*arrow*) has been advanced just inside the vertebral body along the posterior margin of the region to be sampled. *F*, Corresponding AP radiograph for E showing the appearance of the needle in the vertebral body. The pedicle (P) projects over the superolateral aspect of the vertebral body. The needle tip (NT) projects over vertebral body just before obtaining the biopsy specimens. *G*, The initial specimen sample is obtained. Lateral radiograph shows the coaxially placed inner cannula (IC) (a 14-gauge Franseen-tipped Elson biopsy needle), which extends into the target zone of the L1 vertebral body beyond the beveled outer cannula (OC) of the Cook M1 biopsy needle. *H*, A second specimen is obtained by placing an 18-gauge Temno (T) semiautomated biopsy needle system coaxially through the beveled outer cannula (OC) of the Cook M1 biopsy needle.

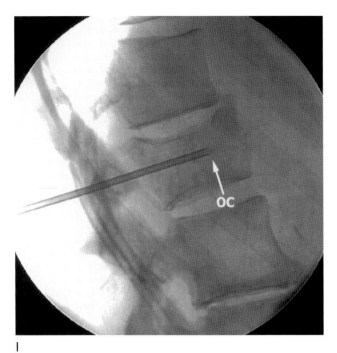
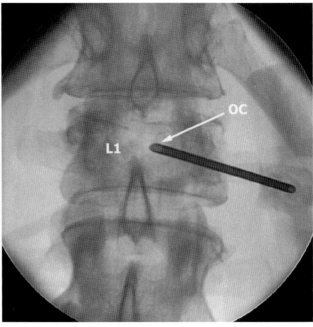

I   J

Figure 7-18 (*Cont'd*) ■ *I,* Lateral radiograph showing position of the Cook M1 larger-caliber outer cannula (OC) after it has been advanced (with syringe suction and without the inner stylet) into the L1 vertebral body for obtaining a third large-core specimen. *J,* Corresponding AP radiograph for I showing position of Cook M1 larger-caliber outer cannula (OC) after it has been advanced into the L1 vertebral body during the application of syringe suction on the needle hub.

Transpedicular Approach: CT Guidance

The only difference between x-ray fluoroscopic guidance and CT guidance is that a radiopaque grid or other radiopaque marker is placed on the skin surface to help localize the lesion. The needle biopsy set used can be identical to that used for the fluoroscopic transpedicular biopsy.

The bone entry site into the pedicle along the posterior surface of the vertebra is a groove formed between the mamillary process medially and the transverse process laterally (Fig. 7-19). If real-time CT fluoroscopy is available on the CT scanner, this can be used to monitor the progress of needle advancement under direct visualization. This method saves considerable time in comparison with the older CT method of obtaining repeated image slices through a region of tissue to observe needle advancement. Local anesthetic should be administered to the periosteum before the needle tip is advanced through the cortex and into the pedicle. Once the needle has been positioned at the proximal margin of the lesion, the biopsy procedure is otherwise identical to that used for fluoroscopic transpedicular biopsy. The outer cannula can be advanced slightly or withdrawn to allow sampling at different positions within the vertebral body with the inner coaxial biopsy needle.

Posterolateral Extrapedicular Approach

This approach is optimally done with CT guidance for direct visualization of small bone lesions that involve only a portion of the vertebral body. The entry site chosen is located more laterally than that for the transpedicular approach (Fig. 7-20). With the use of a single, tandem, or coaxial needle technique, an 11- to 16-gauge bone biopsy needle is advanced under CT guidance to the periosteal margin. Local anesthetic is deposited at the periosteum. The stylet is then placed into the biopsy needle cannula. The goal is to position the needle along the posterolateral vertebral body margin so that the needle is perpendicular to the curving vertebral body cortex. A perpendicular entry into the cortex will prevent the needle tip from sliding anteriorly.

The greatest difficulty encountered is in penetrating the vertebral cortex. A diamond-pointed stylet needle tip often facilitates passage of the needle through the cortical bone and into the vertebral marrow cavity. Depending on the needle set used, considerable manual effort may be required to push and twist the needle through the cortex, even in situations in which the marrow cavity appears completely replaced by tumor on MR imaging or CT. For this purpose, bone biopsy needle sets usually come with various designs of handles or knobs to allow the operator sufficient grip for torquing and advancing the needle through the cortex.

Once the large needle has been positioned in the bone to be sampled, it is preferable to obtain several smaller core tissue samples with a smaller-caliber, longer biopsy needle (e.g., SureCut, Temno or Elson) placed coaxially through the larger bone biopsy needle and then to finish by obtaining a large-core specimen with the outer cannula of the bone biopsy needle. In this way, multiple bone samples can be obtained without multiple needle passes through tissue; damage to paraspinal soft tissues is thereby minimized. The outer cannula can be slightly advanced or withdrawn to allow biopsy at different positions within the vertebral body lesion with the inner coaxial biopsy needle. Previously described bone biopsy/aspiration techniques for single-needle or coaxial systems are then performed.

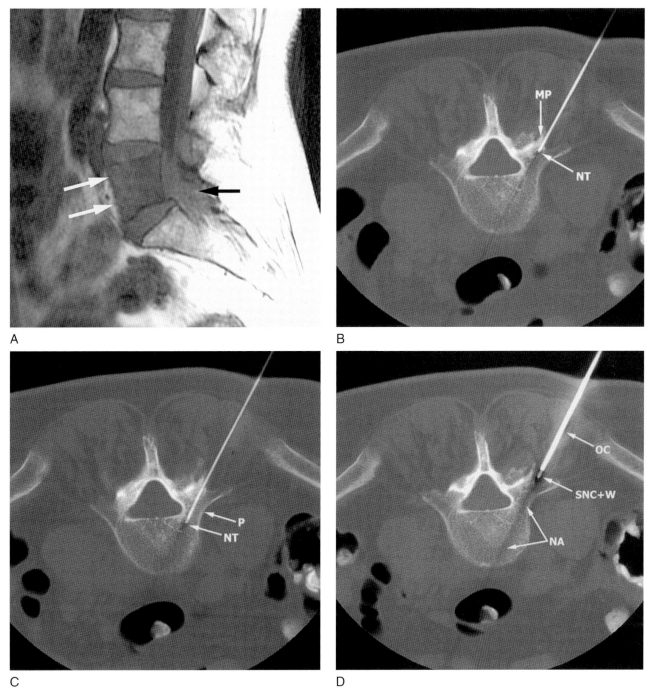

Figure 7-19 ▪ CT-guided L5 transpedicular biopsy. Large cell lymphoma. *A,* T1 sagittal spin-echo MR image. A diffuse marrow-infiltrating process (*white arrows*) involves the entire L5 vertebral body. Epidural soft tissue mass (*black arrow*). *B,* A transpedicular biopsy of the right L5 pedicle with a 17-gauge needle that enters the pedicle in a groove just lateral to the mamillary process (MP). NT = needle tip. *C,* The needle tip (NT) has been advanced into the posterolateral portion of the vertebral body just before obtaining the specimen. P = pedicle. *D,* An additional biopsy is performed with the Elson needle system. Elson biopsy needle with the skinny needle and wire (SNC+W) projecting from the outer cannula (OC). Note that the needle artifact (NA) projects along the expected needle trajectory into the vertebral body.

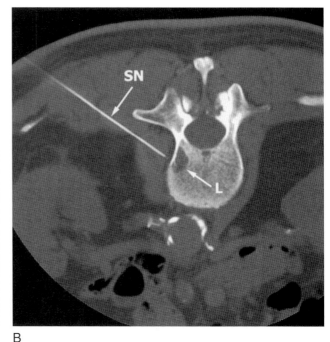

A

B

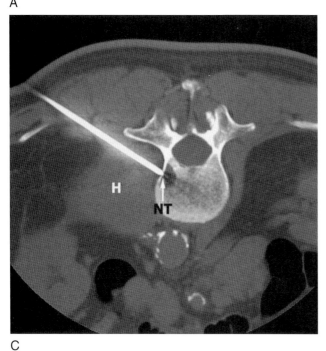

C

Figure 7-20 ■ CT-guided biopsy of a small L1 vertebral body lesion with a posterolateral approach. *A,* The skin surface grid has been applied for localization purposes. The trajectory (T) from skin entry site (S) to target lesion (L) in left lateral margin of L1 vertebral body. P = psoas muscle. *B,* The skinny needle (SN) has been inserted with its tip adjacent to the left lateral cortex of the vertebral body. L = target lesion. *C,* The Elson biopsy needle tip (NT) penetrates the vertebral body cortex just before the needle is advanced into the target lesion. H = psoas muscle hematoma.

Paraspinal Soft Tissue Mass Biopsy

Paravertebral soft tissue masses are readily sampled with the use of the same techniques and needle systems described for vertebral biopsies (Fig. 7-21). Using almost any of the spine biopsy sets available, it is possible to retrieve adequate tissue cores or aspirates from soft tissue masses. In general, a large-caliber (11- to 16-gauge) needle is not required for biopsy of a paraspinal soft tissue mass, but it certainly can be used if a large core sample is desired. Superficially located soft tissue masses are readily sampled with a single-needle technique with an 18- to 22-gauge SureCut or semi-automatic biopsy gun-type biopsy system (e.g., Temno). Large, deep paravertebral masses can also be sampled with relatively small caliber needles; the Geremia system also works well, especially for biopsy of deep soft tissue paraspinal masses. CT guidance is recommended for the vast majority of paraspinal soft tissue mass biopsies because CT provides direct visualization of the needle, target tissue, and surrounding normal structures.

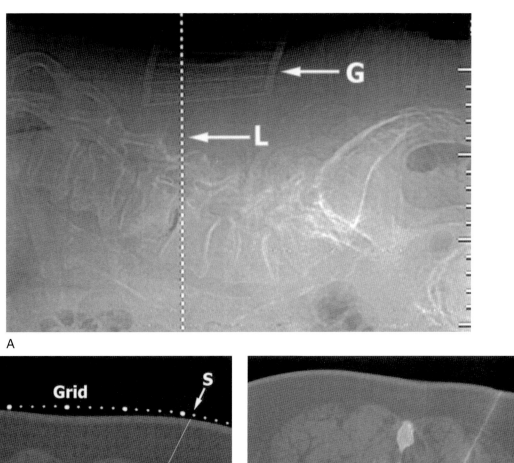

A

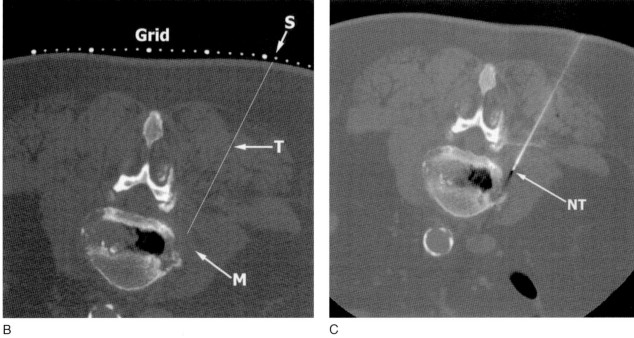

B

C

Figure 7-21 ▪ CT-guided paraspinal soft tissue mass biopsy at the L3 level with a posterolateral approach. *A*, A lateral digital radiograph with a surface localizer grid (G) and a localizer line (L) overlies the grid at the L3 level. *B*, Axial CT image corresponding to localizer line slice location in A. Localizer grid is on the skin surface. The trajectory (T) extends from the skin entry site (S) to the paraspinal soft tissue mass (M). *C*, CT image with 18-gauge biopsy needle tip (NT) located in a paraspinal mass.

Posterior Vertebral Arch and Epidural Soft Tissue Masses

CT guidance is mandatory for biopsy of the posterior verte-bral arch and for biopsy of epidural soft tissue masses (Fig. 7-22). Real-time CT "fluoroscopy" is ideally suited to this category of spine biopsy. The goal is to position the needle safely into the target lesion without damaging the spinal cord or nerve root and to avoid producing an epidural hematoma. If another spinal target lesion is available, epidural biopsy should be avoided. If an epidural tumor is chosen for biopsy, a small biopsy needle should be selected and the number of tissue samples obtained should be kept to a minimum. We do not recommend the use of a semiauto-mated or automated throw-needle biopsy device for sampling masses in the epidural space or neural foramen.

When an epidural biopsy is performed, a surgeon should always be consulted and be readily available in the unlikely occurrence of an epidural hematoma. Once the needle has been positioned within the mass, the tissue sample may be obtained by using gentle suction on a syringe attached to the biopsy needle, as in other types of biopsy. Vigorous advancement or translation of the needle tip should be avoided. A relatively small tissue sample or aspirate is often sufficient to make the diagnosis.[31]

Another application of the epidural fine-needle tech-nique is drainage of symptomatic synovial cysts. These are best approached with CT or MR guidance (Fig. 7-23).[32] Synovial cysts contain gelatinous or serosanguineous liquid. Repeated needle drainage procedures may be necessary for treatment.[33]

The fine-needle aspiration technique may be valuable in evaluating patients who have suspected septic arthritis involving the facet joints.[34] We believe MR imaging is also valuable in diagnosing noninfectious inflammatory facet synovitis. These patients often present with localized pain

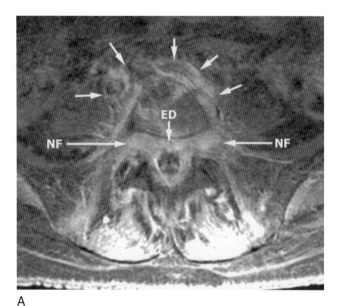

A

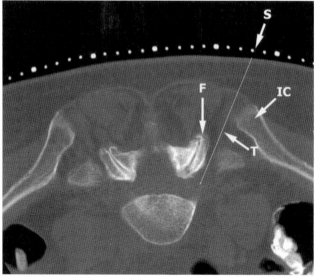

B

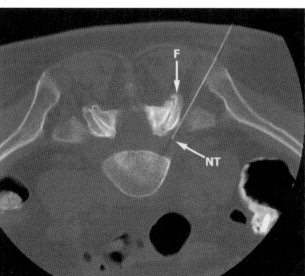

C

Figure 7-22 ■ Biopsy of a mass (lymphoma) in the right L5-S1 neural foramen. *A,* Axial T1-weighted gadolinium-enhanced MR image demon-strates ill-defined enhancing soft tissue in the neural foramen (NF) bilater-ally. Enhancing epidural tissue (ED) also noted ventral to the thecal sac; an enhancing paraspinal soft tissue mass (*arrows*) is located adjacent to the vertebral body. The anterior aspect of the vertebral body on the right is also involved by tumor. *B,* With the skin surface grid in place, the skin entry site (S) is noted. The needle trajectory (T) is for single-needle biopsy placement into the right L5-S1 neural foramen. The needle trajectory is located lateral to the superior articular facet (F) of S1 and medial to the right iliac crest (IC). *C,* A 21-gauge Chiba needle has been placed lateral to the superior articular facet (F) of S1 on the right with the needle tip (NT) positioned in the L5-S1 neural foramen on the right.

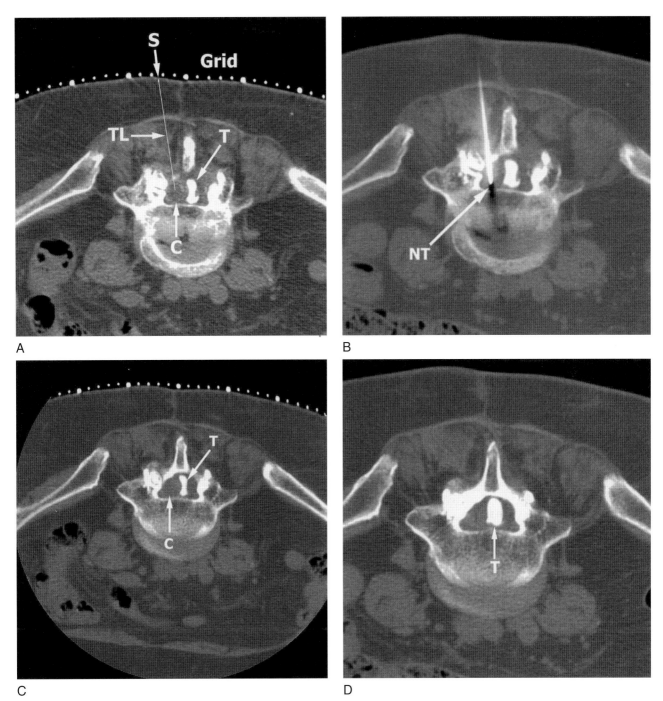

Figure 7-23 ▪ CT-guided synovial cyst aspiration. *A,* With the surface grid localizer in place, the trajectory line (TL) is drawn on the CT image from the desired skin entry site (S) to left L4-5 synovial cyst (C). Note the compression of the contrast medium–filled thecal sac (T) by cyst. *B,* Cyst punctured with 18-gauge spinal needle. NT = needle tip. *C,* A large synovial cyst (C) compresses the thecal sac (T) on the CT image, obtained before biopsy. *D,* CT image showing less compression of the thecal sac (T) after the cyst has been partially drained.

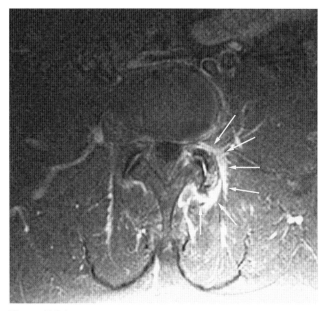

Figure 7-24 ▪ MR image of facet synovitis and periarticular inflammatory process. Axial T1-weighted spin echo image obtained with fat saturation technique after intravenous gadolinium paramagnetic contrast agent has been administered demonstrates enhancement in the left L4-5 facet joint and surrounding articular facets (*arrows*) owing to an inflammatory process, infectious or noninfectious.

over the affected joint, and an MR study with fat saturation technique reveals abnormal signal intensity or enhancement in the facet joint and in the soft tissues surrounding the facets (Fig. 7-24). The soft tissue signal alterations in and around the abnormal facet may not be apparent on conventional MR images unless fat saturation techniques are employed. The signal abnormalities in and adjacent to the involved facets are shown best on T2-weighted fast-spin echo images with fat suppression and gadolinium contrast agent–enhanced T1-weighted images obtained with fat suppression. If these MR imaging sequences are included in routine MR imaging protocols, inflammatory facet synovitis is frequently observed in everyday practice. Therefore, we do not routinely perform needle aspiration in the majority of patients with MR signal abnormalities involving the facets unless indicated by clinical findings. In our experience, unless a paraspinal abscess is present, the majority of patients with these MR imaging findings have a sterile synovitis rather than an infected facet joint.

Disc Aspiration/Biopsy

We prefer the fluoroscopic approach for lumbar aspiration/ biopsy of the intervertebral disc space, and we often use it in the setting of discitis/vertebral osteomyelitis to obtain tissue for microbial culture. Small- or large-caliber needles can be effective in recovering the desired tissue sample. Because most disc space aspirations are obtained for evaluation of infection, it is often not necessary to obtain a large core sample; therefore, smaller (18- to 22-gauge) needles are sufficient to obtain the tissue sample. Of course, larger-caliber needles are easy to place, and they allow coaxial placement of smaller biopsy needles and thus provide the

opportunity to obtain multiple tissue samples. If one positions the needle in the center of an infected disc where necrotic debris exists, a negative microbial culture may result. It is recommended that tissue aspirates be obtained from the disc center, the outer disc margin, and the inflammatory paraspinal mass, if present, when a disc space infection is suggested.

L1 to L4 Disc Aspiration/Biopsy

Needle aspiration of a suspected infected intervertebral disc is performed with patient positioning and needle puncture techniques similar to those used for discography.[27] The only difference is that the target for disc aspiration in the setting of spondylodiscitis is often not the disc centrum but rather the more peripheral portion of the disc, where tissue for viable culture is more likely to be found. If C-arm fluoroscopy is unavailable, a sponge is positioned under the patient's lower abdomen/upper pelvis to elevate the patient and facilitate needle placement. The C-arm (or patient) is rotated until the superior articulating process (ear of the "Scotty dog") arising from the vertebra below and overlying the disc space to be punctured is centered midway between the anterior and posterior aspects of the vertebral body above (Fig. 7-25). If the target is in a more lateral portion of the disc, the superior articulating process is positioned only part of the way between the anterior and posterior aspects of the vertebral body above. During fluoroscopy, the superior endplates of the vertebral body just below the disc to be punctured should superimpose. With the use of this needle trajectory, the possibility of contacting the exiting nerve root or passing through a vital structure is minimal. Contact with the posterolateral margin of the disc is made with the needle tip. The patient often describes mild or moderate pain as the needle passes through Sharpey's fibers in the outer disc margin, although some patients with disc infection have an exaggerated pain response or no pain when the needle passes into the disc.

A large- or small-caliber biopsy needle system can be used to biopsy the disc (Fig. 7-26). Placement of a 16-gauge needle into the disc with a 20-gauge coaxially placed biopsy needle will allow collection of tissue from several biopsy sites with only one pass of the larger biopsy needle. The tissue is sent for Gram stain, culture, and sensitivity (anaerobic and aerobic) and also for cytologic examination.

If the goal of the disc aspiration is not only to culture the intervertebral disc space material but also to aspirate the disc contents for therapeutic reasons in the case of spondylodiscitis, use of a large-caliber needle with a transpedicular approach is recommended. There is some evidence that percutaneous discectomy may be beneficial in treating patients with acute disc space infection.[35]

L5-S1 Disc Aspiration/Biopsy

Again, the positioning of the patient and the fluoroscope are identical to that used for discography, and x-ray fluoroscopic guidance is preferred over CT. For needle insertion into the L5-S1 disc, significant caudocranial beam angulation (image intensifier above the patient, angled toward the patient's head) is required for optimal visualization. The C-arm is rotated into a posterior oblique position. The opening the

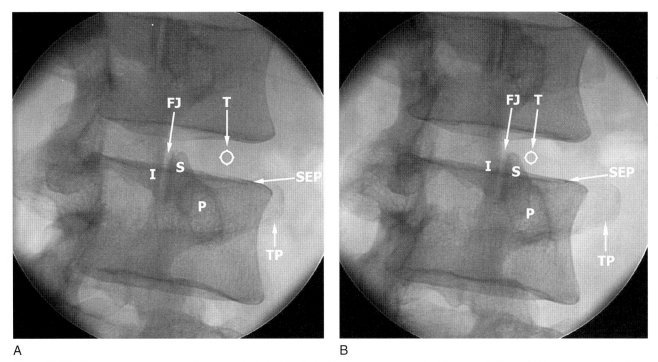

A   B

Figure 7-25 ■ Radiographs demonstrating two methods for identifying ideal target zone for typical fluoroscopically guided lumbar intervertebral disc aspiration (L3-4 level). Both methods place the target zone at the junction of the middle and outer thirds of the disc space. *A*, The x-ray beam (or patient) is rotated until the superior articular process (S) of the vertebral body below projects over the midportion of the intervertebral disc. Superior end plates (SEP) of the vertebral body just below the intervertebral disc should be parallel so that they superimpose. I = inferior articular process of vertebral body above intervertebral disc; FJ = facet joint space; P = right pedicle of vertebra body below target disc space; TP = transverse process. *B*, Same labeling as in A. This time the fluoroscope (or patient) has been rotated until the superior articular process is positioned more laterally overlying the disc space junction of middle and outer thirds of the disc space. The target zone (T) is then positioned adjacent to the lateral margin of the superior articular process.

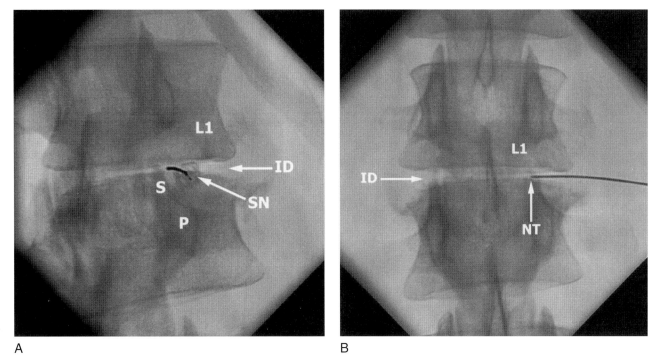

A   B

Figure 7-26 ■ Fluoroscopically guided L1-2 intervertebral disc aspiration in patient with suspected discitis. *A*, LAO radiograph. The superior articular process (S) of L2 is positioned over the disc slightly more lateral than in Figure 7-25. A 22-gauge skinny needle (SN) enters the disc at the junction of the middle and the outer thirds of the disc. P = right pedicle L2; ID = L1-2 intervertebral disc space. *B*, Corresponding AP radiograph for A showing position of the skinny needle tip (NT) relative to the L1 intervertebral disc (ID).

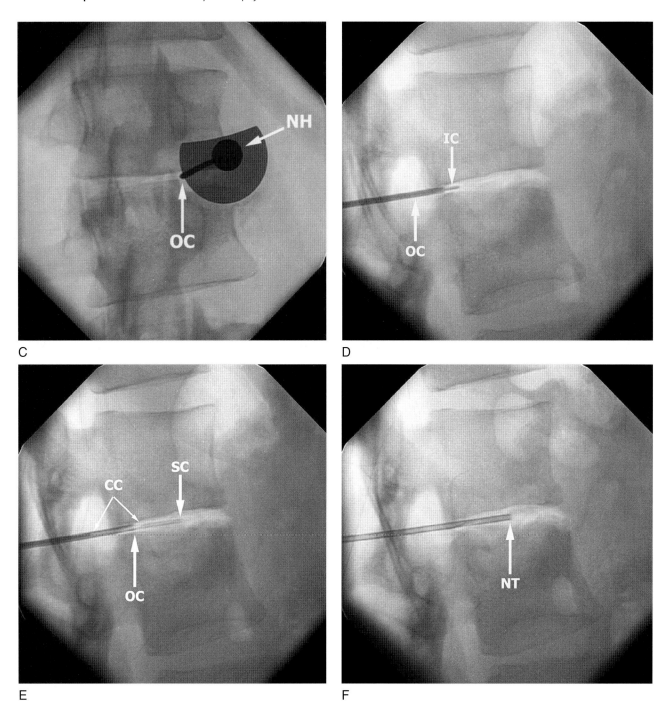

Figure 7-26 *(Cont'd)* ◼ *C*, LAO radiograph of the Geremia needle biopsy system (16-gauge biopsy needle cannula and coaxial 17-gauge introduction cannula) after the skinny needle cannula and stiffener wire have been removed. NH = hub of introduction cannula and outer biopsy cannula superimpose; OC = outer cannula tip projects over disc space. *D*, Lateral radiograph showing Geremia biopsy needle outer cannula (OC) with tip of the introduction cannula (IC) extending 5 mm beyond the end of the outer cannula into the disc. *E*, Lateral radiograph. A 19-gauge SureCut needle has been placed coaxially through the 16-gauge outer cannula of the Geremia needle. The end of the SureCut (SC) extends out the end of the Geremia outer cannula (OC). The specimen collection chamber (CC) of the SureCut remains largely within the outer cannula. Subsequently, the SureCut needle was advanced farther into the intervertebral disc, with fluoroscopic monitoring before obtaining the specimen. *F*, Lateral radiograph. After the SureCut needle has been removed, the 16-gauge Geremia needle outer cannula is seen alone with its Franseen-type needle tip (NT); the needle has been advanced into the intervertebral disc for obtaining the final core-biopsy specimen.

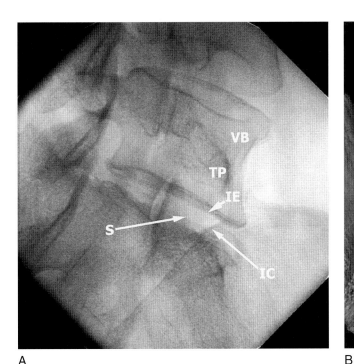 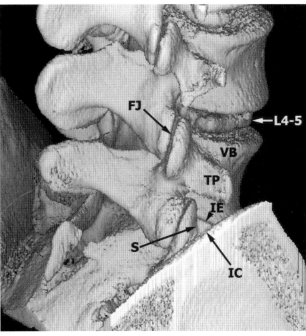

A   B

Figure 7-27 ▪ The target triangle for the L5-S1 disc biopsy is the same as that used for accessing the disc for an intradiscal electrothermal therapy (*IDET*) procedure. *A*, LAO projection, with steep caudocranial x-ray beam angulation. The target triangle is formed by the inferior end plate (IE) of the L5 vertebral body (VB) superiorly, the lateral margin of the right S1 superior articular process (S) medially, and the iliac crest (IC), laterally. TP = right transverse process of L5. *B*, View of the spine on a three-dimensional CT image corresponding to *A*. Steep LAO craniocaudal view of lower lumbosacral spine showing the "target triangle" for accessing the L5-S1 disc with labels as in A. The L4-5 intervertebral disc and the right L4-5 facet joint (FJ) are labeled.

needle must pass through is represented on the fluoroscopic image by a triangle formed by the inferior end plate of L5, the superior articulating process of S1, and the iliac crest. In a small percentage of patients, the iliac crest may impede needle placement into the disc regardless of the angle of approach used. If it is not possible to achieve a position that places the superior articulating process at the midpoint of the vertebral body, one obtains the best possible angle that allows visualization of the triangular opening into the disc (Fig. 7-27).

Placing the needle into the lateral portion of the L5-S1 disc margin is easier than central intradiscal placement, because the iliac crest causes less obstruction to the usual needle trajectory. Caudocranial x-ray beam angulation is usually necessary to optimally visualize the trajectory into the L5-S1 intervertebral disc. Generally, with appropriate beam angulation and patient positioning, it is not necessary to bend the needle tip to facilitate access to the L5-S1 disc as some advocate. Inserting a needle with a bent tip may cause more discomfort to the patient and may interfere with the proper operation of the needle biopsy system and therefore is not recommended.

With the needle in the desired position, disc aspiration biopsy is performed as previously described (Fig. 7-28). If a larger core sample of disc is desired or a paraspinal phlegmonous mass is being sampled, a larger-caliber biopsy needle set (11- to 16-gauge) is preferred, without or with a smaller-gauge needle placed coaxially.

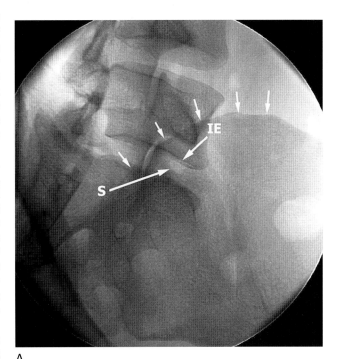

A

Figure 7-28 ▪ "Opening" the L5-S1 target triangle. *A*, In this case, a prominent iliac crest (*arrows*) prevents direct visual access of the target triangle into the L5-S1 disc. S = lateral margin of S1 superior articular process; IE = inferior endplate of L5.

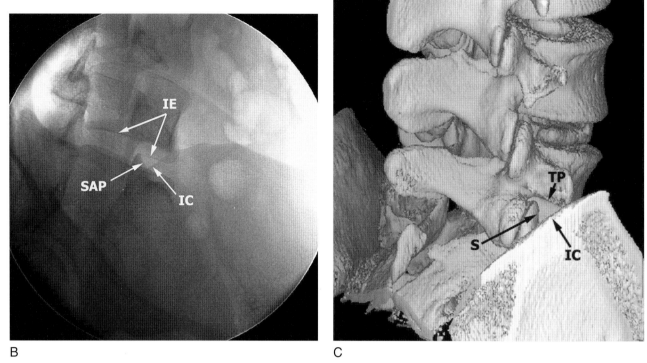

B   C

Figure 7-28 (*Cont'd*) ■ *B*, Accentuated caudocranial x-ray beam angulation and positioning the fluoroscopic tube (or patient) in greater degree of obliquity "opens up" the target triangle by allowing direct visualization of the triangle over the iliac crest (IC). Note that the inferior end plates (IE) of L5 no longer superimpose in this projection. SAP = superior articular process of S1. *C*, In this case, the inferior margin of the L5 transverse process (TP) overlies the inferior end plate of L5 on this three-dimensional CT image with steep obliquity. The target triangle into the L5-S1 disc is now visible.

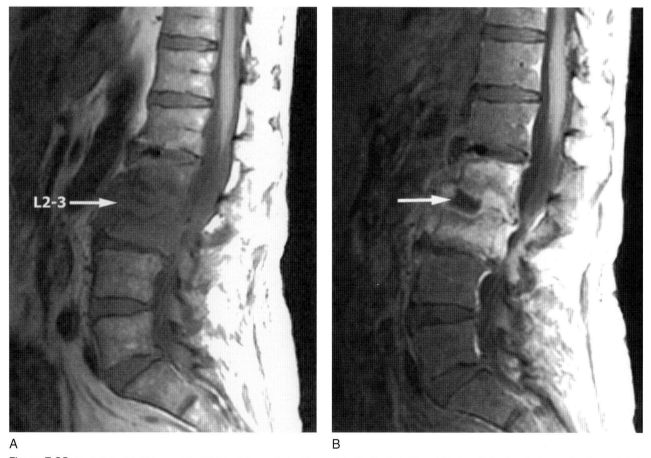

A   B

Figure 7-29 ■ A CT-guided biopsy at the L2-3 level in a patient with spondylodiscitis. *A*, A T1-weighted sagittal spin echo image showing end plate destruction at the L2-3 level (*arrow*) and diminished signal intensity in the L2 and L3 vertebral bodies, representing spondylodiscitis. *B*, Contrast medium enhancement of the L2 and L3 vertebral bodies, end plates, and portions of the L2-3 intervertebral disc. A nonenhancing region of necrosis is seen as a markedly hypointense region in the disc (*arrow*).

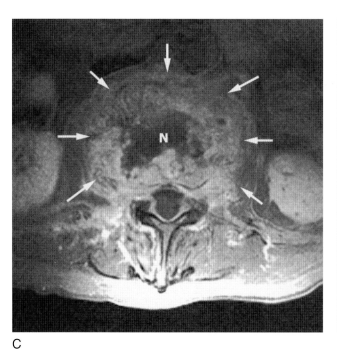

C

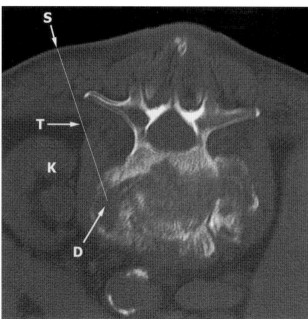

D

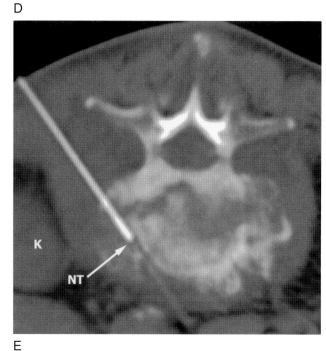

E

Figure 7-29 (*Cont'd*) ■ *C*, Axial gadolinium-enhanced T1-weighted MR image demonstrates peripheral enhancement of the L2-3 disc (*arrows*) with a nonenhancing region of central necrosis (N). *D*, Axial CT image obtained through the L2-3 intervertebral disc level shows desired needle trajectory (T) from the skin entry site (S) into the left lateral aspect of the disc (D). Note that the needle trajectory is medial to the left kidney (K). *E*, CT image shows a 16-gauge SureCut needle that has been inserted using a left extrapedicular posterolateral approach with a single-needle pass. The needle passes medial to the left kidney (K). The biopsy needle tip (NT) is positioned in the intended target in the lateral portion of the disc. Note the extensive bone destruction in the adjacent end plates.

CT-guided disc aspiration can be an equally effective technique for disc space aspiration, especially when real-time CT is employed. Entry into the L5-S1 disc space can be more difficult with this approach because it is necessary to angle the CT gantry, and repeated CT scans are necessary to follow the progress of needle advancement into the disc (Fig. 7-29). CT fluoroscopic guidance may expedite needle placement. Regardless of the disc being sampled, the gantry angle of the scanner is optimally selected to allow one to see an image parallel to the disc. Rather than direct visualization, a localizer grid is placed on the patient's back to help determine the skin entry point. Otherwise, the choice of needle biopsy set and technique for obtaining the tissue sample is the same as for the x-ray fluoroscopic approach.

THORACIC SPINE BIOPSY PROCEDURES

Thoracic spine or paraspinal biopsy can be performed with x-ray fluoroscopy or CT-guided assistance. CT-guided biopsy is believed to be safer in the thoracic region to help avoid

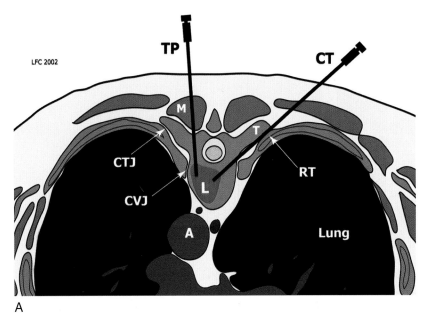

A

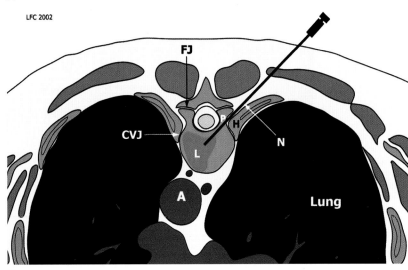

B

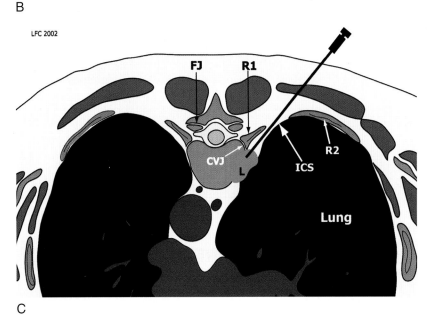

C

Figure 7-30 ■ Illustrations of the thoracic needle biopsy approaches. *A*, Illustration of the transpedicular and posterolateral costotransverse joint approaches. A biopsy needle (TP) has been inserted with a transpedicular approach, through the posterior paraspinal muscles (M), into the left pedicle along its long axis, and into the vertebral body target lesion (L). The biopsy needle labeled CT has been inserted with a right costotransverse approach, extending between the right transverse process (T) and tubercle of the rib (RT); the needle traverses the right costotransverse joint, thereby avoiding the lung. CTJ = left costotransverse joint; CVJ = costovertebral joint; A = descending thoracic aorta. *B*, Illustration of the posterolateral costovertebral groove approach. The needle has been inserted below the level of the transverse process at the level of the facet joint (FJ). Using this approach, the biopsy needle (N) is inserted between the head of the rib (H), and the pedicle (P). *C*, An illustration of the posterolateral intercostal approach obtained one level below that of B. The facet joint (FJ) is still visible. A biopsy needle has been inserted between two adjacent ribs, *R1* and *R2*, in the intercostal space (ICS) and anterior to the head of the rib R1 at the right costovertebral joint (CVJ). The needle passes very near to the posteromedial margin of the lung. L = target lesion.

inadvertent puncture of the pleura. Real-time CT fluoroscopy is a great advantage, allowing direct visualization of the needle in relation to nearby normal structures.

Thoracic Vertebral Body Biopsy

The thoracic spine vertebral body can be sampled with the use of a ***transpedicular*** approach[36–38] or an ***extrapedicular posterolateral*** vertebral approach,[39] with CT or fluoroscopic guidance (Fig. 7-30). In general, CT guidance is preferable to x-ray fluoroscopy, to reduce the incidence of complications in thoracic vertebral biopsies.[29]

Because it is sometimes more difficult to visualize the thoracic pedicle with x-ray fluoroscopy, especially when the bones are demineralized, CT guidance is recommended for

transpedicular biopsy of thoracic vertebral body lesions. Either x-ray fluoroscopic or CT guidance methods are adequate for biopsy of lesions occupying the entire vertebral body. For visualizing posterior vertebral arch lesions or paraspinal soft tissue masses, CT is necessary.

Transpedicular Approach

The transpedicular approach affords a short needle trajectory into the vertebral body compared with the posterolateral approach (Fig. 7-30A). This approach is especially useful when the vertebral body lesion is located within or just anterior to the pedicle or when the lesion occupies the entire vertebral body (Fig. 7-31). The thoracic transpedicular biopsy is performed in a fashion identical to that for lumbar transpedicular biopsies. The thoracic transpedicular biopsy

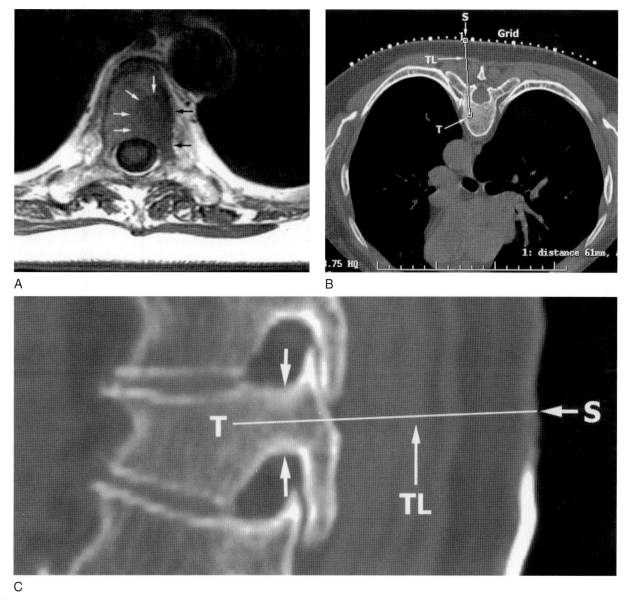

A

B

C

Figure 7-31 ▪ CT-guided transpedicular biopsy in a patient with a left T6 vertebral metastasis. *A,* Axial T1-weighted spine echo MR image. A hypointense lesion (*arrows*) involves the left posterolateral portion of the T6 vertebral body and pedicle. *B,* Axial CT image with skin surface localizer grid in place. The trajectory line (TL) extends from skin entry site (S) through left T6 pedicle into the target lesion (T) in the left posterolateral aspect of the vertebral body. *C,* A sagittal reformatted CT image through left T6 pedicle displays the trajectory line (TL) extending from skin entry site (S) through pedicle (*between arrows*) and into vertebral body at target (T).

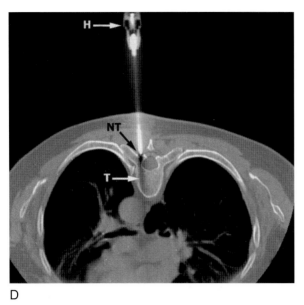
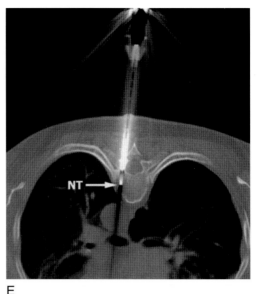

D   E

Figure 7-31 (*Cont'd*) ■ *D*, Axial CT scan obtained after insertion of an 11-gauge Cook biopsy needle with the needle tip (NT) positioned in the groove posterior to the left T6 pedicle. T = desired target; H = needle hub. It is important to obtain a CT scan before penetrating the cortex to ensure that the needle does not disrupt the medial cortex of the pedicle. In this case, the needle tip shown should be directed slightly more laterally to enter the central portion of the pedicle. *E*, Axial CT scan after a coaxial needle system (a 14-gauge Elson needle coaxially inserted into an 11-gauge Cook needle) directed slightly more laterally and advanced through the pedicle. The Elson needle tip (NT) is positioned at the desired target point within the vertebral body.

usually requires an 11- to 16-gauge biopsy needle to traverse the intact pedicle. If the pedicle has been destroyed or is osteopenic, a smaller-gauge needle may be sufficient. The Geremia or Elson needle biopsy system can be used for thoracic spine biopsies using the transpedicular or the paraspinal approach.[40] There is less room for error when performing a thoracic transpedicular biopsy, because the thoracic pedicle has a smaller transverse diameter than the lumbar pedicle,[41] and therefore could fracture more easily. The thoracic pedicle will generally accommodate a needle up to 11 gauge if required, but we prefer to use smaller needles (16 gauge or smaller) for thoracic vertebral biopsy. Again, a coaxial technique placing a smaller-caliber biopsy needle (e.g., 18- to 20-gauge Temno or SureCut) coaxially through a larger biopsy cannula will yield greater amounts of tissue and thus increase biopsy sensitivity.

Extrapedicular Posterolateral Approaches

There are three extrapedicular posterolateral approaches for percutaneous needle biopsy of the thoracic vertebral body: the **costotransverse joint approach**, the **costovertebral groove approach**, and the **intercostal approach** (see Fig. 7-30). The choice of the approach selected is based on the position of the target lesion in or adjacent to the vertebral body. A disadvantage of any of the posterolateral approaches is that the skin entry site is located farther from midline, and so the needle must traverse a longer pathway through the paraspinal tissues.

COSTOTRANSVERSE JOINT APPROACH

The costotransverse joint approach (see Fig. 7-30*A*) is a good choice for vertebral body biopsy. CT guidance is required for this approach to directly visualize needle placement between the vertebral transverse process and the tubercle of

the corresponding rib. The tubercle on the rib at the costotransverse articulation may appear to impede passage of the needle; however, the needle often slides slightly inferior or superior to the tubercle and allows safe passage into the vertebral body. With this approach, the posteromedial margin of the rib prevents inadvertent placement of the needle across the pleura and prevents the needle from sliding forward along the lateral margin of the thoracic vertebral body cortex. The transverse process prevents passage of the needle into the spinal canal. Care must be taken if the needle is displaced by the rib tubercle superior to the costotransverse joint, because the needle will then traverse the intercostal space (Fig. 7-32). If the needle is displaced inferior to the costotransverse joint, the needle will lie in the costovertebral groove (see later). A theoretical disadvantage to the costotransverse joint approach is that the needle could produce damage to the articulating structures of the joint.

COSTOVERTEBRAL GROOVE APPROACH

The costovertebral groove approach (see Fig. 7-30*B*) is an excellent approach for thoracic vertebral body biopsy, and it is the approach we prefer for thoracic vertebral body biopsy, if possible. With this approach, the needle is inserted slightly below the level of the costotransverse joint in the space (groove) between the vertebral pedicle and the head of the corresponding rib (Fig. 7-33). With this approach, the rib prevents the needle from entering the pleura and the costovertebral groove serves as a funnel, directing the needle into the vertebral body. An additional advantage is that the needle does not enter the costotransverse joint.

INTERCOSTAL APPROACH

The posterolateral intercostal approach is useful for biopsy of paravertebral soft tissue masses or masses that involve the vertebral body and the adjacent paravertebral soft tissues

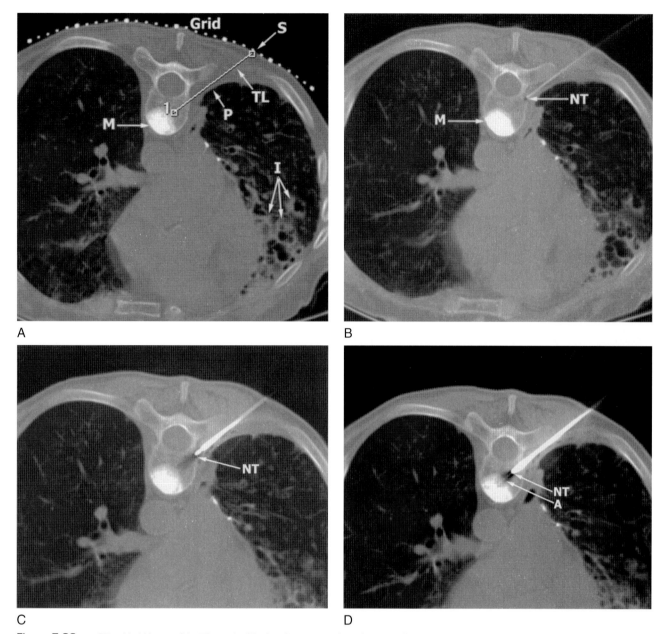

Figure 7-32 ■ CT-guided biopsy of the T9 vertebral body using a posterolateral, extrapedicular approach with the trajectory chosen slightly above the level of the costotransverse joint. Osteoblastic metastatic non–small cell lung carcinoma. *A,* With grid on the surface of the back, a trajectory line (TL) is drawn from the selected skin entry site (S) to the sclerotic target lesion in the T9 vertebral body. Note that the trajectory line passes anterior to the transverse process in the posteromedial aspect of the intercostal space, very near the posterior pleural surface (P) of the right lung. I = right pulmonary infiltrate secondary to bronchiestasis and lung carcinoma; M = osteoblastic vertebral metastasis. *B,* A skinny needle has been inserted using a right extrapedicular posterolateral approach. The needle tip (NT) is located adjacent to the vertebral body cortex, the site where local anesthetic is deposited adjacent to the vertebral body periosteum. M = osteoblastic vertebral metastasis. *C,* The Elson biopsy needle tip (NT) penetrates the vertebral cortex. *D,* The biopsy needle tip (NT) is inserted further into the vertebral body, just before advancing into the target lesion. Note the needle artifact (A) shows the path that the needle will take when advanced further.

(see Fig. 7-30*C*). The needle is inserted into the posteromedial intercostal space, anterior to the head of the rib and costovertebral joint (see Fig. 7-33). Care must be taken in sampling lesions confined to the vertebral body with this approach (see Fig. 7-32), because the needle trajectory is often more tangential to the vertebral cortex. If the vertebral body cortex is intact, this trajectory tends to deflect the needle anteriorly, and thus carries a higher risk of inadvertent lung puncture. Furthermore, with the intercostal approach, the needle may cause vascular injury to the intercostal vessels or paraspinal veins, which may increase the risk of a paraspinal hematoma.

A single biopsy needle system or a coaxial system can provide an adequate tissue sample for analysis. As always, the coaxial system has the advantage of allowing retrieval of multiple tissue samples. Once the needle has been positioned at the proximal margin of the target lesion, the tissue samples can be obtained in a coaxial fashion, as previously

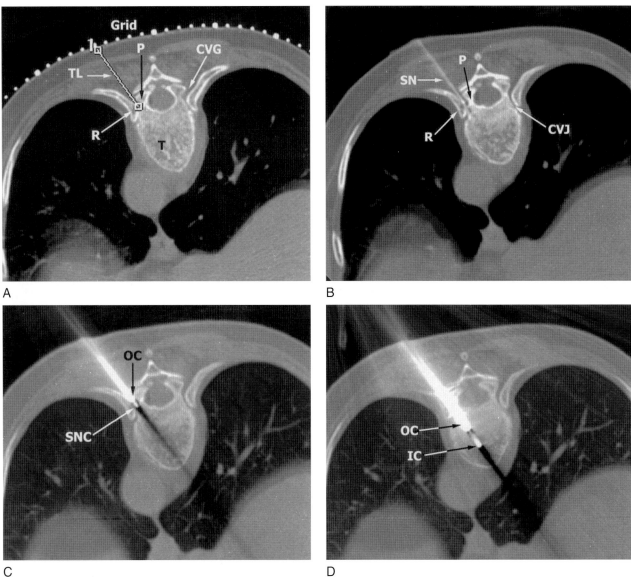

A

B

C

D

E

Figure 7-33 ■ CT-guided costovertebral groove approach. Lymphoma, T9 vertebral body. *A,* With localizer grid on the skin surface, a trajectory line (TL) is drawn from the skin entry site (1) to the costovertebral groove, located between the left T9 pedicle (P) and the head of the left ninth rib (R). CVG = costovertebral groove. *B,* A 22-gauge skinny needle (SN) has been inserted using a left posterolateral approach into the costovertebral groove between the head of the left ninth rib (R) and the left T9 pedicle (P). Note that the costovertebral joint (CVJ) is located anterior to the costovertebral groove. *C,* A 12-gauge Elson coaxial outer cannula (OC) and the inner blunt tip cannula have been advanced, as a single unit, over the skinny needle cannula (SNC) and wire into the left costovertebral groove. *D,* The inner blunt tip cannula has been removed, and the 12-gauge outer cannula (OC) is advanced to the proximal margin of the target lesion. A 14-gauge Franseen-type tipped inner cannula (IC) is inserted coaxially through the outer cannula into the lesion for obtaining the initial biopsy specimen. E, With the inner cannula removed, the 12-gauge outer cannula (OC) of the Elson biopsy needle is advanced into the lesion to obtain a larger core tissue sample.

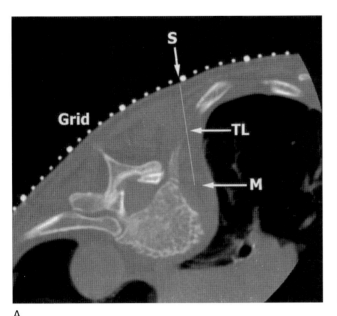

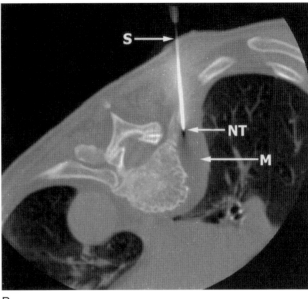

A   B

Figure 7-34 ▪ CT-guided posterolateral intercostal approach. Needle biopsy of a right thoracic paraspinal soft tissue mass. *A*, With the skin surface localizer grid in place, the trajectory line (TL) is drawn from the selected skin entry site (S), through posterior intercostal space on the right, and into the right paraspinal soft tissue mass (M). *B*, An 18-gauge biopsy needle has been inserted to biopsy the right paraspinal soft tissue mass (M). NT = needle tip; S = skin entry site.

described. With any thoracic vertebral body biopsy, care must be taken not to penetrate the anterior cortex of the vertebral body to avoid injury to the aorta, inferior vena cava, or lung.

Disc Aspiration/Biopsy

Again, the main indication for disc aspiration is to obtain a specimen for microbial analysis in the setting of discitis. The thoracic intervertebral disc is sampled using a standard **posterolateral paravertebral** approach with either CT or x-ray fluoroscopic guidance.

X-ray Fluoroscopic Guidance

The technique is similar to that for lumbar disc aspiration. The fluoroscope is rotated in a posterior oblique position around the patient's back. When the bones are well mineralized, the thoracic pedicle can readily be seen to project directly beneath the superior articulating process (Fig. 7-34). The needle tip should always be kept projecting along the lateral aspect of the superior articulating process to avoid entering the spinal canal and medial to the costotransverse junction to prevent the needle from traversing the pleura. It is important to visualize the **three-line configuration** consisting of, from lateral to medial, the anteromedial lung margin, the posterolateral margin of the vertebral body, and the posteromedial lung margin (Fig. 7-35). For lower thoracic levels, patients are instructed to hold their breath in expiration during needle advancement to elevate lung position and decrease the risk of pneumothorax. Insertion of the needle is monitored fluoroscopically in orthogonal planes to ensure intradiscal placement.

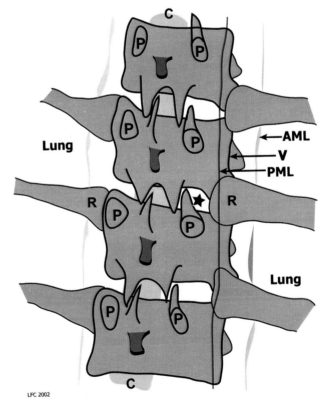

Figure 7-35 ▪ Illustration of LAO thoracic spine radiograph. Landmarks for fluoroscopically guided disc biopsy are identical to that used for discography. The target point (*star*) for needle puncture is at the junction of the middle and outer thirds of the intervertebral disc; the target point is located between the ipsilateral superior articular process and the head of the rib (R). The puncture should be medial to the three lines represented by the posteromedial lung margin (PML), the lateral vertebral margin (V), and the anteromedial lung margin (AML). P = vertebral pedicles; C = spinal cord.

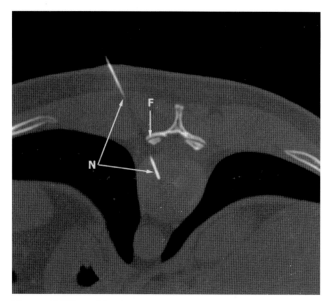

Figure 7-36 ■ CT-guided posterolateral extrapedicular approach for thoracic disc needle aspiration. The biopsy needle (N) passes lateral to the facets (F) and between the ribs in the posterior intercostal space.

CT Guidance

Because the patient population being sampled is usually older, and the bones tend to be more demineralized, CT guidance is often selected for thoracic disc space aspiration (Fig. 7-36). For thoracic disc biopsy, it is usually not necessary to angle the gantry. Often the entire disc is not seen on a single image; therefore, a slice position is chosen where the posterolateral aspect of the target disc is best visualized. An 18- to 20-gauge needle is often suitable for disc aspiration, although larger-caliber needles can be used at the operator's discretion. The needle is inserted with a posterolateral approach and advanced toward the posterolateral annulus, with pauses to obtain CT scans to monitor the progress of each needle advancement. Alternatively, real-time CT fluoroscopy can be used to directly visualize needle advancement, a major advantage in the thoracic region. The operator placing the needle can generally feel a resistance or different tissue consistency when the needle passes through the annulus and a loss of resistance when it enters the nucleus. When the needle is within the lesion, the biopsy sample is collected as already described.

CERVICAL SPINE BIOPSY PROCEDURES

Cervical vertebral biopsies must be carefully planned before the biopsy is attempted, because the risk of potential complications is greater than that for biopsies of the lumbar or thoracic region because of the vital structures surrounding the cervical spine. Possible complications include disc space infection, osteomyelitis, epidural abscess, paraspinal hematoma, epidural hematoma, and associated quadriplegia or myelopathy. Transient recurrent laryngeal nerve damage has been reported.[42] Still, the risk of a serious complication with cervical spine biopsy is very low.

Paraspinal soft tissue masses are often safely sampled by fine-needle (20- to 22-gauge) biopsy needles with the use of a single needle technique. A single pass is often enough to recover an adequate tissue sample. A coaxial technique can also be used if multiple core samples are required from the soft tissue mass. Other neck soft tissue masses can also be sampled with these same techniques with CT or MR guidance.[43]

It was once believed that lesions involving the C1, C2, and often C3 vertebral bodies were usually not amenable to percutaneous biopsy.[44] Accordingly, these lesions were sampled by means of an anterior approach, through the pharynx, by a surgeon, using a large-caliber biopsy needle with the patient under general anesthesia. With careful planning and CT guidance, lesions involving the upper cervical vertebrae can be sampled with percutaneous needle techniques, although care should be taken to select a relatively small-caliber needle (e.g., 20-gauge); this will minimize significant bleeding, which could potentially compromise the spinal cord or other cervical compartments.[45] The lower four cervical vertebrae can readily be sampled with the use of percutaneous needle biopsy techniques.[42] The **anterolateral approach** is used most commonly for biopsy of the mid and lower cervical vertebral bodies or for biopsy/aspiration of adjoining intervertebral discs. The carotid artery is often along the planned trajectory for biopsy of the cervical vertebral body or intervertebral disc. With an anterolateral approach, the carotid artery is manually displaced posteriorly by the operator's fingers by means of the technique originally described by Tampieri and colleagues[46] under fluoroscopic guidance. CT-guided disc aspiration is performed by the same method as that for cervical discography, with the identical anterolateral approach. With either the fluoroscopic or the CT-guided technique, administration of intravenous atropine (0.6 to 1.0 mg) is recommended to minimize the possibility of a vasovagal response from compression of the carotid body.

Single or coaxial needle techniques can be used to sample the mid and lower cervical vertebrae or intervertebral discs with 16- to 20-gauge needle biopsy sets. Cervical vertebral biopsies can be performed with the use of x-ray fluoroscopic guidance, but CT is strongly preferred because it allows direct visualization of the relationship of the needle to adjacent vascular structures and confirms placement of the needle tip in the vertebral lesion. As mentioned previously, real-time CT fluoroscopy is an excellent method for cervical spine biopsy. Administration of an iodinated nonionic, water-soluble contrast agent intravenously can be valuable to opacify the blood vessels, just before insertion of the needle. Lesions involving the entire cervical vertebral body can be successfully sampled with CT or fluoroscopic guidance. Recovery of tissue samples is identical to procedures used in the lumbar and thoracic regions.

Biopsy of the posterior vertebral arch, articular pillars, or a posterior paraspinal soft tissue mass is performed with a **posterolateral approach** and CT guidance. A single-needle technique is usually sufficient to biopsy posterior vertebral arch lesions or posterior paraspinal soft tissue masses.

As mentioned earlier, the cervical intervertebral disc can be sampled with CT guidance. However, it may be easier to sample the cervical intervertebral disc under direct fluoroscopic observation in a manner identical to needle placement

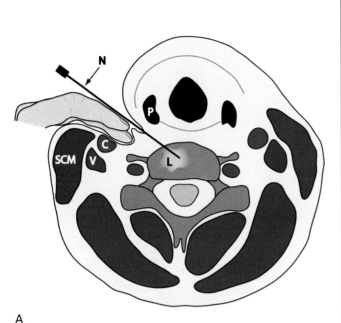

A

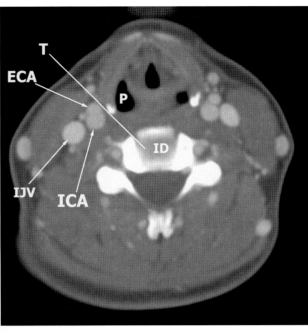

B

Figure 7-37 ■ Method of anterolateral cervical spine biopsy or disc aspiration. *A,* Illustration depicting the anterolateral approach for cervical spine biopsy using manual compression to displace the right internal carotid artery (C), jugular vein (V), and sternocleidomastoid muscle (SCM) posteriorly, allowing insertion of the biopsy needle (N). Note that in this case, the needle is positioned between the right internal carotid artery and the right piriform sinus (P). The needle tip is positioned in the target lesion (L) in the vertebral body. *B,* CT image of the neck. Without manual compression, the internal and external carotid arteries (ICA and ECA) are located very close to the intended needle trajectory (T). A needle placed along this trajectory could produce vascular injury. P = pyriform sinus; IJV = internal jugular vein; ID = intervertebral disc.

for cervical discography. A cushion is placed under the patient's shoulders to slightly hyperextend the neck. The same technique to manually displace the carotid artery posterolaterally is used as for CT-guided biopsy of the cervical vertebral body and for discography. Atropine (0.6 to 1.0 mg) should be administered intravenously to prevent a vasovagal response related to compression of the carotid body receptors.

The C-arm fluoroscope is placed in the AP position initially, and cranial or caudal angulation of the tube is used to optimally visualize the disc space. Needle puncture is made between the carotid sheath and the airway. The carotid pulse at the disc level is palpated with the index and middle fingers, and the carotid sheath structures are displaced posterolaterally by manual palpation (Fig. 7-37). A 20- or 22-gauge, 3.5-inch spinal needle is introduced at a 30- to 40-degree angle in front of the fingertips used to displace the carotid sheath structures. The needle is then positioned with its tip in the center of the disc. Confirmation of the needle tip position should be obtained with AP and lateral radiographs (Fig. 7-38). Once the biopsy needle is in place, the disc tissue sample is obtained as previously described for any disc biopsy.

POTENTIAL COMPLICATIONS

The complication rate for spine biopsy has been variously reported to be less than 10%,[26] but in experienced hands the complication rate for percutaneous biopsy is very small,

probably less than 1% to 3%. Complications include the following:

- Bleeding, usually minimal. Epidural hematoma and psoas hematomas are rare complications.
- Infection, specifically discitis and vertebral osteomyelitis
- Drug-related allergic reactions
- Inadvertent puncture of the thecal sac is usually not associated with any complications but could result in arachnoiditis.
- Headache
- Pneumothorax in the case of thoracic spine biopsy
- Epidural abscess, vascular injury, quadriplegia, and myelopathy
- Vasovagal reaction
- Quadriparesis related to inadvertent spinal cord puncture[47]
- Dissemination of tumor cells or infection along the needle tract is a theoretical risk that is often discussed, but it rarely occurs.[7, 17]

POST-PROCEDURE CARE/FOLLOW-UP

Immediate[27]

1. The patient should be observed for 30 minutes.
2. The patient may sit in a reclining lounge chair; however, if there is significant pain after the procedure or if he or she received intravenous sedation, the patient should be placed at bed rest.

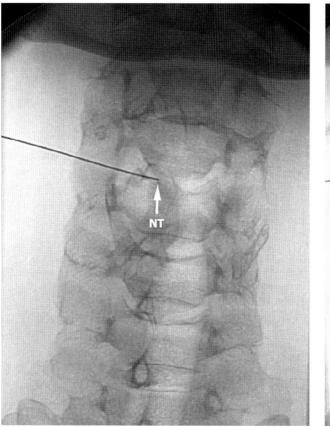

A

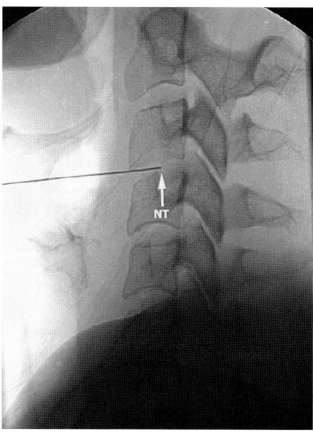

B

Figure 7-38 ■ Fluoroscopically guided C3-4 intervertebral disc space aspiration in patient being evaluated for possible discitis. *A*, Biopsy needle tip (NT) projects over C3-4 disc in AP radiographic view. *B*, Lateral radiograph corresponding to *A*.

3. Blood pressure, pulse, heart rate, and respirations are evaluated immediately after the procedure. If these are stable, no further vital signs are taken. If they are significantly different from baseline, they are checked every 30 minutes until they return to baseline.

Discharge[27]

1. The patient is discharged into the care of a responsible person.
2. The patient is instructed not to drive or perform any other tasks that require clear thought and quick reactions for the remainder of the day, especially if sedation was given.
3. A 2- to 3-day nonrenewable prescription for a narcotic pain reliever and/or a muscle relaxant is given to the patient.
4. Patients are instructed to continue to take their prescription medication, although pain medication may be tapered as indicated.
5. A discharge sheet should be given to the patient outlining the following:
   a. Which procedure was performed and at what levels
   b. Procedurally related symptoms that typically resolve in 7 to 10 days

- Pain at the needle puncture site(s)
- Mild increased back or neck stiffness
- Deep back or neck pain
   c. Treatment for mild post-procedure symptoms
- Rest the affected area for 3 to 4 days.
- Avoid movements that aggravate the pain.
- Apply cold compresses to the area that hurts.
   d. Signs and symptoms of infection
- Fever
- Chills
- Swelling or drainage from the puncture sites
- New back or neck pain that is different from the usual pain
   e. Signs and symptoms of possibly more serious problems
- Stiff neck
- Increasing pain
- Motor dysfunction such as difficulty walking or lifting
- Bowel or bladder dysfunction
   f. Physician name and contact number if the patient has any concerns or if any problems were to arise as a result of the procedure
   g. Advice to schedule a follow-up appointment with the referring physician in 7 to 10 days.

SAMPLE DICTATIONS

Fluoroscopically Guided Disc Aspiration Biopsy and Transpedicular Vertebral Body Biopsy

The procedure and potential complications were explained to the patient, and voluntary informed, signed consent was obtained. The patient was placed prone on the table. Electrocardiogram, pulse oximetry, and blood pressure were monitored during the examination. The patient's back was prepared and draped in sterile fashion.

L3-4 Disc Aspiration

A 22-gauge skinny needle was advanced with a right extrapedicular approach to the margin of the collapsed L3-4 disc along its right posterolateral aspect. Subsequently, a 16-gauge Geremia bone biopsy needle was placed coaxially over the 22-gauge needle and inserted in the right posterior aspect of the L3-4 disc. A 19-gauge, 230-mm SureCut needle was then placed through the 16-gauge Geremia needle, and small bone/disc aspirations were performed, with samples sent for evaluation. Subsequently, a tissue biopsy specimen was obtained with a 20-gauge, 20-cm Temno adjustable throw biopsy device and sent for evaluation. A final biopsy specimen was collected with the 16-gauge needle.

L4 Transpedicular Biopsy

Subsequently, the C-arm was slightly repositioned for entrance to the right L4 pedicle. An 11-gauge, 11-cm Temno needle was advanced into the dorsal portion of the right L4 pedicle. A new 16-gauge Geremia needle was then advanced through the 11-gauge needle and two bone core specimens were obtained, one from the right L4 pedicle and one from the right posterolateral aspect of the L4 vertebral body. The 11-gauge needle was advanced and removed, and this specimen was also sent for evaluation. No complications were observed during or immediately after the procedure.

CT-Guided Thoracic Posterolateral Costotransverse Vertebral Biopsy

The procedure and potential complications were explained to the patient, and voluntary informed, signed consent was obtained. The patient was placed prone on the CT table. A number of 1.25 mm axial CT scans were obtained to localize the T9 vertebral body. The patient's left mid and lower back were prepared and draped in sterile fashion. Lidocaine 1% was instilled into the superficial and deep soft tissues of the patient's left lower back for local anesthesia. With a costotransverse approach, under intermittent CT guidance, a 22-gauge skinny needle was advanced from a left posterolateral approach between the left 9th rib and left T9 transverse process. Subsequently, a 12-gauge Elson bone-cutting needle was advanced coaxially over the skinny needle into the left posterolateral portion of the T9 vertebral body. Two biopsy specimens were obtained with the 14-gauge Elson biopsy needles through the 12-gauge Elson needle, and a final specimen was obtained with the 12-gauge needle. These

needles were then removed. No complications were observed during or immediately after the procedure.

CURRENT PROCEDURAL TERMINOLOGY (CPT) CODES

CPT codes can change and sometimes are only valid for certain states or regions. It is best to consult with CPT coding experts at one's facility to make sure that the coding for the procedures is appropriate for one's practice and location. Below is a sample of codes that are currently being used for spine biopsy.[48]

20220 Biopsy, bone, trocar, or needle; **superficial** (eg, ilium, sternum, spinous process, ribs)

20225 **deep** (vertebral body, femur) (For bone marrow biopsy, use **85102**)

76003 Fluoroscopic guidance for needle placement (e.g., biopsy, aspiration, injection, localization device)

76005 Fluoroscopic guidance and localization of needle or catheter tip for spine or paraspinous diagnostic or therapeutic injection procedures (epidural, transforaminal epidural, subarachnoid, paravertebral facet joint, paravertebral facet joint nerve or sacroiliac joint), including neurolytic agent destruction

76360 CT guidance for needle placement (e.g., biopsy, aspiration, injection, localization device), radiologic supervision, and interpretation

76393 MR guidance for needle placement (e.g., for biopsy, needle aspiration, injection, or placement of localization device), radiologic supervision, and interpretation

76942 Ultrasonic guidance for needle placement (e.g., biopsy, aspiration, injection, localization device), imaging supervision and interpretation

85102 Bone marrow biopsy, needle or trocar

99141 Sedation with or without analgesia (conscious sedation); intravenous, intramuscular or inhalation

References
1. Ball RP. Needle (aspiration) biopsy. J Tenn State Med Assoc 1934; 27:203–207.
2. Robertson RC, Ball RP. Destructive spine lesions: Diagnosis by needle biopsy. J Bone Joint Surg Am 1935; 37:443–464.
3. Siffert RS, Arkin AM. Trephine biopsy of bone with special reference to the lumbar vertebral bodies. J Bone Joint Surg Am 1949; 31:146–149.
4. Ackermann W. Vertebral trephine biopsy. Ann Surg 1956; 143:373–385.
5. Frankel CJ. Aspiration biopsy of the spine. J Bone Joint Surg Am 1954; 36:69–74.
6. Craig F. Vertebral body biopsy. J Bone Joint Surg Am 1956; 38:93–102.
7. Adapon BD, Legada BD Jr, Lim EV, et al. CT-guided closed biopsy of the spine. J Comput Assist Tomogr 1981; 5:73–78.
8. Ottolenghi CE. Aspiration biopsy of the spine: Technique for the thoracic spine and results of twenty-eight biopsies in this region and

over-all results of 1050 biopsies of other spinal segments. J Bone Joint Surg Am 1969; 51:1531–1544.

9. McCollister C. Diagnostic techniques: Closed biopsy of bone. Clin Orthop 1975; 107:100–111.

10. Valls J, Ottolerighi C, Shajowicz F. Aspiration biopsy in diagnosis of lesion of vertebral bodies. JAMA 1968; 136:376–382.

11. Katada K, Anno H, Ogura Y. Clinical experience with real-time CT fluoroscopy (abstract). Radiology 1994; 193:339.

12. Ward JC, Jeanneret B, Oehlschlegel C, Magerl F. The value of percutaneous transpedicular vertebral bone biopsies for histologic examination: Results of an experimental histopathologic study comparing two biopsy needles. Spine 1996; 21:2484–2490.

13. Murphy WA, Destouet JM, Gilula LA. Percutaneous skeletal biopsy 1981: A procedure for radiologists–results, review, and recommendations. Radiology 1981; 139:545–549.

14. Bender CE, Berquist TH, Wold LE. Imaging-assisted percutaneous biopsy of the thoracic spine. Mayo Clin Proc 1986; 61:942–950.

15. Babu NV, Titus VT, Chittaranjan S, et al. Computed tomographically guided biopsy of the spine. Spine 1994; 19:2436–2442.

16. Jankowski R, Nowak S, Zukiel R, Szymas J. [Metastatic vertebral tumors diagnosed by percutaneous needle biopsy]. Neurol Neurochir Pol 1998; 32:831–840.

17. Ashizawa R, Ohtsuka K, Kamimura M, et al. Percutaneous transpedicular biopsy of thoracic and lumbar vertebrae–method and diagnostic validity. Surg Neurol 1999; 52:545–551.

18. Brenac F, Huet H. [Diagnostic accuracy of the percutaneous spinal biopsy. Optimization of the technique]. J Neuroradiol 2001; 28:7–16.

19. Bernardi L, Castellan L. [Percutaneous vertebral biopsy. Assessment of results]. Radiol Med (Torino) 1995; 89:831–834.

20. Vinicoff PG, Gutschik E, Hansen SE, et al. [CT-guided spinal biopsy in spondylodiscitis]. Ugeskr Laeger 1998; 160:5931–5934.

21. Faugere MC, Malluche HH. Comparison of different bone-biopsy techniques for qualitative and quantitative diagnosis of metabolic bone diseases. J Bone Joint Surg Am 1983; 65:1314–1318.

22. Jamshidi K, Swaim WR. Bone marrow biopsy with unaltered architecture: A new biopsy device. J Lab Clin Med 1971; 77:335–342.

23. Jamshidi K, Windschitl HE, Swaim WR. A new biopsy needle for bone marrow. Scand J Haematol 1971; 8:69–71.

24. Avva R, Vanhemert RL, Barlogie B, et al. CT-guided biopsy of focal lesions in patients with multiple myeloma may reveal new and more aggressive cytogenetic abnormalities. AJNR Am J Neuroradiol 2001; 22.781–785.

25. Metzger CS, Johnson DW, Donaldson WF III. Percutaneous biopsy in the anterior thoracic spine. Spine 1993; 18:374–378.

26. Kattapuram SV, Khurana JS, Rosenthal DI. Percutaneous needle biopsy of the spine. Spine 1992; 17:561–564.

27. Fenton D, Czervionke L. Discography. In Williams AL, Murtagh FR (eds). Handbook of Diagnostic and Therapeutic Spine Procedures. St. Louis: CV Mosby, 2002, pp 187–188.

28. Kattapuram SV, Rosenthal DI. Percutaneous biopsy of skeletal lesions. AJR Am J Roentgenol 1991; 157:935–942.

29. Mick CA, Zinreich J. Percutaneous trephine bone biopsy of the thoracic spine. Spine 1985; 10:737–740.

30. Geremia G, Joglekar S. Percutaneous needle biopsy of the spine. Neuroimaging Clin N Am 2000; 10:503–533.

31. Schiff D, O'Neill BP, Suman VJ. Spinal epidural metastasis as the initial manifestation of malignancy: Clinical features and diagnostic approach. Neurology 1997; 49:452–456.

32. Sauvage P, Grimault L, Ben Salem D, et al. [Lumbar intraspinal synovial cysts: Imaging and treatment by percutaneous injection. Report of thirteen cases]. J Radiol 2000; 81:33–38.

33. Imai K, Nakamura K, Inokuchi K, Oda H. Aspiration of intraspinal synovial cyst: Recurrence after temporal improvement. Arch Orthop Trauma Surg 1998; 118:103–105.

34. Douvrin F, Callonnec F, Proust F, et al. [Lumbar interapophyseal septic arthritis: Apropos of 3 cases]. J Neuroradiol 1996; 23:234–240.

35. Arya S, Crow WN, Hadjipaviou AG, et al. Percutaneous transpedicular management of discitis. J Vasc Interv Radiol 1996; 7:921–927.

36. Renfrew DL, Whitten CG, Wiese JA, et al. CT-guided percutaneous transpedicular biopsy of the spine. Radiology 1991; 180:574–576.

37. Pierot L, Boulin A. Percutaneous biopsy of the thoracic and lumbar spine: Transpedicular approach under fluoroscopic guidance. AJNR Am J Neuroradiol 1999; 20:23–25.

38. Hsu WC, Lim KE. Computed tomography-guided percutaneous transpedicular biopsy of the thoracic spine. Chang Gung Med J 2001; 24:368–375.

39. Brugieres P, Gaston A, Heran F, et al. Percutaneous biopsies of the thoracic spine under CT guidance: Transcostovertebral approach. J Comput Assist Tomogr 1990; 14:446–448.

40. Geremia GK, Charletta DA, Granato DB, Raju S. Biopsy of vertebral and paravertebral structures with a new coaxial needle system. AJNR Am J Neuroradiol 1992; 13:169–171.

41. Misenhimer GR, Peek RD, Wiltse LL, et al. Anatomic analysis of pedicle cortical and cancellous diameter as related to screw size. Spine 1989; 14:367–372.

42. Brugieres P, Gaston A, Voisin MC, et al. CT-guided percutaneous biopsy of the cervical spine: A series of 12 cases. Neuroradiology 1992; 34:358–360.

43. Merkle EM, Lewin JS, Aschoff AJ, et al. Percutaneous magnetic resonance image–guided biopsy and aspiration in the head and neck. Laryngoscope 2000; 110:382–385.

44. Ottolenghi CE, Schajowicz F, De Schant F. Aspiration biopsy of the cervical spine. J Bone Joint Surg Am 1964; 4:715–733.

45. Kattapuram SV, Rosenthal DI. Percutaneous biopsy of the cervical spine using CT guidance. AJR Am J Roentgenol 1987; 149:539–541.

46. Tampieri D, Weill A, Melanson D, Ethier R. Percutaneous aspiration biopsy in cervical spine lytic lesions: Indications and technique. Neuroradiology 1991; 33:43–47.

47. McLaughlin RE, Miller WR, Miller CW. Quadriparesis after needle aspiration of the cervical spine: Report of a case. J Bone Joint Surg Am 1976; 58:1167–1168.

48. Derived from CPT 2002, CPT Intellectual Property Services. Chicago: American Medical Association, 2002.

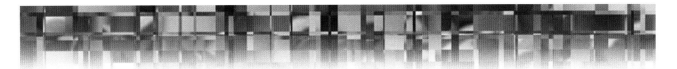

A Spine Surgeon's Perspective

Percutaneous Spine Biopsy

Joseph T. Alexander, MD

Although magnetic resonance imaging is very sensitive in demonstrating spinal disorders, the initial promise of high diagnostic specificity has yet to be realized. Surgeons continue to be consulted regularly to provide samples for pathologic analysis to sort out concerns for neoplasm, infection, and other confounding conditions, to more accurately direct further treatments. Even with newer, less invasive surgical techniques, however, use of open biopsies runs the risk of destabilizing an already diseased spinal segment and thus creating further problems. The concern is the need, with open biopsies, to traverse healthy spinal structures to gain access to the vertebral body or disc, where the pathologic lesion often is located. Percutaneous biopsies can obviate these issues and provide immediate confirmation that the specimen was indeed removed from the area of interest.

As with all biopsies, I always caution the patient and the family that one of the greatest risks is that the specimen will be abnormal, but nondiagnostic. Having worked with various proceduralists over the years, I believe that it is important (1) to utilize the largest possible biopsy needle that can safely be used to maximize the diagnostic yield from this procedure and (2) to be certain that everyone involved knows beforehand exactly which tests are needed for the material that is obtained. At times, such as in the biopsy of a suspected tumor, it may be beneficial for the spine surgeon to specifically discuss the planned trajectory of the needle tract with the proceduralist, so that it could be included in future excisional surgery, if indicated.

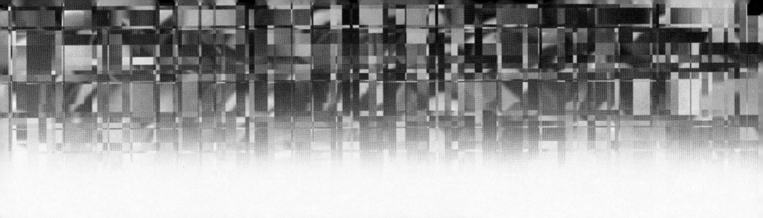

Chapter 8

Vertebroplasty

- David A. Miller, MD
- Douglas S. Fenton, MD
- Jacques E. Dion, MD

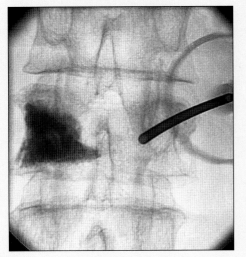

BACKGROUND

Over the years, numerous techniques have been developed to treat pathologic conditions of the spine. As in other areas of the body, less invasive methods for accomplishing this have evolved. Polymethylmethacrylate (PMMA), also called bone cement, has been used as an adjunct to spinal stabilization in open surgical procedures for many years.[1] Percutaneous vertebroplasty was first reported by Deramond and coworkers in 1984.[2] The technique was initially developed for the treatment of aggressive spinal hemangiomas. The initial report described the transpedicular delivery of PMMA to the involved vertebral body. Since then, the indications for vertebroplasty have been expanded to include other tumors of the spine, as well as painful compression fractures resulting from osteoporosis. The procedure was first performed in this country by Jensen and Dion at the University of Virginia in 1993.[3] It has gained widespread popularity in the United States, particularly for the treatment of osteoporotic compression fractures. Osteoporosis, either age-related or resulting from medication or other underlying condition, has been identified in recent years as a major health problem. Reports have shown an incidence of radiographically apparent vertebral compression fractures as high as 26% in women older than age 50.[4] Symptomatic fractures have been reported in one series to be 123 per 100,000 person-years, a rate that exceeded the frequency of symptomatic hip fractures in an elderly population.[5] The increasing popularity of vertebroplasty reflects its high rate of success in selected patients, its low morbidity, and, in most cases, its applicability in an outpatient setting. It offers an alternative for the treatment of painful lesions for many patients who have limited surgical options.

The primary objective of vertebroplasty is pain relief. However, the PMMA also provides some measure of stability. This added stability may be more important in the case of tumors, but it is also of some benefit with osteoporotic fractures, because it halts the possible progression of the fracture and further collapse of the treated vertebral body.

ANATOMIC CONSIDERATIONS

Vertebroplasty targets the vertebral body. The vertebral body, anterior to the spinal cord and thecal sac, is the site of osteoporotic vertebral compression fractures, and it is commonly the major site of involvement of benign tumors such as nonaggressive hemangiomas (aggressive hemangiomas also involve the posterior elements and can have significant soft tissue components). Extrinsic lesions invading the spine may involve the posterior elements or the vertebral body, or both. Patients can benefit from vertebroplasty if a lesion creates fractures and/or collapse of the vertebral body.

Intimate knowledge of vertebral anatomy is essential for the physician performing vertebroplasty. Each vertebra consists of two parts. The anterior portion is the vertebral body. These cylindrically shaped bones, stacked on top of one another, form a pillar for the support of the trunk and head.

With the exception of the arch of C1 and the C2 vertebral body (with the odontoid process), the vertebral bodies of the spine are similar. They become progressively larger from the cervical spine to the lumbar spine. The posterior aspect of the vertebra is the posterior elements or arch. This wishbone-shaped piece of bone, which consists of several pieces, forms a protective arch around the spinal cord and thecal sac. Elements of the arch include the pedicles, which form the lateral portion of the canal, and the laminae, which form the posterior portion of the arch (Fig. 8-1). Other structures of note include the articulating processes, which allow attachment of the ribs in the thoracic region, and articulating facets between the vertebrae.

The transpedicular approach is preferred in the thoracic and lumbar regions (where the majority of compression fractures occur). The pedicles, forming the lateral aspects of the spinal canal, offer a safe route around the spinal canal to the pathologic site. Fractures in the cervical spine require an anterolateral approach because the pedicles are too small to accommodate the needles. A posterolateral approach also carries a significant risk of injury to the vertebral artery.

The venous anatomy of the spine includes an epidural venous plexus located in the anterior epidural space with longitudinal sinuses that extend around the circumference of the spinal canal. This plexus communicates with a basivertebral vein in the central aspect of the vertebral body and with intervertebral and lumbar veins that drain laterally. These veins all eventually drain into the inferior vena cava or into the azygous system (Fig. 8-2). Therefore, spinal and paravertebral veins are a potential source of complications and must be accounted for during any injection of PMMA.

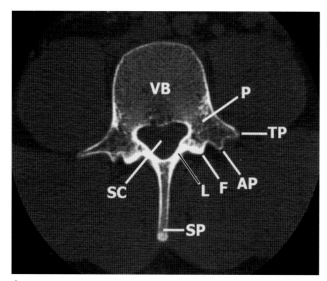

A

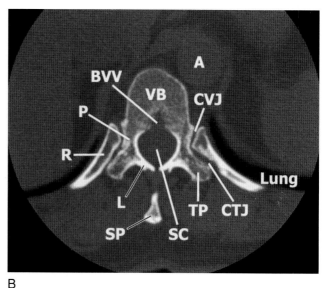

B

Figure 8-1 ▪ Axial CT images of lumbar (*A*) and thoracic (*B*) vertebrae. P = pedicle; L = lamina; VB = vertebral body; SC = spinal canal; TP = transverse process; SP = spinous process; AP = accessory process; F = portion of facet joint; BVV = canal for basivertebral vein; R = rib; CVJ = costovertebral junction; CTJ = costotransverse junction; A = aorta; AP = articular pillar; TF = transverse foramen; AT = anterior tubercle; PT = posterior tubercle; C = common carotid artery; J = internal jugular vein.

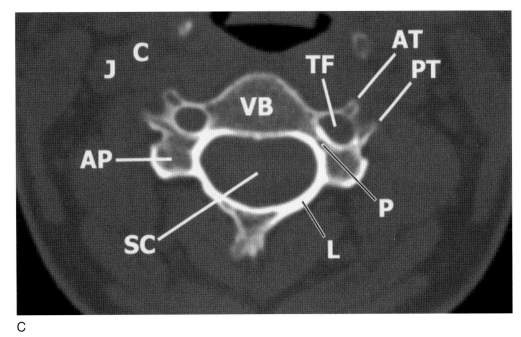

C

Figure 8-1 (*Cont'd*) ■ Axial CT image of cervical (*C*) vertebrae. P = pedicle; L = lamina; VB = vertebral body; SC = spinal canal; TP = transverse process; SP = spinous process; AP = accessory process; F = portion of facet joint; BVV = canal for basivertebral vein; R = rib; CVJ = costovertebral junction; CTJ = costotransverse junction; A = aorta; AP = articular pillar; TF = transverse foramen; AT = anterior tubercle; PT = posterior tubercle; C = common carotid artery; J = internal jugular vein.

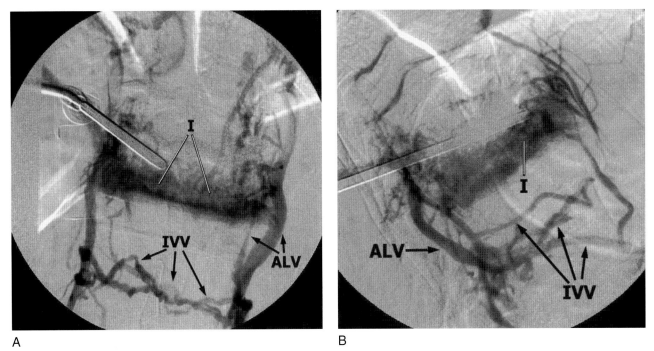

A B

Figure 8-2 ■ Vertebral venous anatomy during intraosseus venography. AP (*A*) and lateral (*B*) venograms demonstrate the initial intratrabecular opacification (I) with subsequent filling of the paravertebral veins. IVV = intervertebral veins; ALV = ascending lumbar veins.

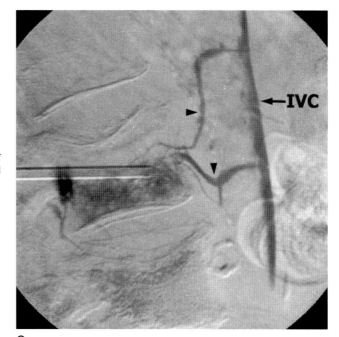

C

Figure 8-2 (*Cont'd*) ■ (*C*) Lateral venogram demonstrates filling of lumbar veins (*arrowheads*) and the inferior vena cava (IVC). AP (*D*) and lateral (*E*) venograms demonstrate filling of the azygous vein (AV).

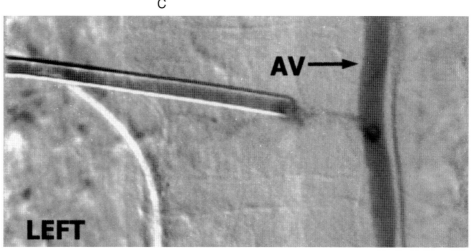

D

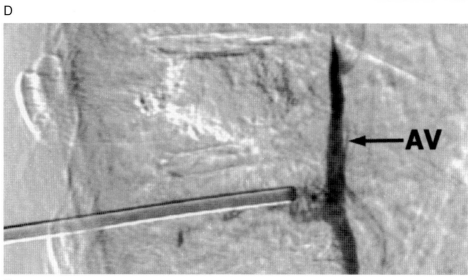

E

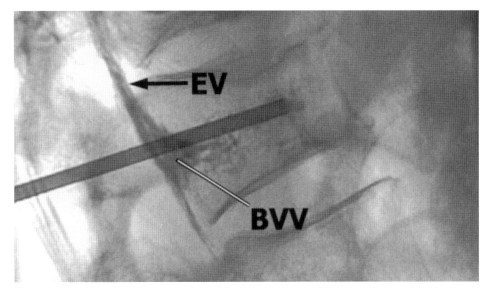

Figure 8-2 (*Cont'd*) ■ (*F*) Lateral venogram demonstrates filling of the basivertebral vein (BVV) and ascending and descending epidural venous plexus (EV).

F

PATIENT SELECTION

Patient selection for vertebroplasty, as for most other procedures, is the most critical factor in predicting a satisfactory result. Back pain is a very common complaint among patients of all ages and can be multifactorial. In addition, different syndromes can present with similar symptoms. This procedure is very effective, but only in appropriately selected patients. Careful review of pertinent imaging, clinical consultation, and a physical examination are necessary not only to identify those patients who are likely to benefit from the procedure but, more importantly, to identify those who are unlikely to obtain pain relief.

History

A thorough history can often identify patients who are unlikely to benefit from vertebroplasty. Often, this history can be obtained by nursing or medical support staff through phone interviews or from the referring physicians' offices. This can limit what could be a flood of back pain referrals with potentially low yield. In treating osteoporotic lesions, the ideal patient is one who has sustained a recent compression fracture. The general rule has been that the more recent the fracture, the greater is the likelihood that vertebroplasty will be beneficial. In the past, patients with fractures more than 2 years old were not considered good candidates for this procedure. Recent evidence from Kaufman and colleagues[6] refutes the theory relating fracture age to clinical outcome. These researchers suggest that whereas greater age of the fracture may increase the amount of analgesia that the patient requires during the procedure, clinical outcome is more dependent on evidence of nonhealing on bone scan and magnetic resonance (MR) imaging and on the degree of persistent pain. In our practice, patients with more remote fractures have been treated, although the success rate appears to be somewhat less than that of patients with more recent fractures.

A careful history usually pinpoints the onset of the patient's pain. Associated trauma (however minor) is a common complaint. However, in many cases there is no specific antecedent event and patients claim that they "just woke up with the pain" or began to notice pain that worsened over several days. Typically, pain from a compression fracture is very severe initially. Patients report being unable to get out of bed or unable to walk, and they often visit the emergency room or are hospitalized for pain control. The pain generally subsides in severity over 1 week to 10 days, becoming somewhat manageable with pain medications and restricted activity.

The longer-term symptoms are often described as a deep ache that is exacerbated by changing position, twisting or moving quickly, or performing tasks that require lifting or bending. Pain is often worse as the day progresses and if the patient has been on his or her feet for any length of time. Reclining or lying flat in bed can improve or alleviate the symptoms. By the time they are seen, these patients have usually had narcotic analgesics prescribed for them. These agents can be effective, although patients are often unable to discontinue using them. Patients describe being reduced to walking with a walker or a cane and being unable to go shopping or even to go out to visit friends because of the discomfort.

A history of documented osteoporosis is a decided advantage when one is dealing with suspected osteoporotic compression fractures. The history should include evidence of conditions that predispose a patient to osteoporosis, such as increasing age, female sex, chronic steroid use, radiation to the spine, and smoking. Bone mineral density testing has recently become a standard practice for the evaluation of osteoporosis and is easily obtained. Still, multiple compression fractures in an elderly patient and a history of a recent fracture from minor trauma are ample evidence that the fracture is due to osteoporosis. Similarly, new onset of back pain in a patient with a history of cancer or with known metastatic disease should raise the suspicion of a neoplastic

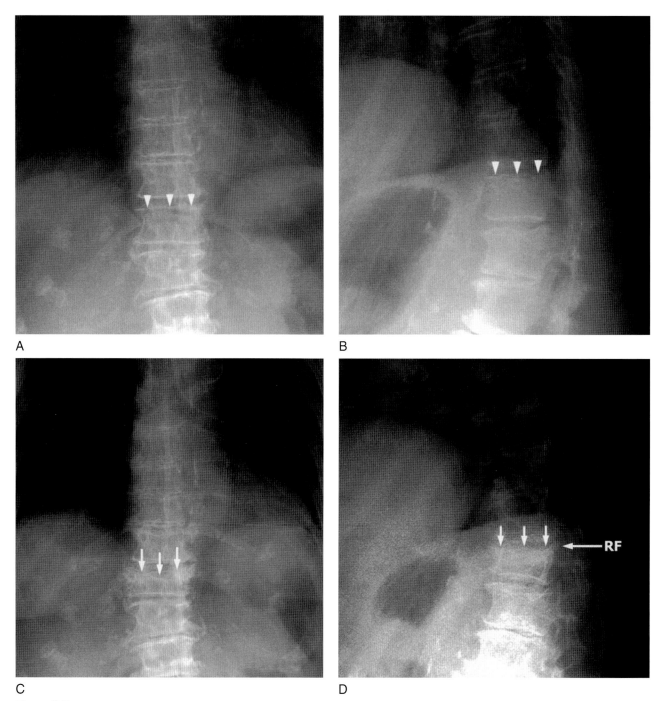

A

B

C

D

Figure 8-3 ■ AP (*A*) and lateral (*B*) chest radiographs demonstrate normal height of the T12 vertebral body (*arrowheads*). AP (*C*) and lateral (*D*) radiographs obtained 1 week later demonstrate compression of the superior end plate of the T12 vertebral body (*arrows*) and some posterosuperior retropulsion of bone (RF) into the spinal canal.

compression fracture. Furthermore, the physician evaluating a patient with a new compression fracture may be the first to uncover an undiagnosed malignancy.

Pain in the lower extremities, especially pain radiating down from the spine, suggests a more complicated compression fracture and should be viewed with concern. Radicular symptoms are generally not caused by uncomplicated compression fractures. They suggest some other pathologic process, such as a retropulsed fragment in the spinal canal or neural foramen compressing the neural elements and causing irritation. Spinal stenosis or a disc herniation, possibly unrelated to the compression fracture, can also be a cause of radiculopathy. In these cases, the patient is not a candidate for vertebroplasty and further evaluation is indicated to consider other treatment, possibly surgical decompression. Any recent change in bowel or bladder habits should also be pursued, with particular attention to signs of urinary retention. In obtaining this history, one must remember that many persons become constipated when taking narcotic analgesics, and that many elderly men have urinary frequency because of prostatic hypertrophy. These disorders should not be confused with dysfunction caused by spinal cord or thecal sac compression.

The history should also document a complete list of the patient's medications, including analgesics that have been tried, those that are currently being taken, previous and present use of steroids, and any calcium or biphosphonate supplements. It is also prudent to document what forms of therapy have been attempted and with what degree of success. This would include physical therapy, chiropractic therapy, bracing, acupuncture, or other conservative measures. In some locations, and for some payers, patients must have failed to respond to conservative therapy to be eligible for vertebroplasty.

Physical Examination

A physical examination is performed to localize the level of the patient's pain, to evaluate neurologic function, especially with regard to signs of spinal cord or conus medullaris compression; to rule out other causes of back pain such as facet disease; and to determine whether the patient can tolerate the vertebroplasty. The patient's pain should be at the level of the fracture or within one vertebral body inferior or superior to the fracture. Although localizing back pain is not always easy, with prompting and patience most patients can point to the area where the pain is located or to the area of greatest pain. One must often carefully question the patient when examining the back. The consulting physician should focus on the pain that has prompted the patient to seek medical attention at this time. There should be a palpable area of tenderness over the spinous process of the fractured vertebra. There may be paraspinal muscle tenderness in the region, and this can extend several levels up or down from the lesion.

The association of the level of the pain and the level of the compression fracture may be confirmed by placing the patient in the left lateral decubitus position on a fluoroscopy table and directly palpating the area of the patient's discomfort. This procedure is coordinated with radiographic visualization of the level. Such an approach is very helpful in identifying the symptomatic levels in a patient who has multiple fractures.

Some patients with thoracic compression fractures have pain radiating around the chest wall. We have seen several patients in whom radicular-like pain around the chest wall was a significant component of their symptoms. They had no radiographic signs of nerve root compression. In most cases, pain was relieved after vertebroplasty.

Imaging

In this era of medicine, most patients present with images in hand, having had plain film radiographs, computed tomography (CT), bone scan, MR imaging, or any combination of these modalities for their initial complaints of back pain. Imaging is crucial in the evaluation of these patients. However, cross-sectional imaging (CT, MR) is not always necessary to make the diagnosis. In general, these fractures can be diagnosed with plain radiographs and remote studies can be compared to evaluate fracture age and progression (Fig. 8-3). A bone scan is extremely helpful in establishing the age of the fractures by detecting activity that suggests recent fracture and/or absence of fracture healing (Fig. 8-4). Maynard and colleagues[7] and, more recently, Kaufman and associates[6] have established a strong link between positive bone scans and pain relief in their vertebroplasty patient population. If cross-sectional imaging is available, an MR imaging study can demonstrate recent fractures, eliciting evidence of bone marrow edema and inflammatory changes, which are particularly obvious with fat saturation techniques (Fig. 8-5). MR imaging also permits the evaluation of other conditions that may be contributing to the patient's symptoms, particularly in the case of infiltrative lesions such as myeloma and lymphoma and of unsuspected metastatic lesions. MR imaging can aid in the diagnosis of spondylosis,

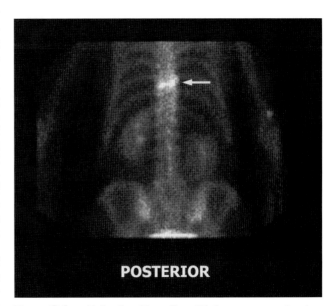

Figure 8-4 ■ Technetium-99m radionuclide bone scan, posterior view. There is a focal region of increased radiotracer uptake involving approximately the T10 vertebra (*arrow*).

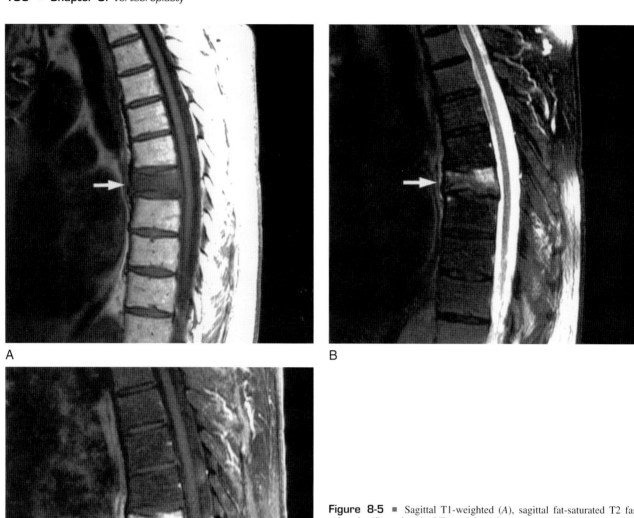

A

B

C

Figure 8-5 ■ Sagittal T1-weighted (*A*), sagittal fat-saturated T2 fast spin echo (*B*), and sagittal T1-weighted fat saturated (*C*) MR images of the thoracic spine demonstrate abnormal signal intensity involving a midthoracic vertebral body (*arrow*).

facet disease, disc disease, and spinal stenosis. We routinely obtain MR imaging in patients whose history and physical suggest another cause for their back pain or when a retropulsed fragment is suspected. In patients who cannot undergo MR imaging (e.g., because of a pacemaker or severe claustrophobia), a limited CT scan through areas of fractures with two-dimensional reconstruction can help evaluate spinal canal compromise from a retropulsed fragment and identify mass lesions (Fig. 8-6). Bone density measurements are supportive data in making the diagnosis of osteoporosis, but they do not contribute much to the direct evaluation of the fractures in candidates for vertebroplasty.

Laboratory Evaluation

Only a few tests are necessary before vertebroplasty. The patient's coagulation status, prothrombin time, partial thromboplastin time, International Normalized Ratio, and platelet count should be verified as being normal. Serum creatinine studies are not necessary, because the amount of contrast medium utilized in vertebral venography is unlikely to create any significant renal toxicity. Whenever general anesthesia is utilized, an electrocardiogram, a chest radiograph, and a standard preanesthetic evaluation are required.

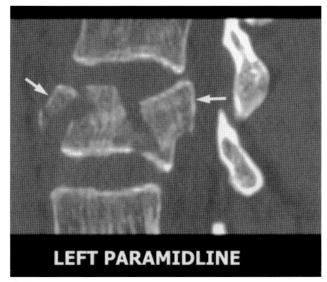

A

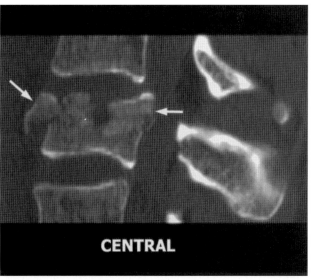

B

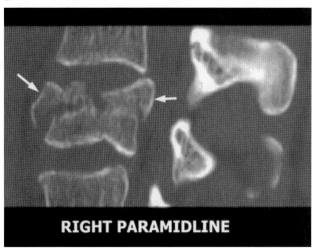

C

Figure 8-6 ■ Sagittal reconstructed images. Left paramidline (*A*), central (*B*), and right paramidline (*C*) sagittal images demonstrate not only significant spinal canal compromise, particularly off midline, but also the presence of free fragments (*arrows*) caused by a burst fracture of the vertebral body. This patient was not a candidate for vertebroplasty.

CONTRAINDICATIONS

There are few absolute contraindications to vertebroplasty. However, certain lesions are much more amenable to treatment than others. In general, fractures with a loss of more than 80% of vertebral body height do not respond well to vertebroplasty. Clinical improvement in patients with vertebra plana is not commonly seen. Some authors have reported limited success with more severe fractures. A series of patients with severe fractures treated by O'Brien and coworkers[8] had a good response to therapy with techniques that confined cement delivery to the lateral aspects of severely fractured vertebrae. In many fractures, there is more residual bone laterally than in the central portions of the vertebral body. Recently, we have successfully treated patients with severe fractures in a similar manner. However, the rate of response is certainly lower than that achieved with less severe fractures.

Fractures resulting in a retropulsed fragment can also be problematic, because injection of cement can cause further migration of the fragment, possibly leading to compression of the spinal cord or other neural elements. We generally do not treat fractures when there is a displaced or retropulsed bone fragment creating more than 30% central spinal canal stenosis. Similarly, fractures caused by tumor infiltration with a large epidural soft tissue component are not very amenable to treatment unless it is performed in conjunction with planned surgical decompression of the spinal canal.

Patients with poorly localized pain or pain that does not correlate with the level of the fracture are generally poor candidates for vertebroplasty. Even though fractures are recent according to imaging studies and appear amenable to treatment, patients whose symptoms cannot be localized rarely experience significant pain relief. As previously mentioned, radicular pain is not usually caused by an uncomplicated compression fracture, and a thorough search should be made for other causes of this type of pain before attempting vertebroplasty.

Patients with medical conditions requiring anticoagulation present a relative contraindication. Although tighter control of the patient's coagulation status can be achieved with conversion to heparin (in hospital) or enoxaparin (outpatient) and reversal with protamine at the time of the procedure, the requirements of maintaining anticoagulation slightly increase the risk of the procedure and can result in longer hospitalization.

Active infection, either systemic or localized to the skin overlying the procedural site, is an absolute contraindication, and any suspicion of infection must be investigated thoroughly before PMMA is introduced. Infection involving the implanted PMMA in the spine is a disastrous complication. Even though there are reports of postvertebroplasty osteomyelitis that have cleared with weeks of intravenous antibiotic treatment,[9] such infections commonly require surgical corpectomy and are associated with a high mortality rate in the geriatric population.

Finally, patients should be able to lie prone, or nearly prone, for at least 30 to 45 minutes to have the procedure performed. Although some adjustments can be made, occasional patients cannot tolerate this positioning. Rarely, general anesthesia is required for patients for whom the required prone position is intolerable, in patients with chronic obstructive pulmonary disease, or in those in whom airway maintenance is an issue.

PROCEDURE

Equipment/Supplies

Styled needles, 11- or 13-gauge or cement delivery system (Fig. 8-7)

- PMMA may be injected through a delivery needle with multiple 1- or 3-mL syringes. Recently, several delivery systems that give greater control and increase the efficiency of the process of PMMA injection have become commercially available.

Codman Cranioplastic Type 1-Slow Set (Codman Cranioplastic, Codman and Shurtleff, Inc., Raynham, MA)

- Polymethylmethacrylate powder (two 30-g packages)
- Liquid methacrylate monomer
- *At the time of this writing, there is no cement that is specifically FDA approved for vertebroplasty.*

Tobramycin powder, 1.2 g (Nebcin, tobramycin for injection, USP, Eli Lilly and Company, Indianapolis, IN)
Sterile barium sulfate powder (Biotrace, Bryan Corp., Woburn, MA)
Syringe, 10 mL, and connecting tube containing non-ionic iodinated contrast medium (320 mg I/mL) for venography
Sterile scalpel and hemostat
Sterile hat, mask, and gloves
Lead apron and C-arm fluoroscopy
Sterile gauze
Adhesive bandages and adhesive strips
Control syringe, 12 mL, with 25-gauge, 1.5-inch needle containing 9.5 mL 1% lidocaine for local anesthesia and 0.5 mL 8.4% sodium bicarbonate injectable (1 mEq/mL) to alleviate burning pain associated with the anesthetic
Spinal needle, 22-gauge, 3.5-inch for deep anesthesia
Prophylactic intravenous antibiotics*

*The role of antibiotic prophylaxis in the performance of vertebroplasty is not uniformly agreed upon. We mix tobramycin powder in the PMMA mixture and believe that this is adequate prophylaxis in most patients. However, in patients who are immunocompromised for any reason or who are particularly debilitated, we do give prophylactic intravenous antibiotics (usually 1 g of cefazolin 1 hour before the initial needle placement) in addition to the tobramycin in the PMMA. We have treated well over 300 patients using this guideline, with a single documented infection 4 weeks after the procedure, which was likely caused by a central venous line placed 3 weeks after the vertebroplasty. Some authors utilize intravenous antibiotics routinely, with or without tobramycin in the PMMA mixture. There is no body of literature to support either practice, beyond the reports of low infection rates with either regimen

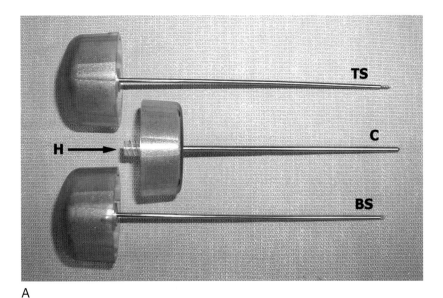

A

Figure 8-7 ▪ Parallax™ EZ*flow* cement delivery system (Scotts Valley, CA). *A,* AccuThread™ access needles include a bevel stylet (BS), a threaded stylet (TS), and a diamond point stylet (*not shown*). These stylets screw into the hub (H) of the cement delivery cannula (C). *B,* DynaTorque Injector system components. The threaded proximal end of the reservoir (R) accepts the mechanical plunger (P). The plunger is advanced mechanically by rotating the knob with one hand while the other hand supports the device by gripping the handle. *Arrows* depict the direction of cement flow from the cement reservoir (R) into the LC connecting tube (CT). *C,* Distal portion of cement delivery system. End of the LC connecting tube (CT) attaches with a Luer-lock connection (LL) to the hub of the cement delivery cannula. Long arrow represents the direction of cement flow into the vertebral body. (*The Parallax™ delivery system is marketed in the United States for the percutaneous delivery of bone cement. Cement delivery system photographed with permission of Parallax™ Medical, Inc., Scotts Valley, CA. Parallax™, DynaTorque™, and AccuThread™ are trademarks of Parallax Medical, Inc.*)

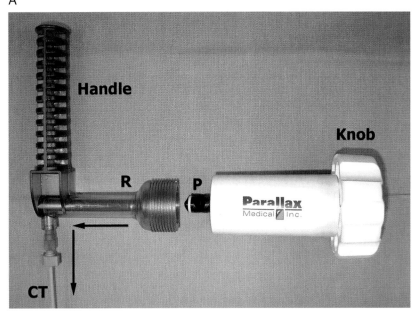

B

C

and the general literature on surgical prophylaxis. We believe that some form of antibiotic is prudent. Whatever prophylaxis is comfortable or customary for each physician or hospital should be adequate. One should, however, err on the conservative side, given the difficulty in dealing with infections involving the implanted PMMA and the consequences of infection in this area.

Sterile Technique

Because vertebroplasty entails injecting a foreign substance permanently into the vertebral body, the practitioner must perform the procedure with the utmost sterility. This includes a surgical scrub, hat, mask, sterile gown, and sterile gloves. The procedural site is scrubbed with povidone-iodine (Betadine) and alcohol three times each and then draped with sterile sheets. Sterile covers are placed over the image intensifier(s), x-ray tube(s), and fluoroscopy control panel.

Methodology

As with any procedure, there are many ways to accomplish the same result. Vertebroplasty techniques vary greatly. We describe the basic method that is used in our institution and the principles that should be observed to perform a safe and technically successful vertebroplasty. Obviously, each operator will modify the technique to what is comfortable for him or her. The description that follows is not a substitute for hands-on training in vertebroplasty. We strongly recommend that physicians wishing to perform vertebroplasty attend a recognized training course or spend time with physicians who are experienced with vertebroplasty before they treat patients on their own. There is no substitute for hands-on training in these kinds of invasive techniques.

Thoracic and Lumbar Procedures

PATIENT POSITIONING

Informed consent is obtained and off-label use of PMMA is disclosed to the patient. A minimum of electrocardiography, pulse oximetry, and blood pressure monitoring is performed during and immediately after the examination. The procedure is generally performed with the patient in the prone position. This allows the best access to the pedicles, which is the preferred access route in the thoracic and lumbar spine. In general, we place patients on "jelly rolls" on the angiogram table, with pillows under the shoulders and head for support. This allows slightly more room for the patient to move his or her head and lie in a comfortable position. The chest and stomach are allowed to hang slightly, which permits more efficient respiration and can decrease venous bleeding that can occur with increased abdominal pressure in the prone position. Some patients are not comfortable on the "jelly rolls" and do better with towels or simple pillows. Some cannot lie in a prone position and are placed three-quarter prone. The flexibility of the C-arm system allows the operator to adjust for these differences without difficulty. Comfortable patient positioning that allows easy access to

the vertebra is extremely important. This procedure can be accomplished in an efficient manner if the patient is comfortable and remains quiet. This can be a challenge, especially in the older patient population. Also important is careful and gentle movement of the elderly patient onto the table. These patients are often extremely osteoporotic, and fractures of the ribs and occasionally other bones can occur when mobilizing any patient. With attention to proper positioning, the use of sedation can be dramatically reduced and the procedure time can be significantly shortened.

SITE PREPARATION

The patient's back is prepared in a sterile fashion with povidone-iodine and alcohol and draped; a wide area of the back is prepared because angles of approach can vary. Entry points can be significantly superior or inferior to the level of the affected vertebral body or significantly off midline. The point of entry and angle of approach are affected by factors such as the degree of scoliosis and kyphosis, the degree and number of compression fractures, and the patient's overall body habitus. A mild sedative and analgesic (midazolam, 1 to 2 mg; fentanyl, 100 to 150 μg) can be administered during the procedure to make the patient more comfortable.

NEEDLE PLACEMENT

Planning for the initial needle placement is one of the most critical steps in the procedure. A multitude of small adjustments can be made when advancing the needle to ensure proper positioning. However, these maneuvers often cannot compensate enough for a poorly chosen entry position or an ill-conceived needle angle. In the "classic approach," the vertebral body is aligned in the straight anteroposterior (AP) and lateral projections. The superior and inferior end plates are aligned to a single line on the AP view, with both pedicles visible and the spinous process in the midline (Fig. 8-8*A*); the ribs, pedicles, neural arches, and posterior aspects of contiguous vertebral bodies are aligned on the lateral view (see Fig. 8-8*B*). This positioning generally allows a good view of both sides of the vertebral body for needle placement. If a single-plane system is being utilized, we recommend that the coordinates for the C-arm be noted in both the AP and lateral planes at the beginning of the procedure to increase the efficiency in switching from one view to the other during the case. One must realize that patients often move slightly without warning. This trend continues and increases in frequency as the procedure progresses and the patient becomes progressively more tired and restless. Continued adjustment of the C-arm angle is required to ensure proper needle position.

We employ a slightly different positioning strategy, utilizing an oblique angle down the pedicle. This approach applies the general concept of an oblique view of the pedicle and facet advocated elsewhere in this book. The C-arm is initially rotated craniocaudad to superimpose the pedicle with the mid to upper third of the vertebral body. The C-arm is then rotated obliquely to a point just before the medial cortex of the pedicle cannot be confidently visualized (Fig. 8-9). This oblique view provides for an excellent view of the pedicle (most importantly the medial cortex of the pedicle) during the entire phase of needle advancement. The other

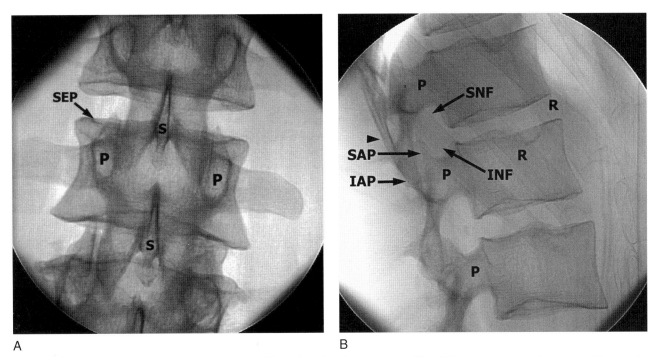

A   B

Figure 8-8 ▪ *A*, AP positioning. The pedicles (P) are equidistant from the spinous processes (S), and the anterior and posterior portions of the superior end plate (SEP) superimpose. *B*, Lateral positioning. The anterior and posterior vertebral structures superimpose and appear as a single unit. R = anterior ribs; *arrowhead* = posterior ribs; SAP = superior articular processes; IAP = inferior articular processes; P = pedicles; SNF = superior neural foramen; INF = inferior neural foramen.

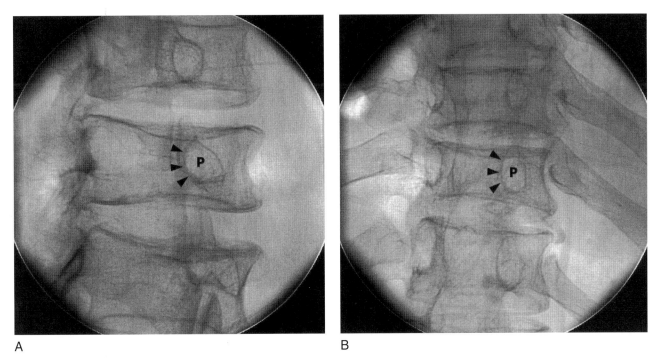

A   B

Figure 8-9 ▪ Lumbar (*A*) and thoracic (*B*) LAO radiographs demonstrate positioning of the pedicle (P) over the mid to upper third of the vertebral body. Note the rounded shape of the pedicle. *Arrowheads* demarcate the medial cortex of the pedicle.

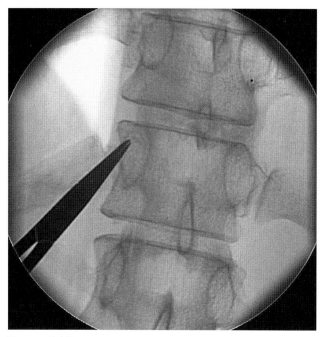

Figure 8-10 ■ Needle entry site. RAO radiograph demonstrates a hemostat overlying the upper outer third of the pedicle.

Once the alignment has been confirmed, and an entry point has been chosen, 1% lidocaine or 0.25% bupivacaine is injected subcutaneously for local anesthesia. The tract of the needle should be infiltrated judiciously to the pedicle, and the periosteum of the pedicle should be liberally anesthetized. When this is accomplished, there is little discomfort for the patient during placement of the larger-caliber vertebroplasty needle. A small skin incision is then made with a scalpel to help facilitate passage of the larger-caliber needle through the skin. The needle is then placed in the mid to upper outer third of the pedicle (Fig. 8-10) and advanced carefully through the pedicle into the vertebral body. The goal of needle placement is to position the tip of the outer needle cannula at the junction of the middle and anterior thirds of the vertebral body, as close to the center (superiorly, inferiorly, and laterally) as possible (Fig. 8-11). Needle path adjustments should be made early, when the needle is still in the pedicle. As the needle progresses deeper, path adjustments are less effective and may result in pedicle fracture from excessive torquing of the needle. Fluoroscopically, the needle should at all times remain lateral to the medial cortical edge of the pedicle until it has passed anteriorly into the vertebral body (Fig. 8-12). Trauma to the thecal sac or the spinal cord or tearing of epidural veins will result when the medial cortex is violated. If the vertebral body collapse is relatively unilateral and mild, the needle may be placed on the involved side. However, if the collapse is severe, it may be necessary to place the initial needle on the side with more residual vertebral body. If there is a severe collapse in the central portion, a single pedicle approach will likely not result in PMMA distribution across the midline. In this case, bilateral needle placement is required (Fig. 8-13).

advantage of this approach is that it offers a greater likelihood that a unipedicular approach will provide cement to both sides of the vertebral body, which obviates a second needle placement. We have reported an 80% to 90% rate of unipedicular injections using this approach.

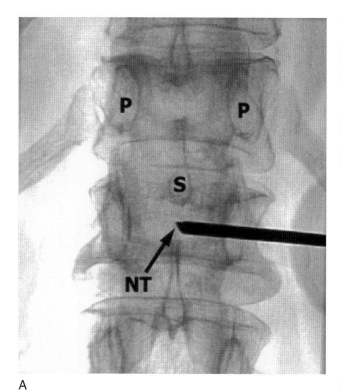

A

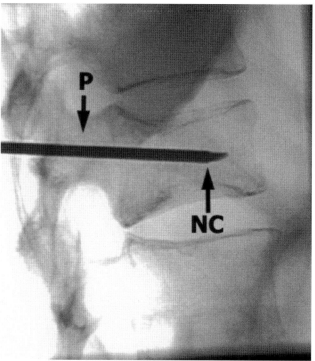

B

Figure 8-11 ■ *A*, AP radiograph. The needle tip (*NT*) is seen in the midline with respect to the pedicles (*P*) and the superior and inferior vertebral margins. S = spinous process. *B*, Lateral radiograph. The tip of the needle cannula (*NC*) is at the junction of the anterior and middle thirds of the vertebral body.

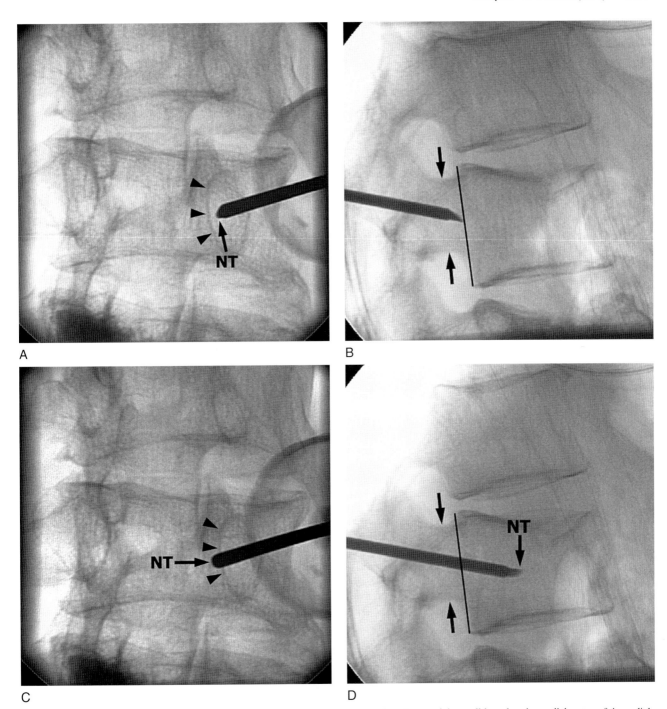

Figure 8-12 ▪ Safe needle placement. *A*, AP radiograph demonstrates the needle tip (NT) remaining well lateral to the medial cortex of the pedicle (*arrowheads*). *B*, Lateral radiograph corresponding to *A* shows the needle traversing the center of the pedicle (bounded by *arrows*) with the needle tip at the posterior margin of the vertebral body (*straight line*). The relationship of *A* and *B* must occur or a breach in the pedicle will have taken place. *C* and *D*, The needle has been advanced into the vertebral body. The needle tip (NT) is now seen medial to the medial cortex of the pedicle (*arrowheads*, C; *arrows*, D), but it remains in a safe position because the needle tip was in proper position before its advancement into the vertebral body.

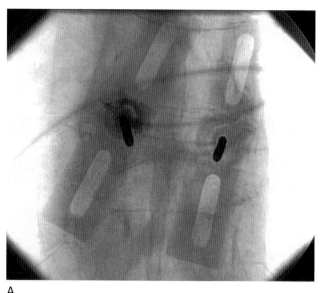
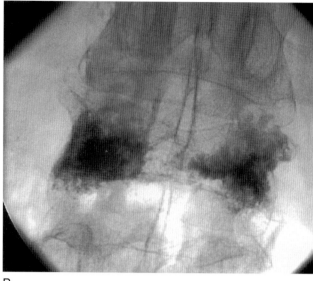

A   B

Figure 8-13 ■ Severe fracture of the central portion of the vertebral body. With this amount of loss of vertebral height centrally, a single needle approach would likely breach the superior or inferior end plate. *A*, A bilateral needle approach was performed with the needles positioned into the lateral portions of each half of the vertebral body. *B*, AP radiograph after bipedicular cement injections. There is good cement distribution in both halves of the vertebral body, with a small amount of cement filling the midvertebral body.

Once past the posterior edge of the vertebral body, with visualization in the lateral plane, the needle can be advanced more rapidly under continuous fluoroscopy. Patients given conscious sedation move during the procedure, and the fluoroscopic image may not reflect a true lateral position. The vertebral body is a rounded structure; when the needle is advanced too far anteriorly, an off-midline needle tip could perforate the ventral cortex. If the needle tip is not advanced past the junction of the anterior and middle thirds of the vertebral body in the lateral projection, even off-midline needle tips should remain within the vertebral body. An errant anterior needle placement has the potential for perforating the aorta and the inferior vena cava, which lie just anterior to the vertebral column in the thoracic and upper lumbar spine.

Cervical Procedures

PATIENT POSITIONING

The approach to fractures in the cervical spine is significantly different from that in the thoracic or lumbar spine. The small size of the pedicles, the vertebral artery, and the geometry of the vertebra do not permit a transpedicular needle placement. The approach to cervical vertebral bodies is antero-lateral, and it requires navigating the needle through the soft tissues of the neck.

Informed consent is obtained, and off-label use of PMMA is disclosed to the patient. A minimum of electrocardiographic, pulse oximetry, and blood pressure monitoring is performed during and immediately after the examination. The patient is placed in a supine position, generally with the head turned slightly contralateral to the side of the needle placement. For the lower cervical levels, the approach can be made with relatively no caudocephalic angulation of the needle. In the upper cervical region, the entry site is often

caudad to the level of the lesion because of the interposed mandible. Having the patient turn his or her head away from the side of entry and thrusting the jaw superiorly lessens some of the angulation.

SITE PREPARATION

The neck is prepared in a sterile fashion with povidone-iodine and alcohol and draped appropriately. A mild sedative and analgesic (midazolam, 1 to 2 mg; fentanyl, 100 to 150 μg) can be administered during the procedure to make the patient more comfortable. A wide field is preferred, centered on the anterior aspect of the sternocleidomastoid muscle.

NEEDLE PLACEMENT

A needle with the smallest possible caliber that will allow delivery of PMMA should be used for cervical vertebroplasty. The technique has been described with 13- and 15-gauge needles. The operator must first palpate the carotid-jugular sheath and displace it posteriorly (Fig. 8-14).[10] Consideration should be given to prophylaxis with atropine (0.6 to 1.0 mg intravenously) before this maneuver because carotid body compression can cause a vasovagal response. The entry site should be at the ventral edge of the sternocleidomastoid muscle. The needle should be advanced slowly, aiming for the junction of the anterior and middle thirds of the target vertebral body, just to the proximal side of the midline. The needle should be advanced slowly into the vertebral body (Fig. 8-15*A* and *B*). Given the complex anatomy and the proximity of important and vulnerable structures in the neck, some operators place the needles in the cervical spine under CT guidance (see Fig. 8-15*C*). This is an easy procedure and can be accomplished with a minimum of risk to the patient. Injection of PMMA is performed under real-time monitoring with fluoroscopy.

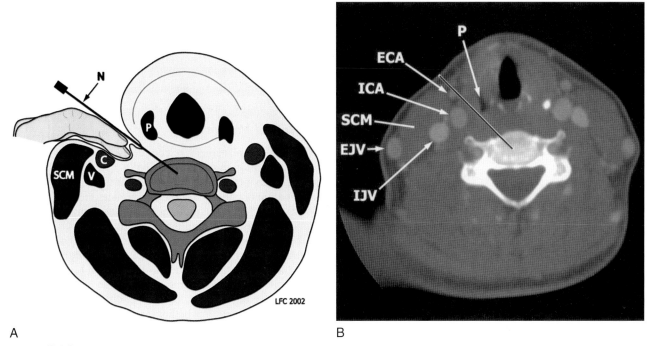

A   B

Figure 8-14 ■ Cervical vertebroplasty needle placement technique. *A*, Axial illustration. The skin entrance is along the anterior border of the sternocleidomastoid muscle (SCM). The discographer's fingers manually displace the vascular structures. The needle (N) is advanced ventral to the fingers. C = carotid artery; V = jugular vein; P = pyriform sinus. *B*, Corresponding axial CT image. The needle trajectory (*line*), in this case, would pierce the right external carotid artery (ECA) if it were not manually displaced posterolaterally. ICA = internal carotid artery; EJV = external jugular vein; IJV = internal jugular vein; P = pyriform sinus.

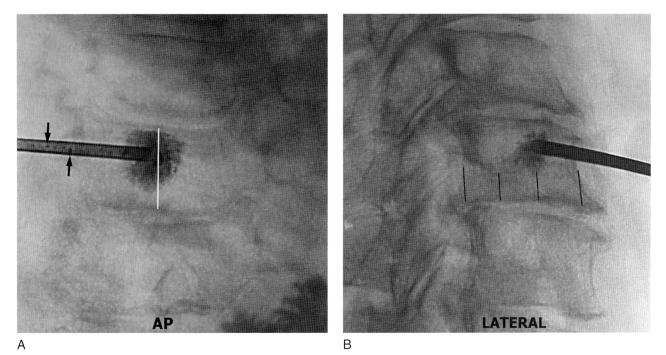

A   B

Figure 8-15 ■ *A*, AP radiograph demonstrates the needle tip just lateral to midline. White vertical line divides the vertebral body into equal halves. Arrows = small clumps of cement in the needle cannula. *B*, Lateral radiograph demonstrates the needle tip at the junction of the anterior and middle thirds of the vertebral body. Black vertical lines divide the vertebral body into three equal parts.

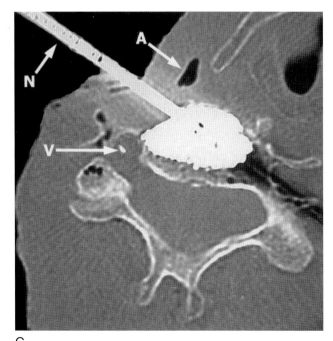

C

Figure 8-15 (*Cont'd*) ■ *C*, Axial computed tomogram demonstrates a needle (N) placed from a right anterolateral approach into the vertebral body. There is good spread of high-density cement throughout the vertebral body without spread to the posterior cortex. A = small amount of iatrogenically introduced air; V = calcification in the wall of the right vertebral artery.

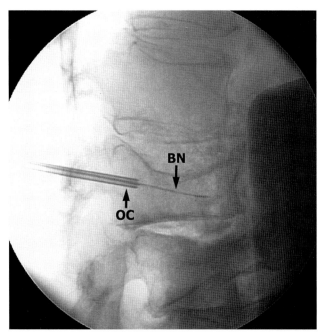

Figure 8-16 ■ Lateral radiograph demonstrates the outer cannula (OC) of the cement delivery system in the posterior aspect of the vertebral body, with a smaller-gauge, longer biopsy needle (BN) passing into the vertebral body to obtain a tissue sample.

Vertebral Biopsy

If the cause of the compression fracture is suspicious, a vertebral biopsy can be performed once the large-caliber needle has been placed. A tissue sample can readily be obtained with a coaxial approach through the large-caliber needle with a longer, smaller-gauge needle (Fig. 8-16).

Vertebral Venography

When needle placement is complete, venography may be performed through the needle (Fig. 8-17). Although not all practitioners perform this step, we believe it gives valuable information of patient-specific venous anatomy and can help determine whether a single needle placement will be adequate. It is easily accomplished, and it adds very little time to the procedure. We generally use 3 to 5 mL of half-strength contrast agent (50:50 mixture of iodinated nonionic contrast and normal saline). The most important function of the venography is to determine whether the needle is in or immediately adjacent to the basivertebral vein or another large draining vein or whether it is within a fissure continuous with the paraspinal structures or adjacent disc spaces. If the needle is in or directly adjacent to a vein, the initial methacrylate bolus could easily be injected into that vein, into the epidural venous plexus, or even into the inferior vena cava, and venous embolism and pulmonary infarction could result. Knowledge of positioning within a vein allows one to reposition the needle slightly and adjust the initial delivery to avoid this circumstance.

Contrast agents and PMMA have significantly different flow characteristics. However, if the venogram shows unilateral drainage without any flow to the opposite side, the chances of a successful unipedicular approach are less (Fig. 8-18). Therefore, the operator may choose to place a second needle before mixing the cement and inject both needles with 1 mixture of methacrylate. Resistance to the flow of contrast medium or extravasation of contrast medium through fractures in the vertebral body cortex alerts the operator to the potential for difficult deposition of cement or for extravasation of PMMA. Strategies for changing the consistency of the methacrylate mixture and changing the speed or other parameters of cement delivery can be devised to achieve the optimal deposition of cement without excessive leakage.

Cement Preparation

Although the cement-mixing procedure is quite straightforward, many variations are used by different practitioners. Our preparation of cement for injection combines PMMA powder, tobramycin powder, and barium sulfate or tantalum powder (for opacification). These ingredients are mixed in aliquots with liquid methacrylate monomer to provide an injectable solution. Thirty grams (1 package) of the methylmethacrylate polymer is mixed with 1.2 g of tobramycin and 12 g of barium sulfate. The powder is carefully mixed to remove any large clumps. Caution should be used not to mix too aggressively, because the presence of small barium clumps is helpful in fluoroscopically visualizing the cement mixture as it moves down the needle during the injection (Fig. 8-19). Aliquots of 20 mL of the powdered mixture are

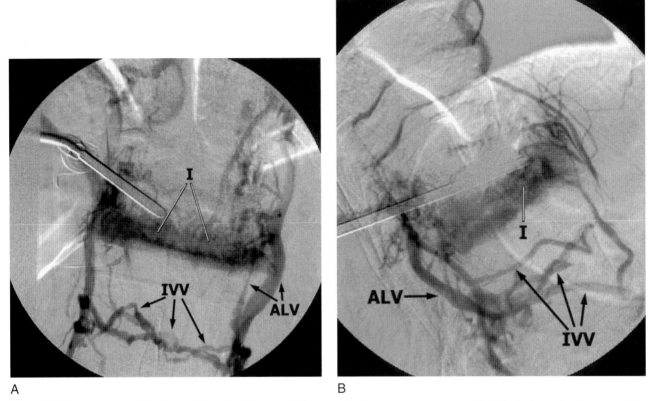

Figure 8-17 ■ AP (*A*) and lateral (*B*) radiographs during vertebral venography demonstrate contrast material within the intratrabecular spaces (I) as well as the paravertebral veins. ALV = ascending lumbar veins; IVV = intervertebral veins.

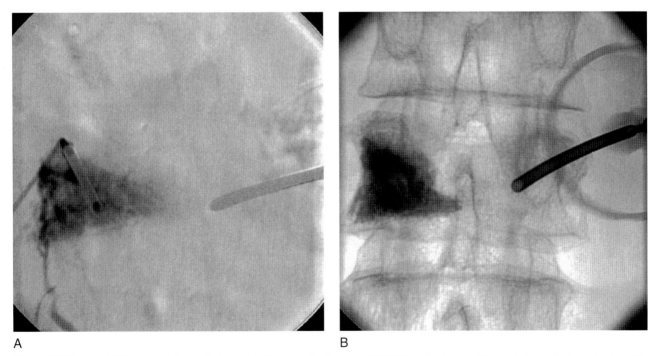

Figure 8-18 ■ *A*, AP fluoroscopic image during vertebral venography through a left-sided needle placement demonstrates contrast agent only within the left half of the vertebral body. *B*, Image in same patient after methacrylate injection demonstrates cement only within the left half of the vertebral body. A right-sided needle placement was performed to fill the right half of the vertebral body.

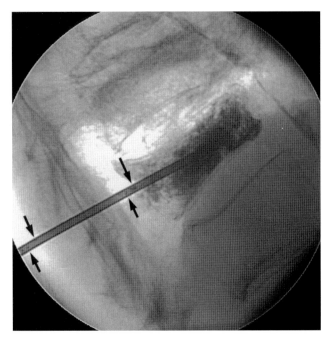

Figure 8-19 ▪ Small clumps in the cement mixture (*arrows*) help the physician evaluate whether there is forward flow of the cement.

room (because the reaction is exothermic, a colder room temperature prolongs the working time of the cement) and the type of containers used to hold the cement. When 1-mL syringes are used, the effective working time is usually shorter than when a commercially available large-reservoir delivery system is used.

Cement Injection

Delivery of the methacrylate mixture is accomplished under direct fluoroscopic visualization. Most of the process should be viewed in a true lateral projection with particular attention to extravasation of methacrylate posteriorly into the basivertebral vein or through a fissure into the epidural space. Complications from methacrylate in the epidural space and the neural foramina are of the greatest concern. The ease of injection and the distribution of the contrast agent encountered during the venography give the operator a clue as to the initial distribution of the methacrylate. Still, the method of injection continuously changes during a procedure, and the distribution of the cement depends on many factors, including the continuous polymerization of the cement in the bone, the presence of fissures or fractures in the vertebral body, and positional changes of the needle during injection. Some patterns of filling can be predicted from the venogram (as described earlier), especially when the vertebral body contains large fissures. Filling of a large central cavity can be problematic when there is a connection to the end plates or the paravertebral space. Extravasation may be difficult to control. Pausing during the injection to allow some curing of the cement in the cavity, combined with repositioning of the needle, can sometimes stop the extravasation and allow further filling of the vertebral body. However, this must be done carefully, because such maneuvers may not always

placed in a plastic bowel, and liquid monomer is slowly added while stirring. The monomer is added until the mixture has the consistency of a thick pancake batter or syrup. In general, 8 to 9 mL of the monomer is required per 20 mL of aliquot of powder. Quantities and ratios are different with other brands of cement. Working time for the mixture varies with the type of delivery system, the brand of polymer and monomer used, and such variables as the temperature of the

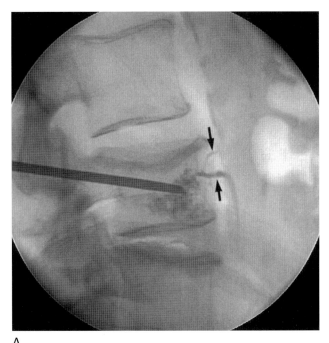

A

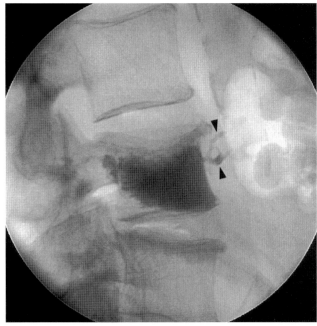

B

Figure 8-20 ▪ *A*, Lateral radiograph during vertebral venography demonstrates contrast medium within the substance of the vertebral body and filling of two small anterior draining veins (*arrows*). *B*, Lateral radiograph after cement injection demonstrates cement within the same two draining veins (*arrowheads*). This patient had no complications caused by the cement.

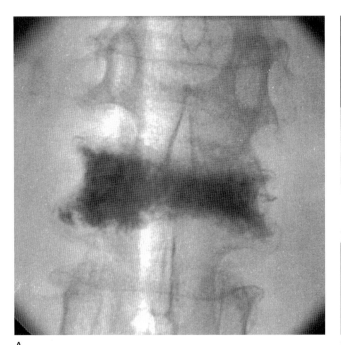

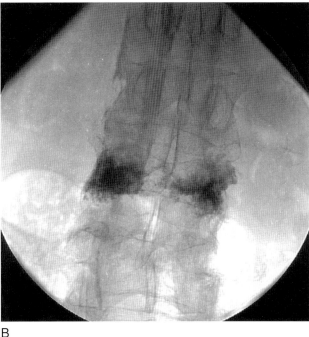

A

B

Figure 8-21 ■ Two patients after vertebroplasty, AP radiographs. *A*, Cement is seen in both halves of the vertebral body and across the midline. *B*, Cement is seen in both halves of the vertebral body, with only minimal amounts in the midline. Both results are radiographically acceptable, and both patients had excellent pain relief.

stop the leak. Fractures that extend to the end plates or to the paravertebral space are common, even if there is no large central cavity. Also, draining veins may fill even if they are not apparent initially (Fig. 8-20).

Recently at our institution we have employed a method to control the rapid flow of cement into these veins in the event the needle is positioned in or adjacent to such a structure. When mixing the liquid PMMA monomer into the PMMA polymer powder, there is a stage when the mixture has the consistency of paste, as opposed to the much more liquid form that is ultimately injected (usually when 6 to 7 mL of monomer has been added). We take a small amount of this paste and place it in the cannula with a spatula. The paste is then pushed through the cannula of the vertebroplasty needle with the stylet until the paste is extruded into the vertebral body. At times a second small aliquot of cement is necessary. The intravertebral cement will polymerize and form a solid plug, while we finish the cement preparation and load the remainder of the PMMA into the reservoir of the injector. The cement plug will impede additional flow into the vein and allow smooth filling of the vertebral body. Care must be taken to ensure that the PMMA plug is pushed entirely out of the cannula so that it does not block further injection and that the stylet is not left in place so long that it is cemented into the cannula. This principle can also occasionally be applied to needles adjacent to large fissures; however, the control of PMMA injection into fissures is somewhat more complex.

An increase in the amount of polymer deposited should be discernible in at least one plane with each small increment of polymer delivered. If it is not, there is a good chance that polymer is not being injected within the vertebral body but outside it. Injecting slowly and purposefully is the best way to control extravasation.

The end point of injection varies among different operators, and appreciation of this point comes with experience. **Avoiding deposition of cement at the posterior aspect of the vertebral body is paramount.** Complete coverage of the vertebral body with the polymer is not required for a good clinical outcome. The following few rules may be applied as general guidelines. There should be cement in both halves of the vertebral body (Fig. 8-21). However, the

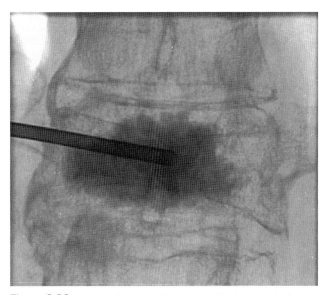

Figure 8-22 ■ AP radiograph with single needle placement in the center of the vertebral body. Cement is seen within the central and medial portions of both halves of the vertebral body. This is a radiographically acceptable result, and the patient had excellent pain relief.

presence of any cement across the midline is generally sufficient (Fig. 8-22), and little is gained in clinical outcome by placing a second needle into the vertebra. A small amount of extravasation into the adjacent disc space is sometimes unavoidable (Fig. 8-23). If it can be kept to a minimum, it will usually have no clinical effect. However the presence of PMMA in the disc space theoretically increases the chances of fracture of the adjacent vertebral body. Nothing is gained in continuing to deliver polymer as

the needle is withdrawn posteriorly into the pedicle; if a pedicular fracture was present, extravasation into the central canal or neural foramen could occur.

Once the needles have been withdrawn, AP and lateral final control radiographs are taken (Fig. 8-24). A small amount of pressure on the skin incision may be required to stop oozing of blood. Adhesive strips and sterile dressings are applied. The patient is turned onto his or her back, kept supine, and transferred to a recovery area.

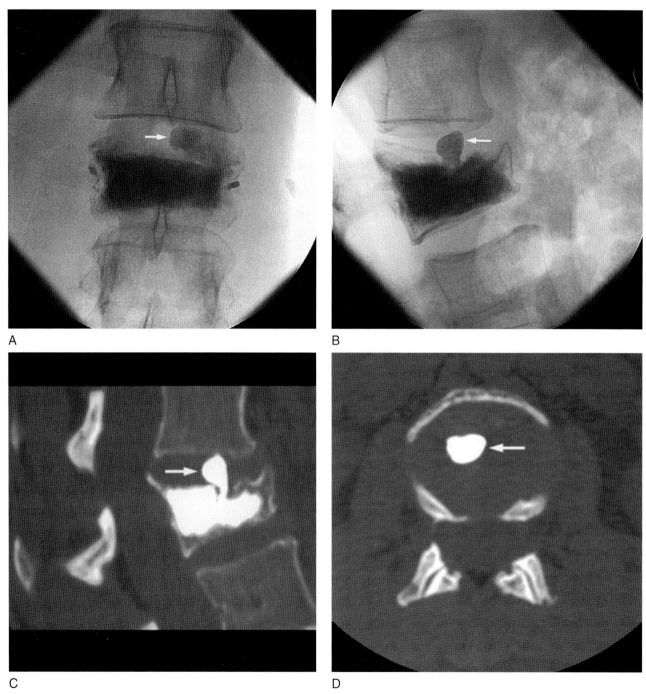

A

B

C

D

Figure 8-23 ■ AP radiograph (*A*), lateral radiograph (*B*), sagittal reformatted CT image (*C*), and axial CT image (*D*) after cement injection demonstrate a small amount of cement (*arrow*) penetrating the disc space above. The patient had excellent pain relief after vertebroplasty.

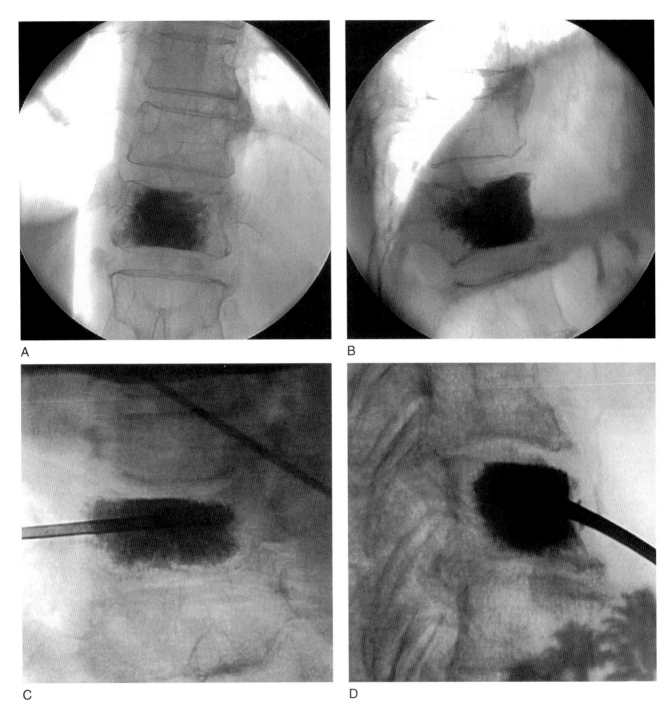

A

B

C

D

Figure 8-24 ■ AP (*A*) and lateral (*B*) radiographs after thoracic vertebroplasty demonstrate an excellent radiographic result. There is cement coverage from pedicle to pedicle in the AP plane (*A*) and good anterior to posterior coverage on the lateral image (*B*) with very minimal cement extending to the posterior cortex. *C* and *D*, There is a similar excellent radiographic result after cervical vertebroplasty.

ALTERNATIVE METHOD FOR VERTEBRAL BODY STABILIZATION

Kyphoplasty is a recently developed method for treating compression fractures of the spine in which a balloon is placed coaxially through a needle into the vertebral body to reduce the fracture, followed by cement augmentation. The technique shares many features with vertebroplasty, including similar transpedicular and extrapedicular approaches. However, kyphoplasty requires larger (9- or 10-gauge) needles and a bipedicular approach. This limits the procedure to the midthoracic and lumbar levels. Balloons are coaxially placed and inflated under fluoroscopy to reduce the compression fracture and create a pocket for the PMMA.

Very thick PMMA is layered into the cavity under very low pressure. The proponents of kyphoplasty believe that the restoration of height improves the biomechanics of the spine and in some cases can improve the kyphosis. They also believe that the introduction of the PMMA under low pressure reduces the chances of extravasation of cement into the epidural space and neural foramina. Early studies of this technique have been encouraging. Lieberman and associates[11] studied a group of 30 patients in a phase I evaluation of kyphoplasty. In that series, some height was restored in 70% of cases, with an average restoration of lost height of 46.8%. The rate of extravasation was 8.6%, less than that reported by many authors performing vertebroplasty. The rate of symptomatic complications from the extravasation, however, is comparable. Rates of pain relief reported in this and other series are in the range of 70% to 90%, similar to those reported for vertebroplasty. The goal of restoration of vertebral body height and possible reduction of kyphosis is intriguing. The technique is somewhat more complicated than that of vertebroplasty, and appropriate candidates are fewer. It requires bilateral needle placement and coordination of balloon inflation in the vertebral body. Kyphoplasty appears to be a viable and potentially useful additional method for treating vertebral compression fractures.

POTENTIAL COMPLICATIONS

The risk of complications with vertebroplasty is very low when basic rules are followed. Good technique allows the operator to perform safe vertebroplasty in almost any situation. However, there are pitfalls, and rare severe complications have been reported.

Complications Associated with Needle Placement

Transpedicular Approach

The most immediate and potentially most severe complication associated with the transpedicular approach can occur during the initial portion of the procedure. Both posterior approaches require advancing the needle past the spinal canal, which contains the thecal sac, the spinal cord, and the cauda equina. If the needle breaches the medial cortex of the pedicle, it enters the spinal canal. Direct injury to the spinal cord or nerve roots is possible. Also possible (and perhaps more likely) is tearing of the epidural or intradural venous plexus, with resulting hematoma. This can lead to sudden and progressive spinal cord, conus medullaris, or thecal sac compression, requiring urgent surgical decompression. This complication can be avoided by carefully selecting the entry point in the outer quadrant of the pedicle and always making sure that the needle remains lateral to the medial cortex as it passes through the pedicle until the needle tip can be seen anterior to the spinal canal on the lateral image. The other major complication with transpedicular needle placement is fracture of the pedicle. Although generally not destabilizing, a pedicle fracture is not very amenable to PMMA placement. It will heal but is quite painful and can remain so for many weeks.

Extrapedicular Approaches

The **posterolateral** approach has the potential for pneumothorax in the thoracic spine and for psoas muscle hematoma in the lumbar region. Although neither of these complications is common, pneumothorax can be a very serious and even life-threatening complication. The **anterolateral** approach, utilized in the cervical spine, has the potential for puncture of the jugular vein, the carotid artery, the vertebral artery, or numerous other structures in the neck. The sequela of such vascular injuries ranges from local hematoma to dissection and stroke. In the cervical area, the needles should be advanced very cautiously. Good patient cooperation or adequate sedation is necessary to avoid complications.

Complications Associated with Cement Injection

Of most concern among complications associated with the injection of the PMMA is extravasation of the cement into the epidural space. This can result in nerve root or spinal cord compression, with persistent radicular syndromes or even paralysis. This potentially devastating problem can be easily avoided by careful attention to preparation of the PMMA and to careful technique during injection. The key is proper visualization under fluoroscopy during the injection. Excellent fluoroscopy is an absolute requirement for the procedure, and attempts to perform vertebroplasty without it have had disastrous outcomes. Most important is the lateral projection, which should allow the operator to readily see the material flowing into the vertebral body. If there is a fracture line in the vertebral body, PMMA can migrate immediately in that direction. The injection should be terminated when the PMMA begins to reach the posterior fifth of the vertebral body. This is especially important when injection devices are employed, because often some residual pressure is present in the system, and a small quantity of cement can continue to flow passively. If an attempted needle placement is unsatisfactory, some authors recommend leaving that needle in place while placing and injecting PMMA through a second, contralateral needle. This measure helps avoid extravasation of PMMA through the tract of the first needle.[12]

In some cases, the fracture lines extend to the superior or inferior end plate. PMMA may migrate into the disc spaces or paraspinal spaces through these clefts. Extravasation through these fracture lines is not as critical as material moving posteriorly into the epidural space; however, it, too, should be avoided. The third location of PMMA extravasation is into the venous system. The movement of PMMA into the veins can be visualized at the time of injection. This event is better predicted when a venogram has been obtained and the operator knows where to look. A little extravasation into the paravertebral veins is not of great concern; however, extravasation into the epidural venous plexus can lead to spinal cord infarction or compression. Still, if the PMMA is not well opacified or if the operator is not alert, significant venous involvement can occur. A clinically significant pulmonary embolus was reported in one instance when a patient returned after a vertebroplasty with pleuritic chest pain and shortness of breath.[13]

Other Procedural Complications

Infection, a rare but very serious complication, requires specific mention. The potential for infection with vertebroplasty is very low. However, the consequences of such an infection are very serious indeed. Several weeks of intravenous antibiotics will be required at least, and surgical débridement and corpectomy is often required. Therefore, vertebroplasty should be performed under strict sterile conditions. In any patient who is immunocompromised, prophylactic intravenous antibiotics should be used in addition to the tobramycin in the PMMA mixture. We inform transplant and other immunocompromised patients of the slightly increased risk associated with the presence of the foreign PMMA material.

Bleeding complications are also a possibility. In general, the PMMA seals most of the bony needle tract, and this should alleviate most of the problem. Still, a fracture of the pedicle or tearing of a vein in the proximity of the spinal canal could lead to a large hematoma in a patient with a bleeding diathesis. This can be avoided easily by verifying that coagulation studies and platelet levels are normal before the procedure.

Vasovagal responses to medications, pain, or portions of the procedure such as PMMA injection are potentially very serious in older adults with diminished cardiovascular reserve. Close monitoring of the patient's vital signs by experienced nurses is required.

In the cervical area, the anterolateral approach also has the potential for laceration or dissection of large vascular structures, laceration of the thyroid gland, and perforation of the trachea or esophagus. Injury to the carotid artery or stimulation of the carotid body can occur with manipulation.

All in all, however, complications are rare and are easily avoided with attention to a few details.

POST-PROCEDURE CARE/FOLLOW-UP

Immediate

1. The patient is carefully rolled from the prone position on the fluoroscopy table to a supine position on a stretcher. He or she is transferred to a regular medical-surgical bed for observation.
2. The patient is kept flat supine for the first hour and then allowed to raise the head of the bed to 30 degrees.
3. The patient is observed over the next hour, with frequent neurologic checks, and is advanced in activity with nursing supervision as tolerated.
4. Generally, the patient is allowed out of bed with assistance at 2 hours after the procedure.
5. When the patient is ambulatory (assuming the patient was ambulatory before the procedure), is taking feedings by mouth well, and feels able to go home, he or she is discharged.

This process applies to the majority of patients, because vertebroplasty is usually an outpatient procedure.

Occasionally, a patient is slow to recover from the conscious sedation or is too fearful to be discharged. In

these cases, the patient is observed overnight in a medical-surgical bed as a 23-hour admission.

All patients are examined and ambulated before discharge. Attention is paid to complaints of chest, back, or leg pain and shortness of breath, which could be a sign of pulmonary embolism, deep venous thrombosis, or nerve root irritation from PMMA extravasation. A neurologic examination is performed to detect any new deficits. Signs of a complication should be aggressively sought before discharge. One should not hesitate to perform imaging of the patient with CT to determine whether there has been extravasation of PMMA, especially as it pertains to the neuraxis.

Discharge

1. All ambulatory patients are discharged to the care of a responsible adult.
2. In general, all patients who receive conscious sedation are encouraged to limit activities for 24 hours and are told not to drive or to make important decisions or conduct significant business during this time.
3. Patients being transferred to another facility or a supervised-care situation can be sent with specific discharge instructions and an appropriate nursing report.
4. Wound care is straightforward.
   a. Wounds consist of 2-mm incisions at each level treated.
   b. These are closed with adhesive strips, covered with sterile gauze, and sealed with a clear adhesive tape at the completion of the procedure.
   c. Patients are asked to keep the dressing dry for 2 days, after which they can shower or bathe.
   d. If the adhesive strips come off and the incision is not closed, a bandage should be placed after showering.
   e. Patients should not take a bath or swim (i.e., soak the area) for 5 days. The incisions are small, but deep, and can open up with soaking.
5. Incisional pain can be handled with nonsteroidal anti-inflammatory agents or acetaminophen. Heat or ice to the paraspinal muscles can also be helpful if there is spasm. We discourage the use of narcotic analgesics; these should not be necessary, and they make assessment of the effectiveness of the procedure difficult.
6. Restrictions of activity are individualized; however, patients can usually return to their normal activities as tolerated the day after the procedure.
   a. Walking is particularly encouraged in the first few days after the procedure. Even patients with incisional pain will benefit from this activity.
   b. Return to more strenuous activities should be gradual. Often, patients feel so much better that they attempt to do too much too soon. Lifting that accompanies many of the chores or hobbies that patients resume can lead to fracture of another vertebra. Falls also occur in patients who have not been walking for some length of time and may result in fractures of the hip and other bones.

Follow-Up

Follow-up in our patients varies but is easily accomplished in a variety of ways. We often follow up with a phone call at

1 week after the procedure. Patients are counseled before the procedure that pain relief may be immediate, although this is not always the case. In general, we inform the patients that their symptoms should be improved by 1 week after the procedure. This allows enough time for resolution of procedural pain. It also permits patients to return to their routine daily activities. At 1 week, clinical improvement can be assessed. Patients who have not improved are encouraged to return at the 1-week interval for reassessment. Any patient who has significantly increased pain or who experiences a neurologic deficit, fever, drainage, or other sign of infection is instructed to contact the physician's office immediately. Follow-up for patients who live a long distance away can be achieved in conjunction with the patient's primary care physician. The main thrust of long-term follow-up is treatment of the underlying disease (malignancy or osteoporosis), avoidance of activities that can lead to further fractures, strengthening of the back, and physical and occupational therapy if necessary to restore the ability to carry out functions of daily living.

CLINICAL OUTCOMES

The initial experiences with vertebroplasty were from Europe. Early reports evaluated vertebroplasty for the treatment of a variety of pathologic processes.[14–18] Deramond and colleagues[14] reported rapid resolution of pain in 35 of 38 patients with aggressive vertebral hemangiomas without radicular symptoms. Similar results were seen in patients with more aggressive lesions requiring combined treatment with ethanol embolization or surgical removal of an associated soft tissue component. Overall, there were only two complications in more than 50 patients, both intercostal neuralgias. This same group reported a significant analgesic effect and an improved quality of life (ability to ambulate, etc.) in more than 80% of 101 patients with metastatic lesions of the spine, including many patients with significant vertebral body destruction. Weill and associates[17] demonstrated marked improvement (the ability to end narcotic medication) in 24 of 33 (73%) patients with painful spinal metastases. Another 7 patients had moderate relief, with decreased narcotic requirements and increased activity levels. These results were stable 6 months after the procedure in the majority of patients. Almost all patients who had persistent or recurrent pain had other metastatic lesions. These authors reported transient sciatica in 3 patients and transient difficulty with swallowing in 2 patients. Cyteval and coworkers[19] evaluated 20 patients with acute compression fractures treated within 1 month of the onset of symptoms. They reported complete relief in 15 patients (75%) and partial relief in 3 (15%). There was one case of cement leakage into the neural foramen, with transient radicular pain.

The experience in the United States has been similar. Jensen and associates[20] reviewed a series of 47 osteoporotic compression fractures in 29 patients treated over a 3-year period. They demonstrated complete pain relief and increased mobility in 26 patients (90%) immediately after the procedure. The only reported complications in this series were new rib fractures in 2 patients, likely related to patient positioning during the procedure. Barr and colleagues[21] reported a 95% success rate for pain relief in 38 patients treated for osteoporotic compression fractures. They demonstrated continued pain relief in 94% of the patients, with a mean follow-up of 18 months. These authors also treated 8 patients with malignant lesions, with somewhat less impressive results. Although they demonstrated technical success and professed to have added stability in 88% of the patients, only 50% of this group received any analgesia. The complication rate for all patients in this series was 6.4%, and all complications were minor.

Thus, a number of authors have reported great success with vertebroplasty in a variety of pathologic processes. In most reported series, a high percentage of patients have had a dramatic initial response to therapy, regardless of the underlying cause of the fracture. Certainly, many series involve relatively small numbers of patients, and follow-up times are not long. However, complications are few and generally minor, and the benefits to the patients are very substantial. Issues such as the timing of treatment and long-term benefits need further study. Still, there is little doubt that this technique, in the proper hands, is safe and can be very effective in the treatment of selected patients with compression fractures of the spine.

SAMPLE DICTATION

Procedure:	Vertebroplasty
Date of Procedure:	Month/day/year
Facility:	Name of facility
Clinical Indication:	The patient has chronic low back pain resulting from a vertebral fracture 1 year ago.
Level Treated:	L2
Materials:	Parallax vertebroplasty kit
	Cement mixture (Cranioplastic, tobramycin, barium sulfate)
	Nonionic iodinated contrast medium, 320 mg I/mL (6 mL)
	Bone biopsy needle, 11-gauge, 6-inch

The risks and benefits of vertebroplasty were thoroughly discussed with the patient and informed consent was obtained. The patient was placed in the prone position on the fluoroscopy table. The skin over the lumbar spine was prepared and draped in a sterile fashion. Conscious sedation was provided by the radiology nursing staff. An entry site was chosen over the left pedicle of the L2 vertebral body. Local anesthesia was achieved with subcutaneous and periosteal infiltration of 1% lidocaine. A small skin incision was made, and an 11-gauge needle was placed through the pedicle into the vertebral body under biplane fluoroscopic guidance. A venogram was obtained using 6 mL of half-strength contrast medium. PMMA was injected through the biopsy needle under continuous fluoroscopic visualization. A total of 9 mL of cement was placed into the L2 vertebral body. There was good coverage of the vertebral body with PMMA. Therefore, a right pedicle approach was not performed. There was no extravasation of cement into the epidural space. The needle was removed, and sterile dressings were applied to the wounds. The patient was rolled to a supine position on a stretcher and transferred to the recovery area. The patient tolerated the procedure well.

CASE REPORTS

CASE 1

Clinical Presentation

The patient is a 48-year-old woman with a history of metastatic paraganglioma presenting after 4 months of increasing midthoracic back pain. She describes a deep, aching pain, more on the left side but extending across the back at about the level of the bra strap. The pain was very infrequent initially, but it has increased in frequency until it has become essentially constant. The patient now requires daily pain medication. A neurologic examination was nonfocal. There was tenderness to palpation over the T8 spinous process. Examination under fluoroscopy confirmed the level of the pain at the T8 and T9 levels, extending to the left lateral chest wall.

Imaging and Therapy

A recent bone scan demonstrates abnormal radiotracer accumulation over the left side of the T8 vertebral body (Fig. 8-25*A*). An MR examination reveals a lesion in the posterior aspect of the T8 vertebral body extending into the pedicle on the left (see Fig. 8-25*B* through *E*). A decision was made to proceed with vertebroplasty in conjunction with a transpedicular bone biopsy of the T8 lesion to confirm the diagnosis before radiation therapy. The lesion was approached from the left pedicle. An 11-gauge needle was placed to the posterior aspect of the left T8 pedicle. The stylet was removed and a Temno side-cutting biopsy needle was then placed through the 11-gauge needle. Multiple tissue samples were obtained (see Fig. 8-25*F*). The stylet was reinserted into the 11-gauge cannula and advanced into the vertebral body. The vertebroplasty was then performed. A single pedicle approach was all that was necessary to achieve good coverage with PMMA (see Fig. 8-25*G* and *H*). The biopsy confirmed the diagnosis of metastatic paraganglioma.

Results

The patient received immediate relief after the vertebroplasty. However, the improvement proved temporary, and some pain returned. The patient's spine was then treated with radiation therapy, which also provided some (but not complete) relief. It did stop the growth of the paraganglioma. The PMMA did not interfere with the radiation therapy.

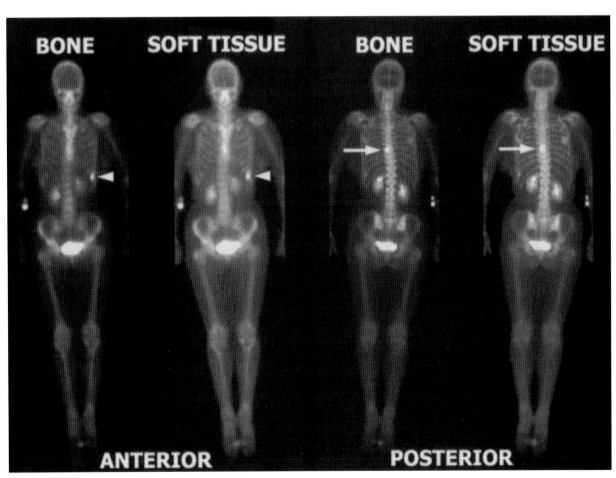

A

Figure 8-25 ■ *A,* Whole-body technetium-99m radionuclide bone scans with anterior and posterior views demonstrate a region of intense radiotracer uptake involving the left posterior spinal elements in the mid to lower thoracic spine (*arrow*).

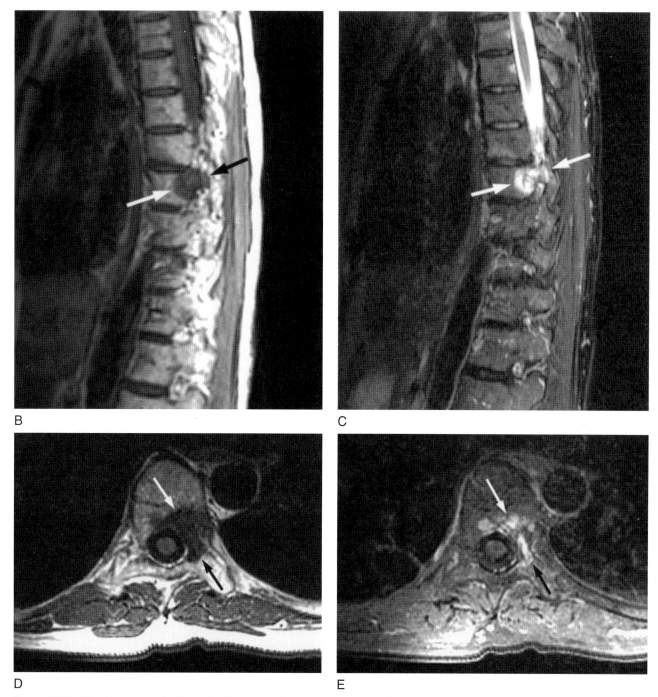

B

C

D

E

Figure 8-25 (*Cont'd*) ■ Note the focus of radiotracer uptake in an anterior lower left rib (*arrowhead*) in a region of recent fracture. Sagittal T1-weighted (*B*) and fat-saturated T2 fast-spin echo (*C*) MR images of the thoracic spine demonstrate abnormal signal intensity involving the left T8 pedicle and posterior vertebral body (*between arrows*). Axial T1-weighted images of the T8 vertebral body before (*D*) and after (*E*) contrast agent infusion demonstrate the extent of the bone involvement (*between arrows*).

Discussion

This case illustrates the ability to combine a diagnostic biopsy with the immediate pain relief that is often achieved with vertebroplasty. PMMA in the vertebral body does not interfere with further treatment with radiation therapy or chemotherapy. Biopsy specimens can be acquired with a variety of needles placed through the large 11- and 13-gauge needles used for this procedure.

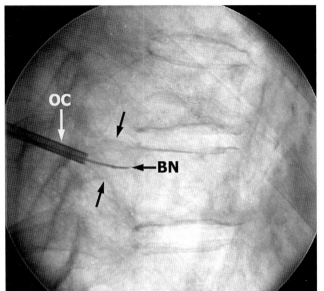

F

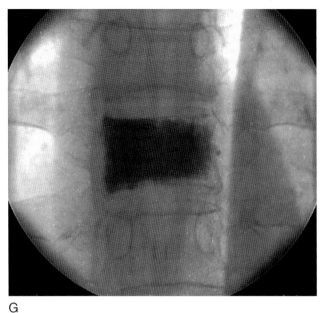

G

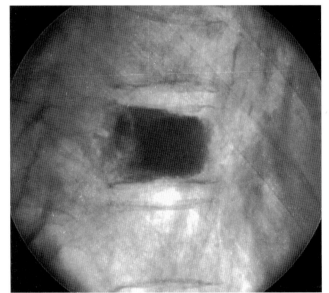

H

Figure 8-25 *(Cont'd)* ▪ *F,* Lateral radiograph demonstrates the outer cannula (OC) of the vertebroplasty needle. A side-cutting biopsy needle (BN) has been placed through the outer cannula to obtain a tissue sample from the pedicle *(bounded by arrows)* before cement delivery. AP *(G)* and lateral *(H)* postvertebroplasty radiographs demonstrate good cement coverage of the vertebral body.

CASE 2

Clinical Presentation

The patient is a 76-year-old man who presents for evaluation of low back pain. He has a long history of diffuse low back pain but describes a more recent onset of severe mid back pain. The patient relates that this pain began 18 months ago, with no specific antecedent event, and increased over a few days to a severe aching pain. This pain has not significantly changed since that time. The pain is described as deep and aching and worse with changing positions or with almost any activity. The pain is only in the back and it radiates to the flank, more on the left side. The pain intensifies the longer the patient is up, and by the afternoon it is often excruciating. The pain is relieved by lying down and is helped a little (though not much) by narcotic analgesics or nonsteroidal anti-inflammatory medication. The patient states that he has had epidural steroid injections twice and has been through a course of physical therapy and a trial of a hard shell brace, all without relief.

Imaging and Therapy

The MR examination demonstrates only a very mild superior end plate compression deformity of the T12 vertebral body. No other spinal pathologic process was seen, with the exception of mild degenerative facet disease. A bone scan with single-photon emission CT (SPECT) imaging of the spine (Fig. 8-26A) demonstrates abnormal increased radiotracer accumulation in the

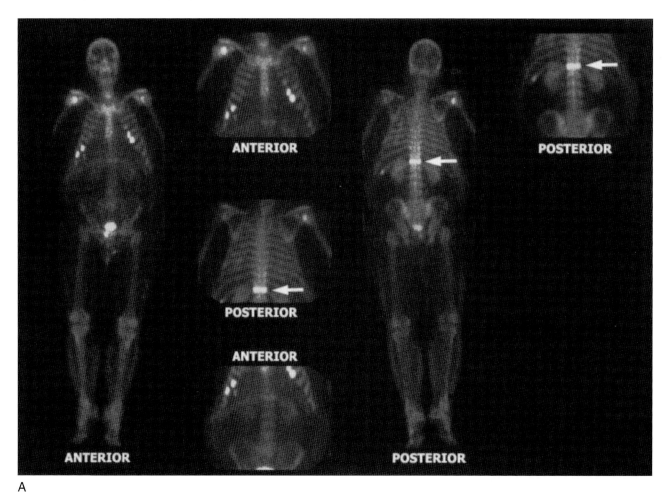

A

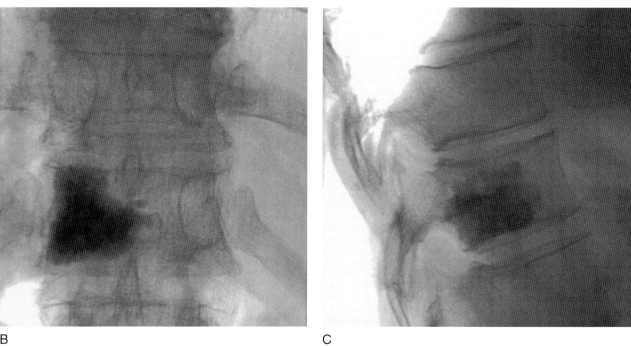

B

C

Figure 8-26 ■ *A*, Technetium-99m radionuclide bone scans demonstrate intense radiotracer uptake in the region of the T12 vertebral body (*arrow*). There are also multiple regions of increased uptake involving anterior ribs, compatible with recent fractures. AP (*B*) and lateral (*C*) radiographs after a left pedicle approach demonstrate cement filling only the left half of the vertebral body.

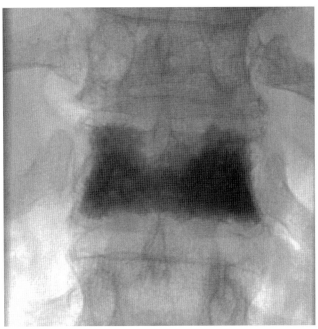
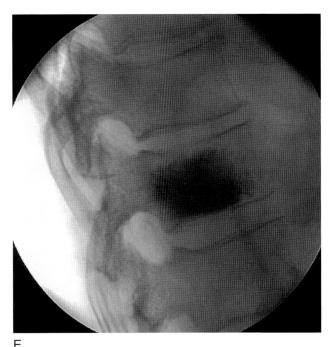

D   E

Figure 8-26 (*Cont'd*) ▪ A right pedicle approach was then performed that demonstrated subsequent filling of the right half of the vertebral body. AP (*D*) and lateral (*E*) radiographs demonstrate the final vertebroplasty result.

T12 vertebral body. No other abnormalities are identified. The patient was placed in a left lateral decubitus position, and the level of the pain was localized under fluoroscopy. This localized the pain to the T11-12 interspace and the T12 spinous process, extending to the right of midline. The patient again mentioned his lower lumbar pain (localized generally from L4 to the sacrum) but admitted that this pain was not as severe as the mid back pain and not of acute concern.

The findings were discussed with the patient and his wife. A decision was made to proceed with vertebroplasty of T12. The initial approach was through the left pedicle. Venography demonstrated the flow of contrast medium across the midline, and an initial deposition of PMMA was made. However, distribution of the cement was limited to the left side (see Fig. 8-26*B* and *C*). Therefore, a second needle was placed through the right pedicle, and PMMA deposition was accomplished on the right (see Fig. 8-26*D* and *E*).

Results

The patient was ambulated 2 hours after the procedure, without pain. He reported essentially complete relief at the 1-week follow-up evaluation.

Discussion

This case demonstrates the usefulness of bone scan in the evaluation of compression fractures. Although it is unusual to have so little compression of the vertebral body, the bone scan is often the most sensitive study for acute or active fracture. As mentioned, Maynard and coworkers[7] have suggested that the age of a fracture is not as important as the appearance of the lesion on bone scan. In our practice, we routinely use bone scans in our evaluations. It is very valuable in determining the pain generator in patients with multiple close or adjacent fractures. This patient was selected for vertebroplasty because his history and symptoms were classic for pain from compression fracture, and the abnormal bone scan corresponding to the fracture identified on MR imaging. Furthermore, the MR examination confirmed a lack of other pathologic processes to explain the symptoms despite the absence of vertebral body collapse.

CASE 3

Clinical Presentation

The patient is a 66-year-old man who presents with a 4-month history of midthoracic back pain that radiates bilaterally around the chest to the sternum, just below the nipple line. No specific antecedent event was associated with the pain, with the exception of an infected sebaceous cyst appearing just before the onset of the pain. This lesion was incised, and the patient received a standard course of antibiotics. However, the pain did not resolve. The patient describes his pain as very sharp, radiating around both flanks from the back and at times creating shortness of breath. It is exacerbated by coughing and hiccuping. The pain is worse with lying down, and the patient is more

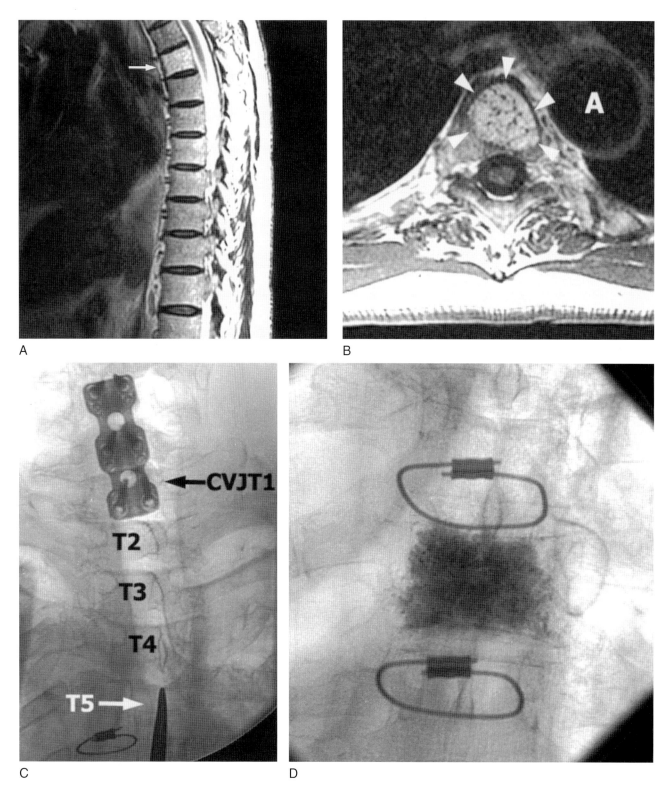

Figure 8-27 ■ *A*, Sagittal T2 fast spin echo MR image demonstrates mottled increased signal intensity involving the T5 vertebral body (*arrow*). *B*, Axial T1-weighted image demonstrates a large region of mottled increased signal intensity (*bounded by arrowheads*) involving much of the vertebral body. Note the focal regions of low signal intensity compatible with the remaining, thickened vertical trabeculae. A = aorta. *C*, AP radiograph before vertebroplasty used to mark the level of the T5 vertebral body. A hemostat is seen overlying the T5 vertebral body. CVJT1 = costovertebral junction of T1. Metallic anterior fixation hardware is seen from C6 through T1.

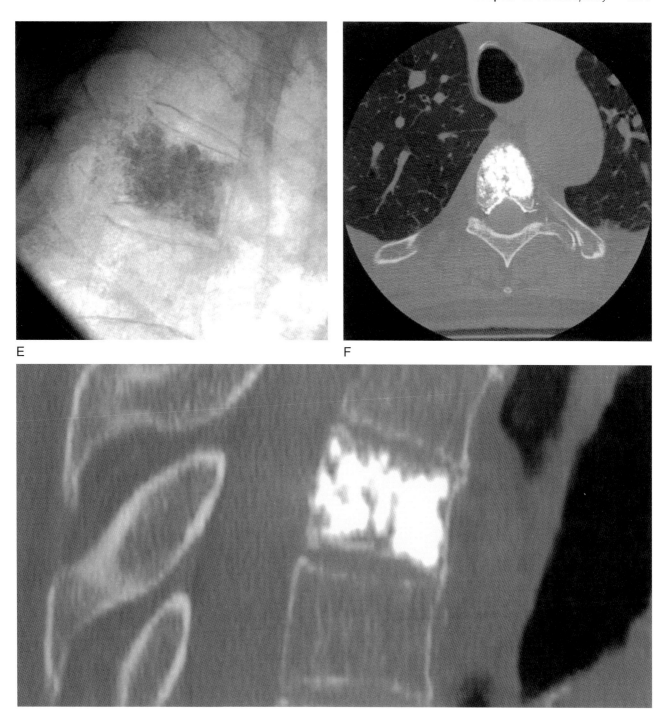

E

F

G

Figure 8-27 (*Cont'd*) ■ AP (*D*) and lateral (*E*) postvertebroplasty images demonstrate good cement coverage of the T5 vertebral body. An axial CT image (*F*) and a sagittal two-dimensional reformatted CT image (*G*) demonstrate adequate cement coverage. There is a small amount of cement in the ventral epidural space bilaterally.

comfortable sitting. The patient was initially evaluated with concern for a cardiac cause, which was ruled out. He was evaluated by a neurosurgeon, and an MR examination was obtained. He was referred for evaluation by the interventional neuroradiology service.

On physical examination, the patient had pain in the T4-5 distribution bilaterally. There was mild tenderness to deep palpation of the T4 vertebral body and some

tenderness over the left paraspinous musculature. The neurologic examination was nonfocal.

Imaging and Therapy

The MR examination revealed a large probable hemangioma, infiltrating at least 80% of the T4 vertebral body (Fig. 8-27*A* and *B*). There was no loss of vertebral height, no cortical disruption, and no significant soft tissue component. Fluoroscopic examination confirmed that the patient's severe midscapular pain was at the level of the T4 vertebral body and the T4-5 interspace. The findings were discussed with the patient and his wife, and vertebroplasty was performed at T4 (see Fig. 8-27*C* through *E*).

Results

Shortly after the procedure, the patient complained of some increased mid-back pain. A CT scan performed to evaluate the area of the vertebroplasty demonstrated good cement coverage with a small amount of cement in the ventral epidural space (see Fig. 8-27*F* and *G*). The patient's pain subsided over the next day and fully resolved after 1 week.

Discussion

This case illustrates the utility of vertebroplasty for control of painful hemangiomas. If there had been a soft tissue component, the procedure could have been combined with transarterial embolization of the soft tissue component with ethanol.

CURRENT PROCEDURAL TERMINOLOGY (CPT) CODES

CPT codes change often and sometimes are valid only for certain states or regions. It is best to consult with coding experts to make sure that coding for one's procedures is legitimate and complete. Below is a sample of codes that are being used for vertebroplasty at the time of this writing.[22]

Vertebral Body, Embolization or Injection

22520   Percutaneous vertebroplasty, one vertebral body, unilateral or bilateral injection; thoracic

22521   Lumbar

22522   each additional thoracic or lumbar vertebral body (List separately in addition to code for primary procedure)

76012   Radiological supervision and interpretation, percutaneous vertebroplasty, per vertebral body; under fluoroscopic guidance

76013   Under CT guidance

99141   Sedation with or without analgesia (conscious sedation); intravenous, intramuscular or inhalation

Other Possible Codes

20225   Biopsy, bone, trocar, or needle; deep (e.g., vertebral body, femur)

76003   Fluoroscopic guidance for needle placement (e.g., biopsy, aspiration, injection, localization device)

76360   Computerized axial tomographic guidance for needle biopsy, radiological supervision and interpretation

76393   Magnetic resonance guidance for needle placement (e.g., for biopsy, needle aspiration, injection, or placement of localization device), radiological supervision and interpretation

References

1. Harrington KD, Sim FH, Enis JE, et al. Methylmethacrylate as an adjunct in internal fixation of pathological fractures: Experience with three hundred and seventy five cases. J Bone Joint Surg Am 1976; 58:1047–1055.
2. Galibert P, Deramond H, Rosat P, et al. Note preliminaire sur le traitement des angiomes vertebraux et des affections dolorigenes et fragilisantes du rachis. Chirurgie 1990; 116:326–335.
3. Jensen ME, Evans AJ, Mathis JM, et al. Percutaneous polymethylmethacrylate vertebroplasty in the treatment of osteoporotic vertebral body compression fractures: Technical aspects. AJNR Am J Neuroradiol 1997; 18:1897–1904.
4. Melton LJ III, Kan SH, Frye MA, et al. Epidemiology of vertebral fractures in women. Am J Epidemiol 1989; 129:1000–1011.
5. Cooper C, Atkinson EJ, O' Fallon WM, et al. Incidence of clinically diagnosed vertebral fractures: A population-based study in Rochester, Minnesota, 1985–1989.
6. Kaufman TJ, Jensen ME, Schweickert PA, et al. Age of fracture and clinical outcomes of percutaneous vertebroplasty. AJNR Am J Neuroradiol 2001; 22:1860–1863.
7. Maynard AS, Jensen ME, Schweickert PA, et al. Value of bone scan imaging in predicting pain relief from percutaneous vertebroplasty in osteoporotic vertebral fractures. AJNR Am J Neuroradiol 2000; 21:1807–1812.
8. O'Brien JP, Sims JT, Evans AJ. Vertebroplasty in patients with severe vertebral compression fractures: A technical report. AJNR Am J Neuroradiol 2000; 21:1555–1558.
9. Chiras J, Deramond H. Complications des vertebroplasties. In Saillant G, Laville C (eds). Echecs et Complications de la Chirurgie du Rachis. Chirurgie de Reprise. Paris: Sauramps Médical, 1995, pp 149–153.
10. Tampieri D, Weill A, Melanson D, et al. Percutaneous aspiration biopsy in cervical spine lytic lesions. Neuroradiology 1991; 33:43–47.
11. Lieberman IH, Dudeney S, Reinhardt M-K, et al. Initial outcome and efficacy of "kyphoplasty" in the treatment of painful osteoporotic vertebral compression fractures. Spine 2001; 26:1631–1638.
12. Depriester C, Deramond H, Toussaint P, et al. Percutaneous vertebroplasty: Indications, technique, and complications. In Connors JJ, Wojak JC (eds). Interventional Neuroradiology. Philadelphia: WB Saunders, 1999, pp 346–357.
13. Padovani B, Kasriel O, Brunner P. Pulmonary embolism caused by acrylic cement: A rare complication of percutaneous vertebroplasty. AJNR Am J Neuroradiol 1999; 20:375–377.
14. Deramond H, Depriester, C, Galibert P, et al. Percutaneous vertebroplasty with polymethylmethacrylate. Technique, indications, and results. Radiol Clin North Am 1998; 36:533–46.
15. Bascoulergue Y, Duquesnel J, Leclercq R, et al. Percutaneous injection of methylmethacrylate in the vertebral body for the treatment of various diseases: Percutaneous vertebroplasty (abstract). Radiology 1988; 169P:372.
16. Martin JB, Jean B, Suigu D, et al. Vertebroplasty: Clinical experience and follow-up results. Bone 1999; 25:11S–15S.

17. Weill A, Chiras J, Simon JM, et al. Spinal metastases: Indications for and results of percutaneous injection of acrylic surgical cement. Radiology 1996; 199:241–247.

18. Cotton A, Dewatre F, Cortet B, et al: Percutaneous vertebroplasty for osteolytic metastases and myeloma: Effects of the percentage of lesion filling and the leakage of methylmethacrylate at clinical follow-up. Radiology 1996; 200:525–530.

19. Cyteval C, Sarrabere MP, Roux JO, et al. Acute osteoporotic vertebral collapse: Open study on percutaneous injection of acrylic surgical cement in 20 patients. AJR Am J Roentgenol 1999; 173:1685–1690.

20. Jensen ME, Evans AJ, Mathis JM, et al. Percutaneous polymethyl-methacrylate vertebroplasty in the treatment of osteoporotic vertebral body compression fractures: Technical aspects. AJNR Am J Neuroradiol 1997; 18:1897–1904.

21. Barr JD, Barr MS, Lemley TJ, et al. Percutaneous vertebroplasty for pain relief and spinal stabilization. Spine 2000; 25:923–928.

22. CPT 2002, CPT Intellectual Property Services. Chicago: American Medical Association, 2002.

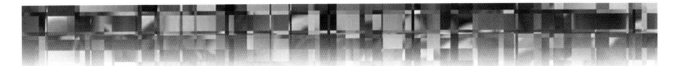

A Spine Surgeon's Perspective

Vertebroplasty

Joseph T. Alexander, MD

The elderly and the very elderly are the fastest growing population groups in the United States, particularly among women. Osteoporosis is common in these groups and is responsible for an estimated 1 to 2 million spinal fractures per year. Better recognition of the risk factors, education on prevention, routine screening, and early, aggressive medical treatment may ultimately reduce the incidence of these fractures, but clinicians are likely to continue to see a rise in numbers for the near term. Although most of these fractures are subclinical or heal with simple, conservative measures, significant morbidity can be associated with the restrictions in mobility caused by the more serious of these fractures. This includes pneumonia, deep venous thrombosis, and pulmonary embolism, not to mention a decreased quality of life. Increasingly, patients are refusing to accept recommendations of prolonged bed rest, limitation of activities, or bracing, and they are demanding better pain control and early return to normal daily and recreational activities.

These fractures present clinically with the new onset of localized pain after a minor event such as a simple fall at home. However, many patients with fractures visualized radiographically have no recollection of a painful episode, suggesting that some of these initial fractures may be asymptomatic. The pain associated with these fractures is generally worsened with activity and ambulation and improved by recumbency. Fortunately, neurologic symptoms and complications are rare, perhaps because the spinal canal is rarely compromised by retropulsed fragments, even in the presence of a severe vertebral collapse. Diagnostic dilemmas for the clinician in this setting include the possibility of primary or metastatic tumors, infectious causes, and symptoms from other types of spinal degenerative disease, because many of these patients are also at risk for these disorders. Conventional imaging often fails to resolve this issue, and percutaneous biopsy of the area of concern may be requested before treatment is started.

Although the pain of a compression fracture can initially be severe, many patients respond in a matter of days or a few weeks to bed rest, analgesics, and anti-inflammatory medications. As a general rule, tolerance of narcotics and muscle relaxants tends to be poor because of the cognitive side effects in this age group; therefore, standard pain management options may be limited. There can also be a role for aggressive osteoporosis treatment in pain management, such as therapy with intranasal calcitonin.

Bracing, particularly for chronic spinal pain, is challenging in this patient population. Many of these fractures occur at or near the thoracolumbar junction, necessitating a plastic thoracolumbar orthosis. Even a custom-fitted orthosis is irritating, cumbersome, and difficult to put on and remove for these often elderly, arthritic patients. As a result, patients with chronic pain are likely to limit their activities significantly rather than wear a brace, perhaps thereby increasing the risk of complications.

Patients with osteoporotic compression fractures who do not respond to simple, conservative treatment, pain management, or bracing have been a considerable challenge for the spine surgeon. The complication rate for surgical stabilization has been relatively high, because of comorbidities and anesthesia risks in this age group and the significant rate of pseudoarthrosis, hardware failure, and adjacent vertebral segment collapse. The problems are compounded because sites such as the iliac crest provide poor stock for autogenous bone harvest. When surgical intervention is necessary, long fusion constructs with segmental fixation at several spine segments above and below the fracture level have the best outcome. These are major surgical procedures, however, and patients face extended hospitalization and recovery even in the best of circumstances. Because of these factors, traditional surgical dogma has been to intervene only in cases with neurologic compromise, although incapacitating pain and nonambulatory status are also valid surgical indications. Thus, many symptomatic patients with moderately severe pain and a diminished quality of life are left without a good treatment option.

Vertebroplasty represents a significant advance in our ability to treat patients who have persistent pain from osteoporotic compression fractures. Although debate continues as to the mechanism of the pain relief after vertebroplasty, in the properly selected patient the clinical results can be clear, rapid in onset, and often dramatic. Although the risks of the procedure, such as spread of the cement into the spinal canal or inferior vena cava, are real and must be discussed with the patient, these risks are of less magnitude than those associated with the conventional surgical options and should not be overstated. The current debate among spine specialists is not over the utility of the procedure but rather over how long to pursue conservative measures before considering vertebroplasty.

On the strength of the early clinical reports of the success of vertebroplasty, as well as attention in the popular press and information available through the Internet, increasing numbers of patients are being referred from their primary physicians to be considered for this procedure or are even self-referring. In some of these cases, the patient may end up seeing a proceduralist directly, without an intermediary evaluation by another spine specialist. The challenge in these cases for the proceduralist is to be certain that the patient has had an appropriate evaluation, that other causes of pain have been excluded, that appropriate conservative measures have been attempted, that the patient's post-procedural course is followed, and that necessary care is arranged in the event the procedure is unsuccessful or complications arise.

Despite the relief of symptoms afforded by vertebroplasty in many cases, some apparently suitable patients fail to gain relief. One theory is that the pain can result from the effect of the local deformity on the paraspinal muscles and ligaments and that restoring spinal alignment would be beneficial. Concerns have also been raised over the possible long-term effects of kyphosis on the adjacent spinal segments, because no long-term outcome studies have as yet been reported for vertebroplasty. Lastly, some vertebral bodies may not be amenable to direct injection of cement, either because of an excessive degree of collapse or because of fractures in the cortex that might allow cement extravasation. To address these concerns, a percutaneous technique utilizing an inflatable "bone tamp" has been developed (Kyphoplasty). The tamps or balloons are deployed into the vertebral body bilaterally through a percutaneous, transpedicular approach. When the tamps are then inflated, a degree of reduction in the deformity is effected. The resulting cavity in the vertebral body is then filled with cement under "low pressure." Although the idea is appealing, published clinical data at this point are limited. The benefits and risks are unknown at this time, as are the indications for this procedure as compared with vertebroplasty.

Chapter 9

Discography

- Douglas S. Fenton, MD
- Leo F. Czervionke, MD

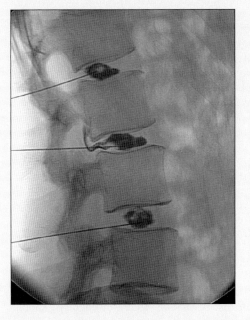

BACKGROUND

In discography, contrast material is injected into the nucleus pulposus of an intervertebral disc by means of a percutaneously placed needle. The discographic procedure is composed of two main elements. First, and most important, is the assessment of the patient's response to pain, which may or may not be induced when fluid is injected into the disc. Second, disc morphology is assessed, with contrast material in the disc, by radiographic imaging and/or computed tomography (CT).

Discography is the only imaging procedure for the assessment of discogenic back pain that directly relates the patient's pain response to the morphologic appearance of the disc.[1, 2] Although magnetic resonance (MR) imaging is considered the primary screening imaging modality for the evaluation of low back pain, discography is more sensitive in the detection of internal disc disruption, including the detection of disc degeneration and annular fissuring. MR imaging may show an area of T2-weighted signal hyperintensity in the annulus referred to as a "high intensity zone" (Fig. 9-1*A*), which has a high correlation with the discogenic pain associated with annular fissures.[3, 4] These "high intensity zones" often enhance (see Fig. 9-1*B*). However, approximately 13% of patients with annular fissures visible on MR imaging are asymptomatic, and discography is more sensitive to the presence of annular fissures (tears).[4]

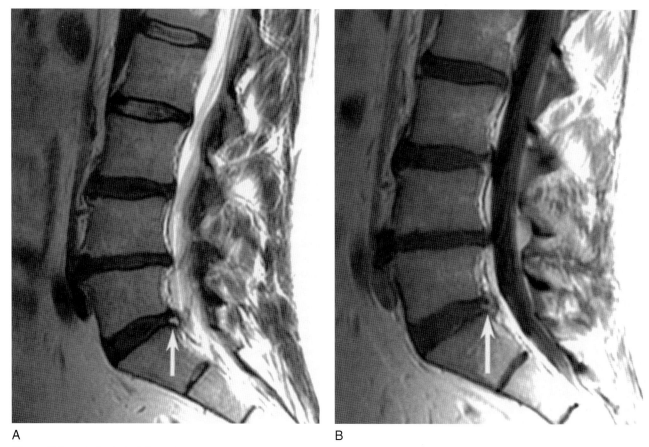

Figure 9-1 ■ *A*, Sagittal T2 fast spin echo MR image. Small focus of increased signal intensity ("high intensity zone") posterior annulus L5-S1 disc (*arrow*) is compatible with an annular tear. *B*, Note enhancement of annular tear (*arrow*).

The causes of back pain are many, and isolating the source of chronic low back pain can be a complex diagnostic challenge, even with the modern imaging tools now available. Nerve endings have been shown to exist in the outer third of the annulus fibrosis, and there are encapsulated nerve receptors along its lateral surface.[2, 5] The posterior longitudinal ligament and the ligamentum flavum are also innervated.[2, 5] Pain can often be elicited by injecting contrast material into a morphologically normal nucleus pulposus. The primary goals of discography are **first** to determine whether discogenic pain is a source of the patient's back pain and **second** to identify the disc level(s) causing the pain before treatment. Whether pain can be elicited by discography is not important. The **critical question to answer** is whether the pain produced by the discography at a given disc level matches the patient's typical pain (concordant) or is different from the patient's pain (nonconcordant).

Discography was first performed in the 1940s by Lindblom.[6] The role of discography in the assessment of back pain has been shrouded in controversy for many years.[1, 2, 7, 8] Holt wrote one of the earliest papers questioning the role of discography in 1965. In his often-cited study, which was performed on young "normal" inmates, there was a high rate of false-positive results, and therefore discography was reported to be an unreliable diagnostic test.[7] This study has been refuted in many papers since that time, but controversy still exists regarding the clinical role of discography.

Simmons and associates[8] revisited Holt's study. They stated that although Holt's study was considered appropriate for its time, it should not be used as the standard for modern discography. They found that several components of Holt's original study should be questioned, including the choice of using inmates with uncertain reliability, suboptimal needle placement, and discrepancies in data. Moreover, there have been technical improvements over the past 20 years, including the use of nonirritating contrast material (Holt used Hypaque, an ionic contrast agent), fluoroscopy, and post-discography CT.

Discography has undergone many refinements in the past 30 years. The criteria for diagnosing a positive discogram have also changed. In Holt's study, a discogram was considered positive in anyone who experienced severe pain on injection. It was originally believed that any severe pain on injection of the disc represented a positive pain response. Today, a positive pain response implies pain **concordant** with the patient's symptoms, elicited by a low-volume injection that often correlates on post-discography CT with radial and/or concentric tears (internal disc disruption). Conversely, demonstration of internal disc disruption alone, without concordant pain, is now considered a negative discographic pain response.[8]

In the early days of discography it was performed to evaluate for possible disc herniation. Today, discography should never be the initial procedure performed for the purpose of diagnosing disc herniation or for the evaluation of the patient with acute low back pain. MR imaging is the procedure of choice for evaluating disc herniation and nerve root involvement in the acute setting. Discography is generally performed as a complementary procedure after other imaging studies have been performed. A discogram should always be performed before IDET (IntraDiscal ElectroThermal) therapy to decide whether therapy is indicated and to help plan the approach for catheter insertion. Discography may have an important role in patients suffering from chronic low back pain for presurgical planning before spine fusion, in the assessment of failed back syndrome, and before chemonucleolysis (still performed in some countries outside the United States).

PATIENT SELECTION

1. Discogenic pain
   a. Back and/or neck pain
   b. Cumulative loading intolerance (can stand for only a short period of time)
   c. Sitting intolerance (can sit for only a short period of time)
   d. Nonradicular extremity, thoracic, or abdominal pain
   e. No nerve root distribution weakness
   f. Equivocal straight-leg raising test (low back pain without leg pain)
   g. No evidence of reflex abnormality
2. Facetogenic, neoplastic, inflammatory, and traumatic pain has been excluded
3. No signs of pain caused by compression of the neural elements (e.g., disc herniation, osteophytes, synovial cysts)
4. To assess level(s) for possible spinal fusion
5. To assess levels above and/or below a possible fusion to include or exclude those levels from the fusion
6. To assess levels at, above, and/or below a fusion in patients with recurrent or residual pain (failed back syndrome)
7. To assess for symptomatic level(s) in patients with minimal or no findings on MR imaging or CT
8. To determine the symptomatic level(s) in patients with multilevel disc abnormalities on MR imaging or CT
9. As a test of exclusion when other minimally invasive tests and therapies have failed to provide an answer
10. As a precursor to other therapies (IDET™, chemonucleolysis)

CONTRAINDICATIONS

1. Coagulopathy (International Normalized Ratio [INR] >1.5 or platelets <50,000/mm^3)
2. Pregnancy (because of teratogenic effects of radiation)
3. Systemic infection or skin infection over the puncture site
4. Severe allergy to any component of the injection mixture (injectate) or other medication
5. A previously operated-on disc, which may yield a false-negative or false-positive result (and thus its evaluation may be difficult)

6. A solid bone fusion that does not allow access to the disc
7. Significant spinal cord compromise at a level to be studied, because there is a theoretical risk of causing or aggravating a myelopathy as a result of the injection producing temporary distention of the disc

PROCEDURE

Equipment/Supplies

Spinal needle, 22-gauge, 6-inch (1 for each level–lumbar and thoracic discography) (Monoject Special Technique Needle With Stylet, Diamond Point, Sherwood Medical, St. Louis, MO)
Spinal needle, 25-gauge, 3.5-inch (1 for each level–cervical or thoracic discography) (Quinke type point, Becton Dickinson & Co., Franklin Lakes, NJ)
Luer-lock syringe, 3 mL (1 for each level)
Control syringe, 12 mL with 25-gauge, 1.5-inch needle containing 9.5 mL 1% lidocaine for local anesthesia and 0.5 mL 8.4% sodium bicarbonate injectable (1 mEq/mL) to alleviate burning pain associated with anesthetic
Povidone-iodine (Betadine) scrub
Alcohol scrub
Sterile drapes
Sterile gauze
Adhesive bandages
C-arm fluoroscopy
Lead apron and sterile gowns
Hat, mask, and sterile gloves

Medications

Lidocaine-MPF* 1% (Xylocaine-MPF* 1%, AstraZeneca LP, Wilmington, DE)
Bupivacaine hydrochloride-MPF* 0.25% (Sensorcaine-MPF* Injection 0.25%, AstraZeneca LP, Wilmington, DE)
Cefazolin† (Ancef, SmithKline Beecham, Philadelphia, PA) 1 g intravenously within 1 hour before procedure
Cefazolin† (Ancef), 10 mg/5 mL normal saline
Clindamycin† (Cleocin Phosphate, Pharmacia & Upjohn, Peapack, NJ), 600 mg intravenously 1 hour before procedure (if cephalosporin or penicillin allergy)
Clindamycin,† 6 mg/5 mL normal saline (if cephalosporin or penicillin allergy)
Nonionic myelographic contrast medium, 300 mg I/mL (Omnipaque [Iohexol] Injection, Nycomed Inc., Princeton, NJ)
Atropine (cervical discography)
Ketorolac tromethamine (Toradol$^{IV/IM}$, Roche Pharmaceuticals, Nutley, NJ)

Injection Mixture (Injectate)

Combine:
2.3 mL nonionic myelographic contrast 300 mg I/mL
0.5 mL cefazolin (10 mg/5 mL)†

*Local anesthetics should be from single-use vials and be free from paraben (MPF) and phenol to prevent flocculation of the steroid.[9] Some preservatives have been implicated as a cause of arachnoiditis if injected intrathecally.

†Discitis is a known complication of discography. It is recommended that an antibiotic be given to decrease the risk of infection. One gram of intravenous cefazolin (Ancef) is given routinely within 1 hour of the procedure. One milligram of cefazolin is also added to the injectate for each disc. Each 3-mL syringe used for disc injection should contain 2.3 mL of nonionic iodinated myelographic contrast medium and 0.5 mL of cefazolin (10 mg/5 mL) for a total of 2.8 mL. This will leave enough space in the syringe to allow drawing back on the syringe to exclude intravascular placement of the needle tip before injection of the mixture. If the patient has a known cephalosporin or penicillin allergy, 600 mg of clindamycin can be given intravenously with 0.6 mg (6 mg/5 mL) added to each disc injection syringe. If the patient has a known allergy to iodine, gadopentetate dimeglumine (MR contrast, Magnevist, Berlex Laboratories, Wayne, NJ) can be substituted.

All medications are used **without** epinephrine because vasocontrictive properties are neither needed nor wanted, particularly because of the risk of vasospasm in the head and neck region.

Methodology

Pre-Procedure

Discography is performed as an outpatient procedure. Patients are instructed to stop using their pain medications on the day of the procedure to allow greater diagnostic accuracy. The patient is instructed to have a driver with him or her after the procedure as well as someone who can be responsible for his or her well-being for the remainder of the day because sedation may be given during the examination. A minimum of electrocardiographic, pulse oximetry, and blood pressure monitoring is performed during and immediately after the examination. Within 1 hour before the examination, an intravenous antibiotic is given.

Lumbar Discogram

Informed consent is obtained. The patient is placed prone on the fluoroscopy table. The patient's lower back is prepared and draped in sterile fashion. Intravenous sedation is optional but is not preferred. A mild sedative and analgesic (midazolam, 1 to 2 mg, and fentanyl, 100 to 150 µg) can be administered during the procedure to make the patient more comfortable; however, the patient must be able to fully understand the questions being asked during the discography and must be able to describe the distribution and quality of the pain produced.

PATIENT AND/OR C-ARM POSITIONING

L1-2 THROUGH L4-5
Proper positioning is the key to an effective discogram. The disc puncture should always be performed contralateral to the patient's more symptomatic side to minimize the chance of a false-positive pain response. A pillow or wedge positioned under the patient to elevate the less symptomatic side will facilitate needle placement. The disc to be punctured is placed in the center of the field of view. The C-arm (image intensifier above the patient) is rotated in a contralateral oblique angle with respect to the patient's more symptomatic side. The C-arm (or patient) is rotated until the superior articulating process (ear of the "Scotty dog"), which has the same number as the inferior vertebrae of the disc space to be injected, is centered midway between the anterior and posterior aspects of the vertebral body. The superior end plates of the same vertebral body should superimpose (Fig. 9-2).

L5-S1
For needle insertion into the L5-S1 level, significant caudal angulation (image intensifier above the patient, obliqued toward the patient's head) is required for optimal visualization. The C-arm is rotated in a fashion similar to that for the upper lumbar discs. Generally, the window that the needle has to pass through is represented on the fluoroscopic images as a small triangle formed by the inferior end plate of L5, the superior articulating process of S1, and the iliac crest (Fig. 9-3). However, the iliac crest may obstruct the approach irrespective of the angle of trajectory used (Fig. 9-4*A*). If one is not able to achieve a position that places the superior articulating process at the midpoint of the vertebral body, one obtains the best possible angle that allows visualization of the upside-down triangle (see Fig. 9-4*B*). The puncture site for L5-S1 is usually higher than that for L4-5 (Fig. 9-5).

A midline L5-S1 puncture where the needle traverses the thecal sac is an alternative to the oblique approach but is seldom required to puncture the L5-S1 disc. This approach carries the added risk of possible arachnoiditis.

PROCEDURE

Local anesthesia is given along the expected path of the needle tract. The spinal needle is then inserted parallel to the x-ray beam and advanced, using intermittent fluoroscopy, so that the needle tip stays just ventrolateral to the superior articulating process and midway between the vertebral end plates (Fig. 9-6). With this needle trajectory, the possibility of contacting the exiting nerve root or passing through any vital structures is minimal. Furthermore, this trajectory will allow placement of the needle tip into the center of the disc.

Contact with the posterolateral margin of the disc is made at various depths. The patient often describes a mild or moderate sharp pain as the needle passes through the disc's outer fibers (Sharpey's fibers). The disc has a firm, gritty feel as the needle passes through the annulus; then, less resistance is felt when the needle passes into the nucleus. The position of the needle tip should be confirmed in straight anteroposterior (AP) and true lateral projections before injection of contrast medium (Fig. 9-7). The needle needs to be positioned with its tip in the middle third of the disc in both planes to ensure intranuclear placement of contrast material. If the needle is too far lateral, ventral, or posterior, an annular deposition of contrast agent may result (Fig. 9-8). With this technique, discographic needle placement should be performed at all other relevant disc levels before injection of contrast material. **It is strongly recommended that at least one other level (preferably a normal-appearing disc by**

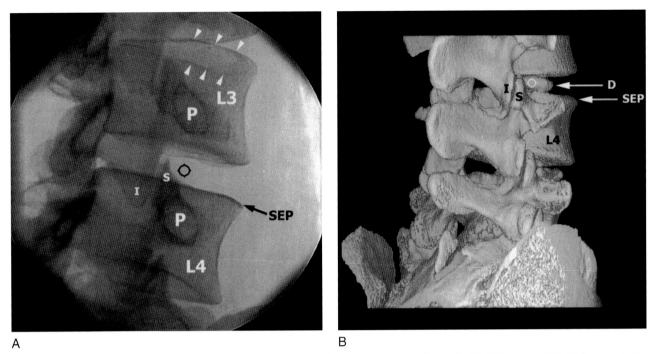

A   B

Figure 9-2 ■ LAO radiograph (*A*) and three-dimensional CT image (*B*) demonstrate proper positioning for L3-4 discogram, right-sided approach. The apex of the right L4 superior articular process (S) is positioned midway between the anterior and posterior aspects of the L4 superior end plate. The superior end plate of L4 (SEP) is flat. Note that the superior end plate of L3 does not superimpose (*arrowheads, A*). The needle should be placed just ventrolateral to the right L4 superior articular process (*black target, A; white target, B*). I = right L3 inferior articular process; P = pedicle.

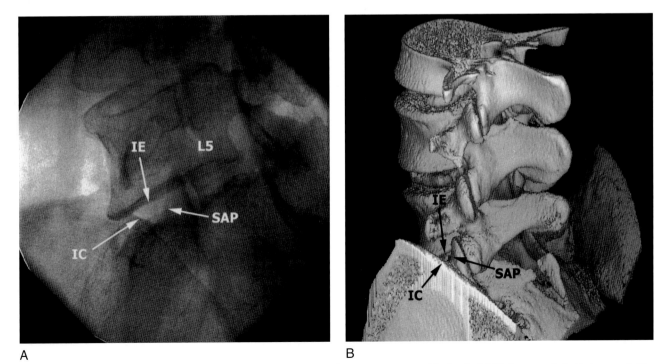

A   B

Figure 9-3 ■ RAO radiograph (*A*) and three-dimensional CT image (*B*) demonstrate proper positioning for L5-S1 discogram, left-sided approach. The apex of the left S1 superior articular process (SAP) is positioned midway between the anterior and posterior aspects of the S1 superior end plate. IE = L5 inferior end plate; IC = iliac crest.

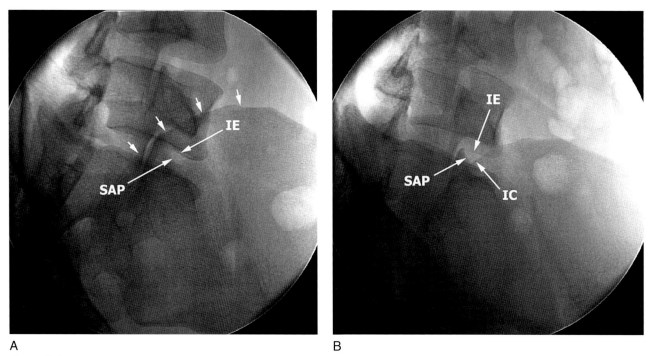

A

B

Figure 9-4 ■ *A*, LAO radiograph. The high-riding iliac crest (*arrows*) obstructs the optimal approach into the L5-S1 disc. *B*, LAO radiograph, caudocranial x-ray beam angulation. This maneuver "lowers" the iliac crest (IC) until the target triangle begins to open, allowing disc access, although it is not the most optimal or facile. SAP = lateral border of the right S1 superior articular process; IE = inferior end plate of L5.

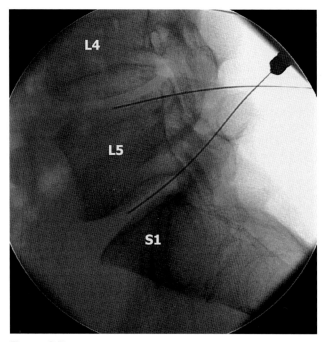

Figure 9-5 ■ Lateral discogram needle placement, L4-5 and L5-S1. Note that the skin entrance for L5-S1 is cephalad to that for L4-5.

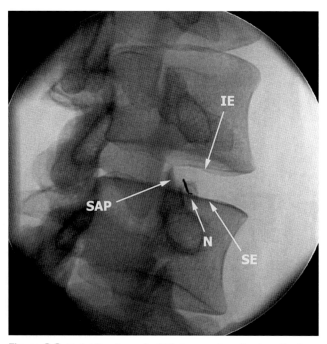

Figure 9-6 ■ LAO radiograph of L3-4, proper intradiscal needle placement. Needle (N) is just ventrolateral to the L4 superior articular process (SAP) and midway between the L4 superior end plate (SE) and the L3 inferior end plate (IE).

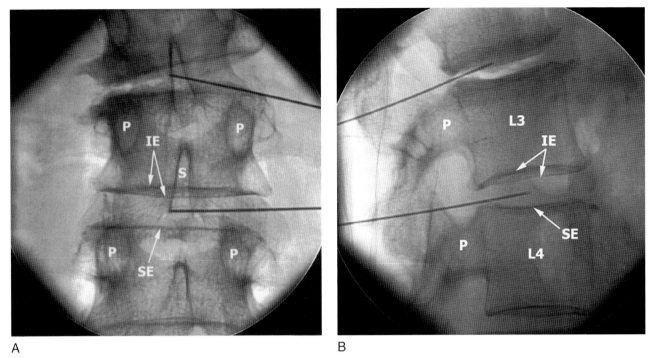

A   B

Figure 9-7 ■ AP (*A*) and lateral (*B*) radiographs L3-4, proper intradiscal needle placement. The needle tip is in the center of the disc, midway between the L4 superior end plate (SE) and the inferior end plate of L3 (IE). S = spinous process; P = pedicle.

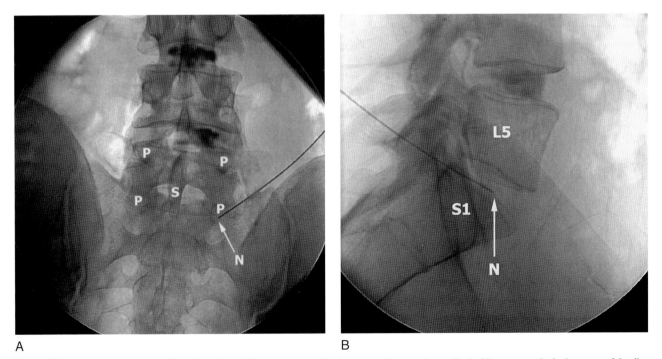

A   B

Figure 9-8 ■ AP (*A*) and lateral (*B*) radiographs L5-S1, improper needle placement. Although the needle tip (N) appears to be in the center of the disc on B; on A, the needle tip is at the level of the mid pedicle (P). S = spinous process.

Discography Pain Form

Pt. Name:		Injection Mixture:		_____
Pt. Number:				_____
Date:		IV Antibiotic		

DISC	Pain Intensity (0–10)		Volume Injected		mL
LEVEL	0 1 2 3 4 5 6 7 8 9 10		Firm Endpoint	Y	N
_____	Location:		Additional Notes:		
	Typical:	Y N			

DISC	Pain Intensity (0–10)		Volume Injected		mL
LEVEL	0 1 2 3 4 5 6 7 8 9 10		Firm Endpoint	Y	N
_____	Location:		Additional Notes:		
	Typical:	Y N			

DISC	Pain Intensity (0–10)		Volume Injected		mL
LEVEL	0 1 2 3 4 5 6 7 8 9 10		Firm Endpoint	Y	N
_____	Location:		Additional Notes:		
	Typical:	Y N			

DISC	Pain Intensity (0–10)		Volume Injected		mL
LEVEL	0 1 2 3 4 5 6 7 8 9 10		Firm Endpoint	Y	N
_____	Location:		Additional Notes:		
	Typical:	Y N			

DISC	Pain Intensity (0–10)		Volume Injected		mL
LEVEL	0 1 2 3 4 5 6 7 8 9 10		Firm Endpoint	Y	N
_____	Location:		Additional Notes:		
	Typical:	Y N			

imaging) adjacent to the disc level of interest be injected to serve as a control for assessing pain response.

Once the needles are all in position, they are injected one at a time without the patient knowing which disc is being injected. We recommend injecting the normal control level(s) first to gain some idea of the patient's pain tolerance and proceeding sequentially to the anticipated symptomatic disc levels in succession. Disc injection is performed by first removing the stylet and then attaching a 3-mL syringe containing the injectate. The fluoroscope is rotated into true lateral with the disc being injected in the center of the field of view. The injection is performed slowly, using continuous fluoroscopy, and should be terminated when firm resistance is met. The annulus is intact if there is a firm endpoint to the injection. It is important to instill an adequate amount of fluid into the disc to distend the annulus in an attempt to provoke pain sensation. If severe pain is elicited at low volumes, that injection is terminated. Also, if there is firm resistance at the beginning of the injection, this may indicate an intra-annular injection. The contrast medium needs to be evaluated in both AP and lateral planes to make sure it is central (intranuclear) and not peripheral (annular). An annular injection can lead to a false-positive pain response.

Some authors believe that a manometer should be used during disc injection and that the disc should be injected until either pain is elicited or a specific atmospheric pressure (4 to 5 atmospheres or 120 to 150 mm Hg) is reached.[10] We believe that, with experience, the discographer will learn what amount of disc pressurization will be necessary by hand injection. Furthermore, many discs have full-thickness tears and cannot be pressurized by hand or manometer. One cannot assume that a patient's pain is not caused by a disc with a full-thickness tear. In these cases, we inject preservative-free local anesthetic into the disc and evaluate the patient's response immediately, at discharge, and for the next several days, with the patient keeping a pain diary. This technique will be discussed later in the chapter.

A normal lumbar disc can receive 1.5 to 3.0 mL of fluid. During the injection, the patient is asked what he or she is feeling. It is best for the discographer to have a pre-printed pain assessment form (see Discography Pain Form) available to be completed by a nurse or technologist assisting in the procedure.

Specifically, the patient is asked whether he or she is sensing any pain or pressure, where the pain is located, its intensity, and whether it is typical of the usual pain or atypical. Often the patient will describe the pain as typical, although the pain is located only along a portion of its usual distribution. This pain is considered concordant and should be noted. Also, any significant body posturing or facial grimacing during injection should be noted. Finally, the volume of the mixture instilled into the disc and whether there was a firm endpoint (intact annulus) should be recorded.

The needles are left in place until all levels have been injected. After administration of contrast medium, at concordant pain levels, local anesthetic can be instilled through the needle. The patient's pain is often diminished or alleviated immediately, a response that further substantiates that particular disc as a pain generator. Anesthetic injection may also serve to diminish a false-positive pain response at a disc level, owing to residual concordant pain from injections at other levels. We like to use a mixture of 0.25 mL lidocaine 1% and 0.25 mL bupivacaine 0.25% because this combines a short-acting and a long-acting anesthetic to allow a longer evaluation period. The needles are then removed, and AP and lateral spot images of all levels are obtained (Fig. 9-9). The patient's back is cleansed to remove the antiseptic agent, and small adhesive bandages are applied to the puncture sites. Additional CT imaging of the injected disc levels is then obtained.

Thoracic Discogram

Thoracic discography is not routinely requested and therefore is rarely performed. However, thoracic disc degeneration can be associated with clinically significant pain and disability, including mid-back, chest wall, visceral, abdominal, and upper lumbar pain. Thoracic discography must be approached with caution because of the possibility of causing a pneumothorax by inadvertent puncture of the pleura. Thoracic discography can be performed equally well with either fluoroscopic or CT guidance.

FLUOROSCOPIC-GUIDED NEEDLE INSERTION

The examination is performed in a fashion similar to lumbar discography, with a few exceptions. A 25-gauge needle is optimal for thoracic discography because it is less traumatic. Many thoracic discs are more superficial than lumbar discs; therefore, 3.5-inch spinal needles can usually be used. It may be difficult to visualize the thoracic superior articulating process with fluoroscopy; however, the pedicle, which is easily visualized, always projects directly beneath the superior articulating process (Fig. 9-10*A*). In the thoracic region, the facet joints are more coronally oriented. Therefore, a steeper angle should be taken into the disc to reach the center of the nucleus. This is achieved by placing the superior articulating process 30% to 40% of the distance across the ipsilateral ventral aspect of the vertebral body (see Fig. 9-10). With a shallower approach, the junction of the rib and transverse process (costotransverse junction) would obstruct the entry point. During needle insertion, it is important to

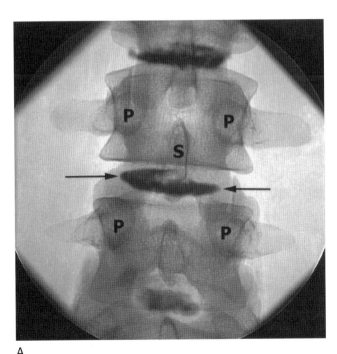

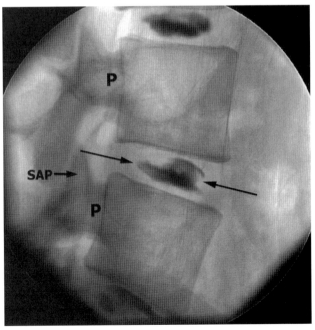

A   B

Figure 9-9 ■ *A*, Contrast agent is within the nucleus at L4-5 (*arrows*). Note proper AP radiographic positioning with the spinous process (S) midway between the pedicles (P) and the x-ray tube angulated to view the disc en face. *B*, Contrast agent is within the nucleus at L4-5 (*arrows*). Note the proper lateral radiographic positioning with the left and right pedicles (P) and the superior articular processes (SAP) overlapping to appear as a solitary unit.

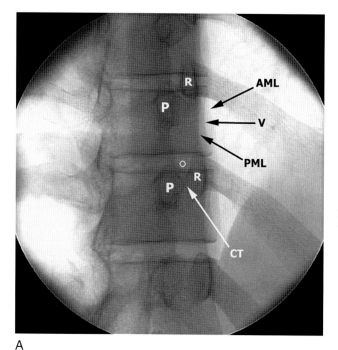

A

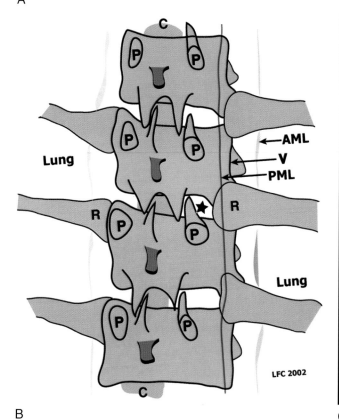

B

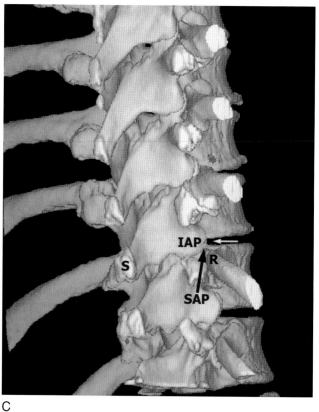

C

Figure 9-10 ■ LAO radiograph (*A*), illustration (*B*), and three-dimensional CT (*C*) showing positioning for thoracic discogram. Pedicle (P) is 35% to 40% of the distance from the anterior vertebral margin. X-ray tube angulation is used to separate the puncture site (*white target, A; black star, B; white arrow, C*) from the costotransverse junction CT. It is crucial to note the three-line configuration composed of anteromedial lung (AML), vertebral margin (V), and posteromedial lung (PML), to lessen the risk of pneumothorax. R = head of rib; S = spinous process; SAP = superior articulating process; IAP = inferior articulating process.

always keep the needle tip along the lateral aspect of the superior articulating process to avoid entering the spinal canal and medial to the costotransverse junction to avoid pleural puncture. It is important to visualize the three-line configuration consisting of, from lateral to medial, the anteromedial lung margin, the posterolateral margin of the vertebral body, and the posteromedial lung margin (see Fig. 9-10A and B). This will ensure that the needle does not pass through the pleura and possibly cause a pneumothorax. For lower thoracic levels, we have the patients hold their breath in expiration during needle advancement to elevate lung position and decrease the risk of pneumothorax. Once the

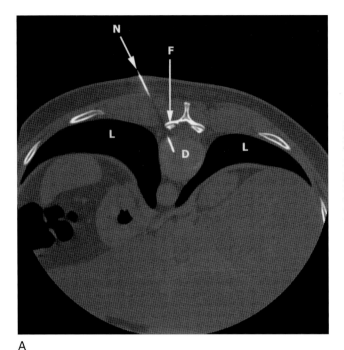

A

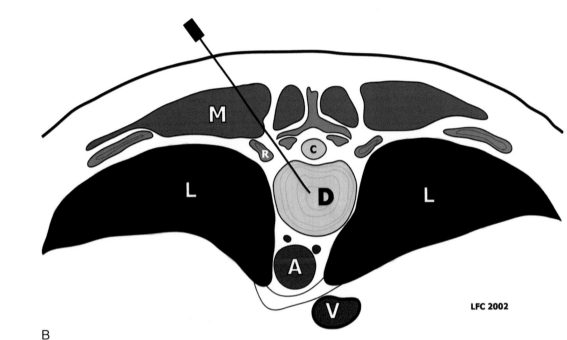

B

Figure 9-11 ▪ *A*, Prone axial CT image, thoracic discogram. The needle (N) is placed from a left posterolateral approach into the disc (D). The projected course of the needle is medial to the lung margin (L) and lateral to the facet joint (F). *B*, Illustration, thoracic discogram, prone position. The needle takes a posterolateral approach through the paraspinal musculature (M), lateral to the facet joint and medial to the head of the rib (R), into the center of the disc (D). This pathway keeps the needle medial to the adjacent lung (L) and lateral to the spinal canal and cord (C). A = aorta; V = inferior vena cava.

needles are in position, injection, patient questioning, and fluoroscopic and CT imaging are performed as described for lumbar discography.

CT-GUIDED NEEDLE INSERTION

Although CT scanning does not allow real-time evaluation of the disc, it still provides the most important part of discography, that being the patient's pain response. One benefit of CT is that it identifies the relationship of the needle tip to the exiting nerve root.

With the patient prone, CT scanning is performed at 3-mm intervals, using helical technique for localization of the entry point(s). The CT scanner gantry is not angulated. Often the entire disc is not seen on a single image; therefore, a slice position is chosen in which the posterior aspect of the target disc is best visualized. The entry points are marked, and the skin is prepared and draped in a sterile fashion. The needle is inserted, using a posterolateral approach, and advanced toward the posterolateral annulus with intermittent CT guidance. When the needle tip contacts the posterolateral annulus, the needle usually deflects into the nucleus. The final position of the needles can be assessed with a single helical acquisition (Fig. 9-11) with sagittal reformatted images to make sure that the needle tip is in the central

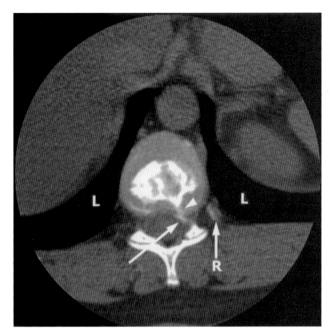

Figure 9-12 ■ A thin band of contrast medium (*arrowhead*) extends posteriorly from the central nucleus toward the left paramidline disc margin, with extravasation into the medial neural foramen (*long arrow*), compatible with a grade 5 tear. R = head of rib; L = lung.

nucleus. These images can also be used to assess for pneumothorax. Once the needles are all in place, contrast medium injection, patient questioning, and CT imaging (Fig. 9-12) are performed in a fashion identical to that for lumbar discography.

Cervical Discogram

Some discographers believe that the information that can be obtained from cervical discography does not outweigh the increased risk of the procedure, and these investigators recommend that cervical discography not be performed. Some authors have reported complication rates as high as 13% for cervical discography.[11] Complications include discitis, epidural abscess, hematoma, quadriplegia, and myelopathy. Localized bleeding is generally minimal, assuming that proper technique is followed. The risk of producing a sizable hematoma is greater in cervical discography. The incidence of infection after cervical discography has been reported to be greater.[12] Predisposing factors for infection include the presence of a beard and a short neck.[12] Therefore, we believe one must carefully consider the risks versus benefits before proceeding with cervical discography.

Informed consent is obtained. The cervical disc cannot be approached posteriorly because of the spinal cord, anteriorly because of the airway, or posterolaterally because of the vertebral artery and the uncinate process. The cervical disc is therefore approached anterolaterally. The patient is placed supine on the fluoroscopy table. A cushion should be placed under the patient's shoulders to slightly hyperextend the neck. The neck skin surface is prepared and draped in sterile fashion. A mild sedative can be administered but is optional and usually not necessary. It is preferable to perform the procedure without sedation to allow the patient to respond to pain sensation in typical fashion. Because cervical discography necessitates manually displacing the carotid artery laterally, the carotid body may be compressed. Therefore, administration of intravenous atropine (0.6 to 1.0 mg) is recommended to minimize the possibility of a vasovagal response.

Ideally, the cervical disc should be punctured on the side opposite the patient's symptoms to reduce the chance of a false-positive response. However, this may be technically difficult, and therefore many authors believe that a right-sided approach should always be used for right-handed discographers, and vice versa. The fluoroscope is placed in the AP position, and cranial or caudal angulation of the C-arm is used to optimally visualize the disc space. As a guide for needle entrance, a sterile metallic mark or needle can be placed on the skin surface and projected over the midline of the disc space to be injected, or the spinal needle can be placed parallel to the disc space and viewed fluoroscopically to guide the level of needle insertion along the medial border of the sternocleidomastoid muscle (Fig. 9-13). Needle puncture should be made between the carotid sheath and the airway. The carotid pulse at the disc level is then palpated with the index and middle fingers, and the carotid sheath structures are displaced laterally by manual palpation (Fig. 9-14). Local anesthesia is given along the expected needle tract. A 25-gauge, 3.5-inch spinal needle is then introduced at a 30- to 40-degree angle in front of the fingertips used to displace the carotid sheath structures. The needle is then positioned with its tip in the center of the disc. Confirmation of needle tip position should be obtained with AP and lateral fluoroscopy (Fig. 9-15).

Needle injection, patient questioning, and fluoroscopic imaging are performed as in lumbar discography, with the

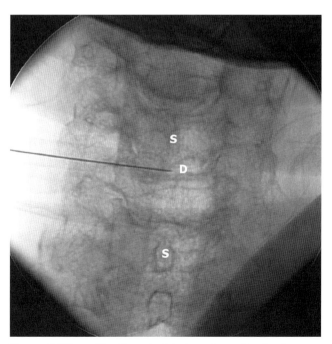

Figure 9-13 ■ AP radiograph. Spinal needle overlies the disc space (D) as a guide for needle puncture. S = spinous process.

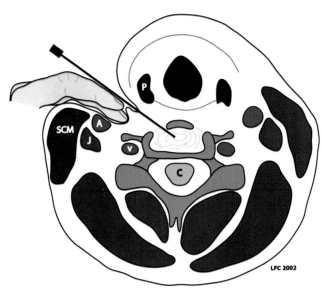

Figure 9-14 ■ Cervical discography technique. The skin entrance is along the anterior border of the sternocleidomastoid muscle (SCM). The discographer's fingers manually displace the vascular structures. The needle is advanced ventral to the fingers. A = carotid artery; J = jugular vein; V = vertebral artery; P = pyriform sinus; C = spinal cord.

exception that the cervical disc holds between 0.5 and 1 mL of fluid. Filling of venous structures during injection is a common occurrence and is believed to be of no clinical significance. Caution should be used not to overfill the disc. Again, up to 0.5 mL of local anesthetic can be injected into a concordant pain disc to evaluate for symptom relief and to further confirm that disc as a pain generator. CT imaging of the injected disc levels is then obtained.

Alternative Methods

DOUBLE-NEEDLE VS. SINGLE-NEEDLE APPROACH

Many discographers still use the traditional double-needle approach for discography, using a shorter 18-gauge needle as a guide to the posterolateral disc margin and placing a longer, 20- or 22-gauge needle through it into the disc. The distal aspect of the smaller-gauge needle is sometimes gently pre-shaped with a curve to facilitate entrance into the center of the disc. Some studies have shown a lower rate of disc infection when the double-needle technique is used,[13] but we have not observed this in our experience. We have performed over 500 patient discograms on approximately 1500 discs with only a 22-gauge, styleted, single-needle approach and have had no cases of discitis. We believe that

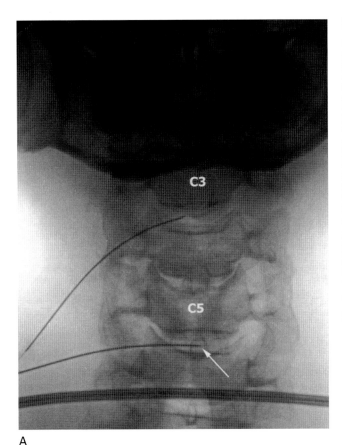
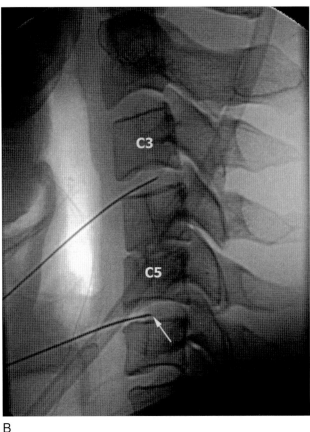

A   B

Figure 9-15 ■ AP (*A*) and lateral (*B*) radiographs demonstrating the needle tip (*arrows*) in the center of the C5-6 disc. (Courtesy of William Greenlee, Jr., MD.)

the double-needle approach is unnecessary. Using the high-quality fluoroscopic imaging now available, with proper technique and patient positioning, we have found no need for a two-needle approach and rarely find it necessary to puncture the disc more than once.

ANTIBIOTIC (INTRAVENOUS VS. INTRADISCAL) VS. NO ANTIBIOTIC

Our earliest cases of discography were performed without antibiotics, and there were no clinical cases of discitis. Studies using sheep demonstrated no evidence of discitis in any sheep inoculated with *Staphylococcus epidermidis* and treated prophylactically with ceftriaxone.[14] Furthermore, the sheep model of discitis suggests that in most cases this process is self-limited. We now routinely administer intravenous antibiotics (1,000 mg ceftriaxone) 1 hour before the procedure as a precaution against infection, even though there is little strong evidence to support the routine use of antibiotics for discography. However, a study by Lang and colleagues[15] demonstrated that although there was good penetration of ceftriaxone into the disc at therapeutic levels from 1 to 4 hours after an antibiotic bolus, the minimum inhibitory concentration effective against *S. epidermidis* (the usual agent responsible for post-discography discitis) was not exceeded. The options then became either to increase the concentration of antibiotics or to give intradiscal antibiotics. We now use intradiscal antibiotics in addition to intravenous antibiotics for all of our discograms.

PATIENT POSITIONING

For lumbar and thoracic discography, the patient is ideally positioned prone with the less symptomatic side slightly up to make it easier for the discographer to place the needle. Some advocate placing patients on their side, although this is usually not as stable a position. Some discographers advocate entering the skin at measured distances lateral to the spinous processes. This is not optimal, because people come in different shapes and sizes. By the use of the landmarks described earlier, needle tip positioning in the nucleus pulposus can be achieved in more than 95% of patients. With this positioning, one should rarely need to resort to transthecal needle puncture to perform discography at the L5-S1 level.

INTRADISCAL LOCAL ANESTHESIA PLACEMENT AFTER CONTRAST AGENT INJECTION

This is an optional technique that we routinely use in two specific situations. First, in patients with full-thickness tears, one is not able to increase the intradiscal pressure. Therefore, in theory, for patients with mechanoreceptor discogenic pain, a false-negative discogram may be obtained. Thus, if this level is suspect, an injection of 1 to 2 mL of bupivacaine 0.5% may relieve these patients of their usual back pain for 1 to 3 days. Second, in patients with intact annuli, once contrast medium has been instilled into the disc, it is difficult to instill further fluid (anesthetic). If this level has questionably concordant pain during discography, we may ask the patient to return 1 week after the discography and we then inject a mixture of 2 mL bupivacaine 0.5% and 0.5 mL nonionic myelographic contrast medium (to confirm needle position) into that disc. In either scenario, the patient is asked to keep a pain diary for 3 days.

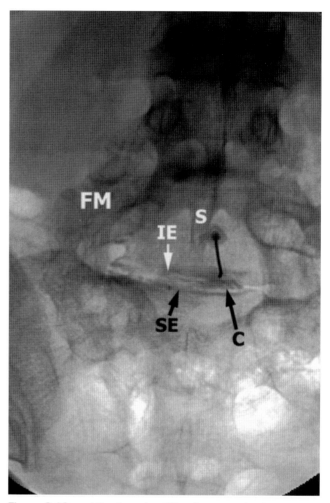

Figure 9-16 ■ AP radiograph, midline disc approach. Bilateral lateral fusion masses (FM) do not allow posterolateral access to the L5-S1 disc. The x-ray tube is angulated to visualize the L5-S1 disc space en face, and, with a transthecal approach, the needle is placed in the middle third of the disc. Contrast agent (C) is seen within the L5-S1 disc. IE = inferior end plate of L5; SE = superior end plate of S1; S = spinous process.

We are finding that relief of concordant discogenic pain after diagnostic anesthetic injection provides valuable information for discographic evaluation before possible IDET or spinal fusion.

MIDLINE L5-S1 APPROACH (TRANSTHECAL)

This approach has been used in the past by some discographers to position the needle in the L5-S1 disc by means of a midline or paramidline puncture when it was difficult to gain access through an oblique approach (Fig. 9-16). We do not advocate this method routinely, because of the theoretical risk of introducing infection into the subarachnoid space and the risk of causing arachnoiditis from a subarachnoid hemorrhage. With the use of the method just described with steep craniocaudal angulation of the x-ray beam, we believe the midline approach is rarely required today.

Post-Discography CT

Post-discography CT is more sensitive in the detection of annular disruption than fluoroscopic evaluation. CT scanning

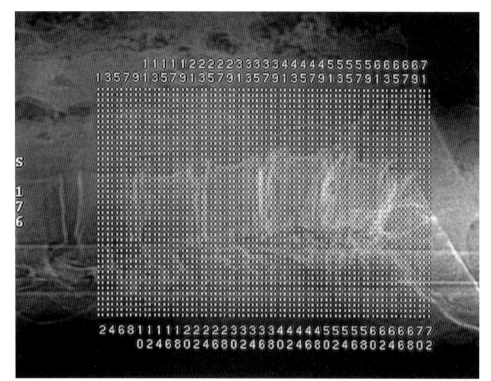

Figure 9-17 ▪ Sagittal CT scout view. Continuous slice acquisition setup from L1-S1.

after discography is obtained in one of two ways. With the patient supine, imaging is performed in a single acquisition using a helical technique to include all injected discs (Fig. 9-17). Axial reformatted images angled parallel to each disc from the pedicle above to the pedicle below can then be obtained as well as sagittal and coronal reformatted images. Alternatively, each disc can be scanned separately from the pedicles above the disc to the pedicles below the disc, with the CT gantry angled to each disc (Fig. 9-18). With either method, slice thickness should be no greater than 3 mm in the lumbar and thoracic spines and 1 mm in the cervical spine.

CT images are valuable in planning for an IDET procedure. Whereas the discogram establishes whether there is

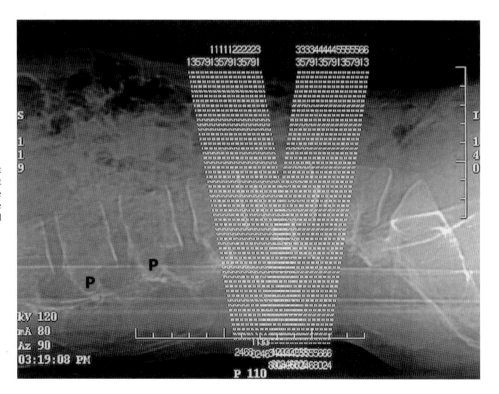

Figure 9-18 ▪ Sagittal CT scout view. Angled disc acquisition setup at L3-4 and L4-5. Continuous slices are obtained angled to each disc from the mid pedicle above the disc to the mid pedicle below the disc.

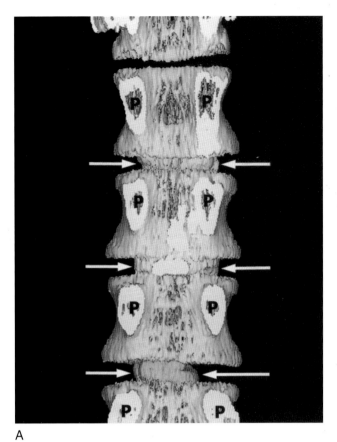
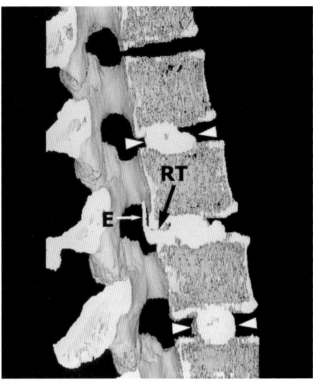

A   B

Figure 9-19 ■ Coronal (*A*) and sagittal (*B*) three-dimensional reconstruction demonstrate the lateral boundaries of the nucleus (*arrows*, *A*) and the anterior and posterior boundaries of the nucleus (*arrowheads*, *B*). P = pedicle; RT = radial tear; E = epidural contrast.

adequate access to the target disc with a straight needle, CT can more readily evaluate the size and shape of the nucleus pulposus. The anterior, posterior, and lateral boundaries of the nucleus pulposus are clearly identified in relation to the bony structures of the vertebrae (Fig. 9-19). This method can be used during the IDET procedure to determine where the IDET introducer needle needs to be positioned to be intranuclear. It is most helpful at L5-S1, where entrance into the more medial aspect of the disc may be obstructed by the iliac crest. The postdiscogram CT may demonstrate that the nucleus extends more lateral than expected, allowing a more lateral needle approach.

POTENTIAL COMPLICATIONS[11, 16, 17]

* Bleeding, usually minimal; although a serious spinal canal epidural hemorrhage is possible
* Infection, specifically discitis and vertebral osteomyelitis
* Drug-related allergic reactions
* Inadvertent puncture of the thecal sac (usually not associated with any complications but could result in arachnoiditis)
* Headache
* Pneumothorax for thoracic discography
* Epidural abscess, vascular injury, quadriplegia, and myelopathy (cervical discography)

* Vasovagal reactions (more commonly reported with cervical discography)

PROCEDURE REPORTING

The discography report should be a compilation of all information obtained from the discogram and post-procedure CT. Each level should be reported separately, including information about the patient's pain response (severity, location, and similarity to the usual pain), the quantity of the mixture instilled into the nucleus, the presence or absence of pain relief after injection of local anesthetic, and disc morphology. **The nature of the pain response is the most important aspect of discography.** A simple system to classify the pain response follows:

1. No pain or pressure
2. Pain reported, but not similar in intensity or distribution to the usual pain (nonconcordant)
3. Pain reported similar to some of the usual pain (concordant)
4. Pain reported entirely identical to the usual pain (concordant)

Disc morphology is assessed from the radiographic and CT images. The various descriptions of the nucleus include

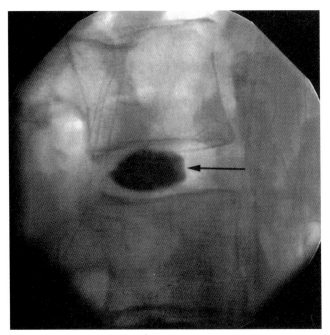

Figure 9-20 ■ Normal nucleogram. Lateral radiograph. Contrast material is seen as an ovoid shape (*arrow*) in the disc nucleus.

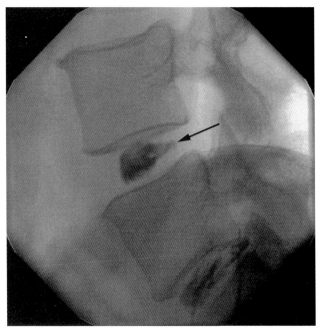

Figure 9-22 ■ Irregular nucleogram. Lateral radiograph. Most of the contrast medium is in the central nucleus, with a focal region of it extending posteriorly into the inner two thirds of the disc annulus (*arrow*).

normal, radial tear, circumferential or concentric tear, transverse tear, or annular injection.

Various stages of disc degeneration have been described to correlate with the fluoroscopic portion of the discogram.[18]

1. Cottonball (Fig. 9-20)
   a. Normal nuclear appearance
   b. Contrast medium remaining central with an oval appearance

   c. Equivalent to grade 0 modified Dallas classification[3, 13]
2. Lobular, hamburger bun, or horseshoe (Fig. 9-21)
   a. Normal mature disc appearance
   b. Intranuclear cleft forms
   c. Equivalent to grade 0 modified Dallas classification[3, 13]
3. Irregular (Fig. 9-22)
   a. Early degeneration
   b. Fissures or clefts seen in the inner two thirds of the annulus

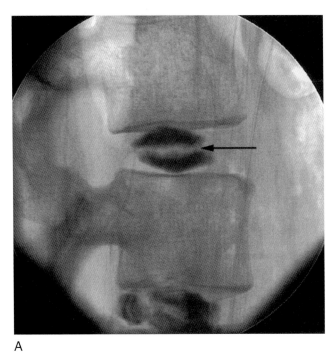

A

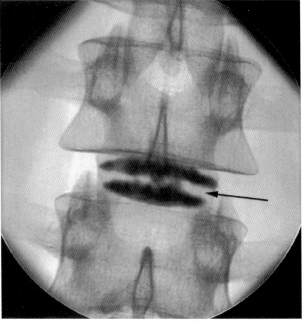

B

Figure 9-21 ■ Normal mature nucleogram. Lateral (*A*) and AP (*B*) radiographs. Contrast material is seen in the disc nucleus separated by a cleft (*arrow*) with a hamburger bun or horseshoe appearance.

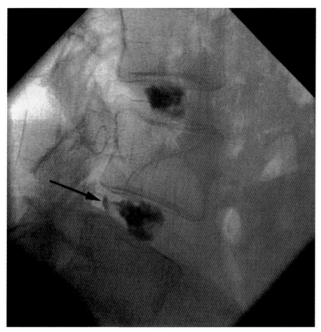

Figure 9-23 ■ Fissured nucleogram. Lateral radiograph. Most of the contrast medium is in the central nucleus, with some extending to the posterior annular margin (*arrow*).

   c. Equivalent to grade 1 or 2 modified Dallas classification[3, 13]

4. Fissured (Fig. 9-23)
   a. Further degeneration

   b. Radial tears or fissures extending to the periphery of the annulus without entrance into the epidural space
   c. Equivalent to grade 3 or 4 modified Dallas classification[3, 13]

5. Ruptured (Fig. 9-24)
   a. Complete radial tear
   b. Contrast medium seen to escape the confines of the disc and perhaps enter the epidural space and/or neural foramen
   c. Can be seen at any stage of disc degeneration
   d. Equivalent to grade 5 modified Dallas classification[3, 13]

If the needle is not placed within the nucleus of the disc, an annular injection will occur with deposition of contrast material within the peripheral fibers of the disc (Fig. 9-25). Although this is not considered serious, it is suboptimal. If firm resistance is met at the beginning of an injection, an annular injection may be occurring. The injection should be evaluated in both AP and lateral planes before proceeding.

Three types of annular fissures or tears have been described, which can occur alone or in combination:

1. Radial tears, either narrow or wide, are those that extend in a linear fashion from the central nucleus various distances toward the peripheral annulus, perpendicular to the circumferential annular fibers.
2. Concentric or circumferential tears occur when the interlamellar collagen bridging fibers are torn. These tears can be associated with normal aging and are caused by delamination or separation of the annular lamellae, leading to annular laxity and generalized disc bulging (Fig. 9-26). They are not believed to be clinically significant.

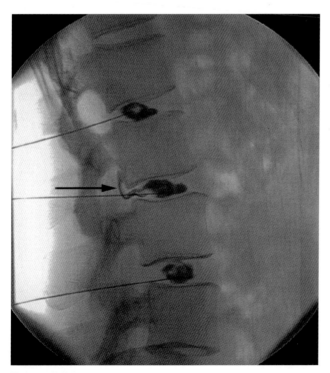

Figure 9-24 ■ Ruptured nucleogram. Lateral radiograph. Contrast medium extends through the posterior annulus with extra-annular extension (*arrow*).

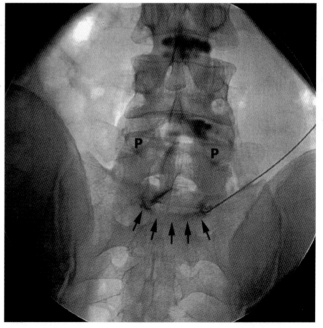

Figure 9-25 ■ Annular injection. AP radiograph. Contrast medium is seen with a curvilinear appearance as it dissects through the annular layers (*arrows*). Note that the needle tip is not within the central third of the disc but at the level of the pedicle (P).

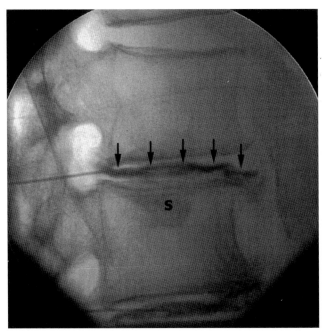

Figure 9-26 ■ Concentric (*circumferential*) tears. Lateral radiograph. Contrast medium spreads throughout the disc with an amorphic appearance (*arrows*). Note disc space narrowing, end plate flattening, anterior vertebral marginal spurring, and Schmorl's node (S) of the superior end plate of the inferior vertebral body.

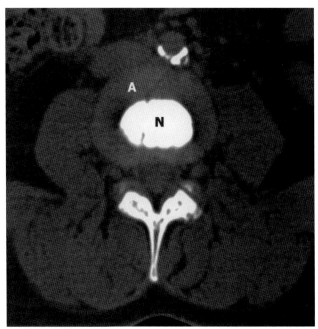

Figure 9-28 ■ Grade 0 radial tear. Hyperdense contrast medium is confined to the nucleus of the disc (N). A = disc annulus.

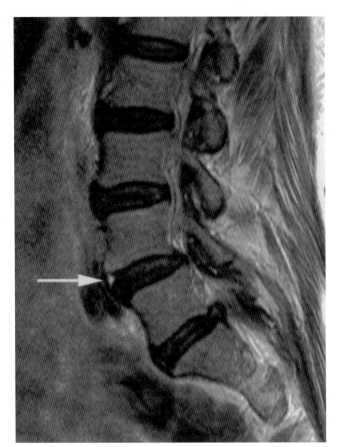

Figure 9-27 ■ Transverse tear. Sagittal MR image T2 fast spin echo. A small focus of increased signal intensity is present at the junction of the anterosuperior L4-5 annulus and the anteroinferior L4 vertebral margin (*arrow*).

3. Transverse tears are avulsions of the peripheral annular fibers at their insertions on the vertebral body ring apophysis (Fig. 9-27).

The radial tear is considered to be most closely related to discogenic pain. Posterior annular fissures are more likely to be associated with pain. The Modified Dallas Discogram Scale[3, 13] is the standard for reporting radiographic and post-discography CT findings in the cervical, thoracic, or lumbar spine, with the following grading system:

Grade 0   Contrast medium confined to a normal nucleus pulposus (Fig. 9-28)
Grade 1   Radial tear confined to the inner third of the annulus fibrosis (Fig. 9-29)
Grade 2   Radial tear extending to the middle third of the annulus fibrosis (Fig. 9-30)
Grade 3   Radial tear extending to the outer third of the annulus fibrosis (Fig. 9-31)
Grade 4   Grade 3 tear with dissection into the outer third of the annulus to involve more than 30 degrees of the disc circumference (Fig. 9-32)
Grade 5   Any full-thickness tear with extra-annular leakage of contrast (Fig. 9-33)

Contrast material within the needle tract may be misinterpreted as a radial tear. On CT images, the opacified needle tract is seen as a thin, straight line of contrast medium extending on an approximately 45-degree angle from the nucleus toward the posterolateral disc margin (Fig. 9-34). Of course, this should be correlated with the actual side of needle puncture and the true direction of the needle path that was imaged during fluoroscopy.

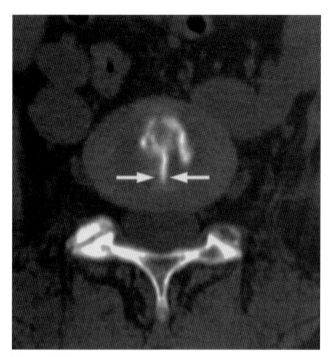

Figure 9-29 ■ Grade 1 radial tear. Contrast medium extends from the central nucleus posteriorly into the inner third of the annulus (*arrows*).

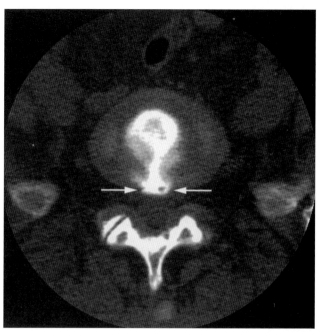

Figure 9-31 ■ Grade 3 radial tear. Contrast medium extends from the central nucleus posteriorly to the posterior disc margin (*arrows*).

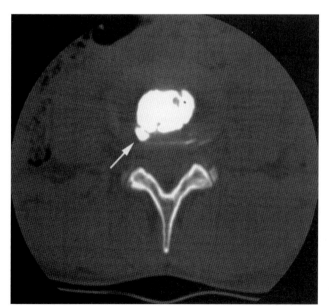

Figure 9-30 ■ Grade 2 radial tear. Contrast medium extends right posterolaterally into the middle third of the annulus (*arrow*).

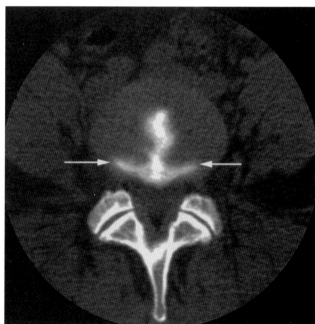

Figure 9-32 ■ Grade 4 radial tear. Contrast medium extends from the central nucleus to the posterocentral disc margin with dissection through the outer annulus of more than 30 degrees of the disc circumference (*arrows*).

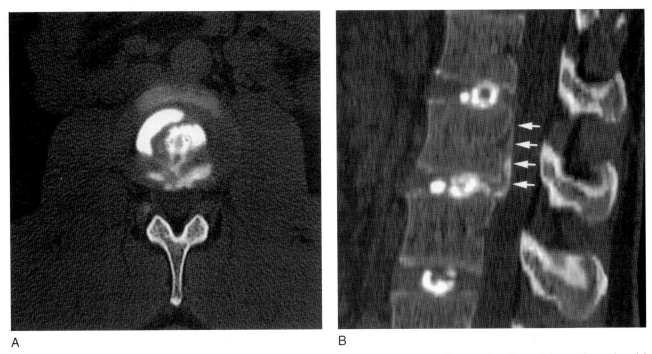

A   B

Figure 9-33 ■ Grade 5 radial tear. Axial (*A*) and sagittal (*B*) reconstructed CT images. Contrast medium extends to the posterior annulus on the axial image; however, the reconstructed image demonstrates epidural extravasation with cephalad extension to the posterior disc margin above (*arrows, B*).

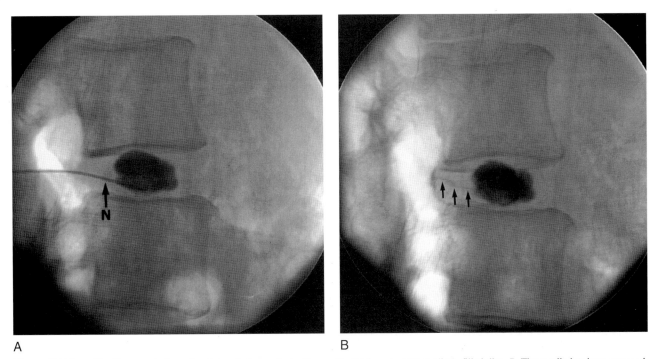

A   B

Figure 9-34 ■ Needle tract. *A*, Lateral radiograph demonstrates the needle (N) in a contrast medium–filled disc. *B*, The needle has been removed. There is a thin linear region of contrast agent (*arrows*) that extends from the central nucleus, along the path of needle in *A*, to the posterior disc margin.

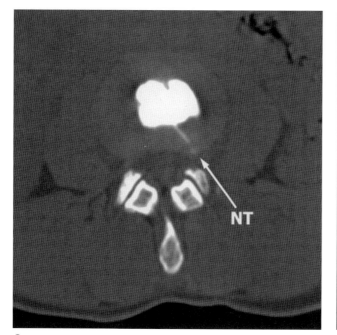

C

Figure 9-34 (*Cont'd*) ■ *C*, Axial post-discography CT image at the disc level demonstrates the needle tract (NT) extending to the left posterolateral margin of the disc.

Figure 9-36 ■ Annular injection. No significant contrast medium is present in the nucleus (N). Contrast medium is seen in a curvilinear fashion dissecting through the circumferential annular fibers (*arrows*).

With aging, complex tears of the disc can be seen. In such severely degenerated discs that have been injected, there is often diffuse spread of contrast agent throughout the entire disc, compatible with full-thickness tears (Fig. 9-35). Contrast medium entering the epidural space can remain subligamentous, or it can extend through the ligament and above and/or below the disc injected, sometimes entering the neural foramen.

If the discography needle is placed too anteriorly, posteriorly, or laterally, an annular injection will occur. On CT, contrast material is seen in a curvilinear pattern in the outer portions of the disc, with minimal or no contrast agent centrally (Fig. 9-36). If enough contrast material is given, a ring is seen around the annulus that is caused by contrast medium dissecting through the annular layers.

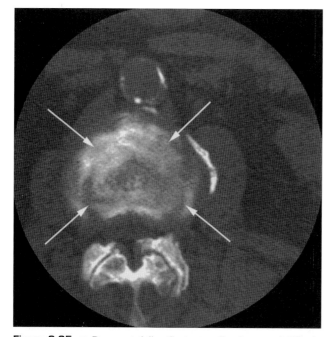

Figure 9-35 ■ Degenerated disc. Contrast medium has spread diffusely throughout the nucleus and annulus (*arrows*).

POST-PROCEDURE CARE/FOLLOW-UP

Immediate[19]

1. The patient should be observed for 2 hours after discography.
2. The patient may sit in a reclining lounge chair; however, if there is significant post-procedure pain or if the patient received intravenous sedation, he or she should be placed at bed rest.
3. Blood pressure, pulse, heart rate, and respiration are evaluated immediately after the procedure. If they are stable, no further vital signs are taken. If they are significantly different from baseline, evaluation is repeated every 30 minutes until the vital signs return to baseline.
4. Toradol[IV/IM]
   a. If the patient is younger than 65 years of age, then a one-time dose of 60 mg is given intramuscularly.
   b. If the patient is older than 65 years of age, renally impaired, or weighs less than 50 kg, then a one-time dose of 30 mg is given intramuscularly.
   c. Toradol[IV/IM] should not be administered if the patient has a contraindication to nonsteroidal anti-inflammatory medications.

Discharge[19]

1. The patient is discharged into the care of a responsible person.
2. The patient is instructed not to drive or perform any other tasks that require clear thought and quick reactions for the remainder of the day, especially if sedation was given.
3. A 2- to 3-day nonrenewable prescription for a narcotic pain reliever and/or a muscle relaxant is given to the patient.
4. Multiple adhesive bandages may be on the patient's back or neck. These should remain dry for at least 24 hours, at which point they can be removed.
5. Patients are instructed to continue to take their prescription medication, although pain medication may be tapered as indicated.
6. A discharge sheet should be given to the patient outlining:
   a. Which procedure was performed and at what levels
   b. Procedurally related symptoms that typically resolve in 7 to 10 days
      * Pain at the needle puncture site(s)
      * Mild increased back or neck stiffness
      * Deep back or neck pain
   c. Treatment for mild post-procedure symptoms
      * Rest the affected area for 3 to 4 days.
      * Avoid movements that aggravate the pain.
      * Apply cold compresses to the area that hurts.
   d. Signs and symptoms of infection
      * Fever
      * Chills
      * Swelling or drainage from the puncture sites
      * New back or neck pain that is different from the usual pain
   e. Signs and symptoms of possibly more serious problems
      * Stiff neck
      * Increasing pain
      * Motor dysfunction such as difficulty walking or lifting
      * Bowel or bladder dysfunction
   f. Physician name and contact number if the patient has any concerns or if any problems were to arise as a result of the procedure
   g. Advice to schedule a follow-up appointment with the referring physician in 7 to 10 days

SAMPLE DICTATIONS

Lumbar Spine

Procedure: Lumbar discogram with post-discography CT
Date of Procedure: Month/day/year
Facility: Name of facility
Levels Studied: L3-4, L4-5, L5-S1
Supplies: Spinal needles (3), 22-gauge, 6-inch

The procedure and potential complications, including the risk of disc infection, were explained to the patient and voluntary informed, signed consent was obtained. The patient was a candidate for conscious sedation. One gram of cefazolin was administered intravenously 30 minutes before the procedure. Electrocardiographic, pulse oximetry, and blood pressure monitoring were utilized during the examination. The patient was placed in a shallow right anterior oblique (RAO) position on the table. The patient's back was prepped and draped in usual sterile fashion. Subcutaneous 1% lidocaine was instilled into the superficial soft tissues of the patient's lower back for local anesthesia. With fluoroscopic guidance, three 22-gauge, 6-inch spinal needles were placed percutaneously, one at a time, using a left posterolateral extrapedicular approach into the L3-4 through L5-S1 discs. The thecal sac was never violated. Under fluoroscopy, after gentle negative aspiration, the needles were injected with a varying amount of solution (as described later) from a mixture of 2.3 mL nonionic myelographic contrast medium (300 mg I/mL) and 0.5 mL cefazolin (2 mg/mL), one at a time, without the patient knowing which disc was being injected. Note was made of the patient's response to the individual injections as to location, quality, and severity of the pain caused by the injections, the amount of solution injected, and whether the annulus was intact. The needles were then removed. Spot AP and lateral images of the discs were then obtained. No complications were observed during or immediately after the procedure. Additional CT disc imaging with sagittal reformatted images was then obtained.

L3-4: Injection was performed with 0.6 mL of fluid. The patient described no evidence of pain or pressure. There was a firm endpoint. During fluoroscopy and CT, the disc had a normal appearance, with the contrast agent remaining centrally within the nucleus pulposus.

L4-5: Injection was performed with 0.8 mL of fluid with a firm endpoint. The patient described severe left low back pain (10 out of a possible 10 on a pain scale) that was identical to his usual back pain. Fluoroscopically, contrast medium was seen to extend posteriorly along the disc margin. Post-discography CT demonstrated a grade 3 left paramidline radial tear.

L5-S1: Injection was performed with 2.8 mL of fluid without firm endpoint. The patient described some left-sided back pain (5 out of a possible 10 on a pain scale) that was not quite typical of his usual pain. Contrast medium was seen to spread more diffusely throughout the disc, compatible with concentric tears. Post-discography CT demonstrated a small linear region of contrast agent extending from the central nucleus posteriorly toward the disc margin but remaining within the posterior third of the disc, compatible with a grade 1 to 2 annular tear, which was slightly right of midline.

Cervical Spine

Procedure: Cervical discogram with post-discogram CT
Date of Procedure: Month/day/year
Facility: Name of facility
Levels Studied: C4-5, C5-6
Supplies: Spinal needles (2), 25-gauge, 3.5-inch

The procedure and potential complications, including the risk of disc infection, were explained to the patient and voluntary informed, signed consent was obtained. The patient was a candidate for conscious sedation. One gram of cefazolin was administered intravenously 30 minutes before the procedure. Electrocardiographic, pulse oximetry, and blood pressure monitoring were used during the examination. The patient was placed in the supine position on the table. The patient's neck was prepped and draped in usual sterile fashion. Before the procedure, 1 mg of intravenous atropine was given to prevent a vasovagal reaction. Subcutaneous 1% lidocaine was instilled into the superficial soft tissues of the patient's neck for local anesthesia. With fluoroscopic guidance, two 25-gauge, 3.5-inch spinal needles were placed percutaneously, one at a time, using a right anterolateral approach, into the C4-5 and C5-6 discs. The thecal sac was never violated. Under fluoroscopy, after gentle negative aspiration, the needles were injected with a varying amount of solution (as described later) from a mixture of 2.3 mL nonionic myelographic contrast medium (300 mg I/mL) and 0.5 mL cefazolin (2 mg/mL), one at a time, without the patient knowing which disc was being injected. Note was made of the patient's response to the individual injections as to location, quality, and severity of the pain caused by the injections, the amount of solution injected, and whether the annulus was intact. The needles were then removed. Spot AP and lateral images of the discs were then obtained. No complications were observed during or immediately after the procedure. Additional CT disc imaging with sagittal reformatted images was then obtained.

C4-5: Injection was performed with 0.5 mL of fluid with a firm endpoint. The patient described minimal (1 out of a possible 10 on a pain scale) central neck pressure, which was not typical of his usual pain. At fluoroscopy and on CT, the disc had a normal appearance, with contrast agent remaining centrally within the nucleus.

C5-6: Injection was performed with 1.5 mL of fluid without a firm endpoint. The patient described severe (9 out of a possible 10 on a pain scale) central neck and left shoulder pain that was identical to his usual pain. At fluoroscopy, contrast agent immediately flowed toward the left posterolateral margin of the disc. On CT images, there was a grade 5 left posterolateral radial tear with contrast medium entering the left anterior epidural space and left C5-6 neural foramen.

CASE REPORTS

CASE 1

Clinical Presentation

The patient is a 21-year-old woman with low back pain and bilateral proximal lower extremity pain, left greater than right. She had a lumbar discectomy 1 year earlier. Her pain is different from her preoperative pain and is nonradicular. Lumbar extension and flexion are full. Straight-leg raising is negative to 90 degrees bilaterally. Motor strength is strong and symmetric.

Imaging and Therapy

Sagittal MR imaging (Fig. 9-37A) demonstrated degenerative low signal intensity in the L5-S1 disc (there was a rudimentary disc at S1-2). There was also a small disc bulge to the left of midline with some increased signal intensity compatible with an annular tear (see Fig. 9-37B). A lateral discogram (see Fig. 9-37C) and a sagittal reformatted post-discogram CT

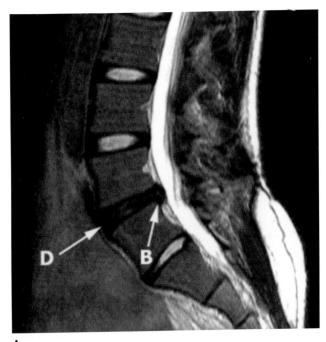

A

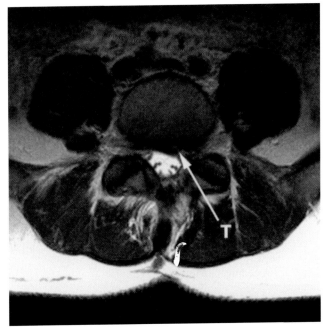

B

Figure 9-37 ■ *A*, Sagittal MR image, T2 fast spin echo. There is decreased signal intensity of the L5-S1 disc (D) with minimal posterior disc bulging (B) compatible with disc degeneration. A rudimentary disc is seen at S1-2. *B*, Axial MR image, T2 fast spin echo. There is subtle increased signal intensity within the left posterolateral disc bulge, compatible with an annular tear (T).

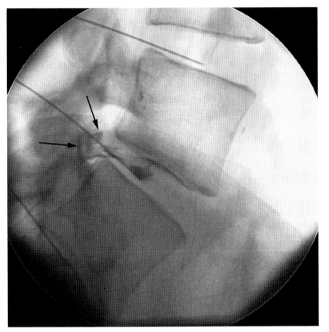

C

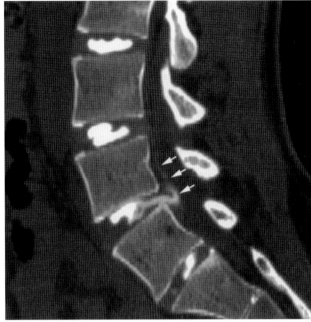

D

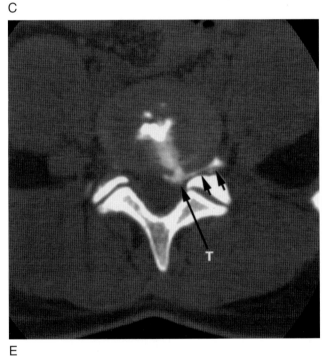

E

Figure 9-37 *(Cont'd)* ▪ *C*, Lateral discogram, L5-S1. Contrast medium is seen centrally within the disc and extending posteriorly, overlying the inferior neural foramen (*arrows*), compatible with a grade 5 tear. *D*, Sagittal reformatted CT image. Another perspective demonstrates contrast medium extravasating through a posterior annular tear and extending cephalad to the mid-L5 vertebral body (*arrows*). *E*, Post-discography axial CT. Contrast medium is seen extending from the central nucleus through an annular tear (T) to the left posterior paramidline disc, with extension into the left neural foramen (*short arrows*), compatible with a grade 5 tear. The L3-4, L4-5, and S1-2 nucleograms are normal.

(see Fig. 9-37*D*) demonstrated contrast medium extravasating posteriorly into the epidural space, compatible with a grade 5 tear. Post-discography axial CT demonstrated a grade 5 tear extending to the left posterior paramidline annulus, with extravasation into the left neural foramen (see Fig.9-37*E*).

Results

Injection of the L5-S1 disc with 0.7 mL of injection mixture (contrast material and antibiotic) reproduced

the patient's entire pain complex. Injection of all other levels reproduced no to minimal pressure or pain that was not consistent with her usual pain. Injection of 1.0 mL bupivacaine (0.25%) into the L5-S1 disc after discography relieved the patient of her pain for a total of 2 days.

CASE 2

Clinical Presentation

The patient is a 44-year-old man with 2 years of low back pain and nonradicular proximal right leg pain. The pain is precipitated by activity and somewhat relieved by sitting. The patient's condition has not improved with medication or physical therapy. He has had facet injections, facet denervations, and epidural steroid injections without benefit. On neurologic examination, gait and strength are normal. He has some discomfort in his back and right buttock at 90 degrees straight-leg raising on the right.

Imaging and Therapy

A sagittal T2-weighted MR image demonstrated foci of increased signal intensity in the posterior aspects of the L3-4 and L4-5 discs, compatible with annular tears (Fig. 9-38*A*). Lateral discogram images demonstrated contrast medium extending to but contained by the posterior longitudinal ligament at L3-4 (see Fig. 9-38*B*)

and extending into the epidural space at L4-5 (see Fig. 9-38*C*). Axial post-discography CT images demonstrated contrast medium and iatrogenically introduced air extending to the posterior central disc margin at L3-4, compatible with a grade 3 tear (see Fig. 9-38*D*) and contrast agent extending to the posterior central disc margin with bilateral lateral spread within the annular layers, compatible with a grade 4 tear (see Fig. 9-38*E*).

Results

Injection of the L3-4 disc with 0.5 mL of injection mixture (contrast material and antibiotic) reproduced the upper portion of the patient's low back pain. Injection of the L4-5 disc with 0.8 mL of injection mixture reproduced the lower portion of the patient's low back pain as well as his right leg pain. Injection of the other levels reproduced no to minimal pressure or pain that was not consistent with his usual pain.

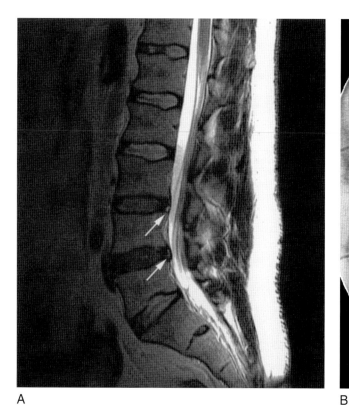

A

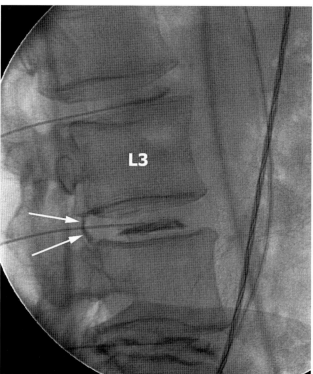

B

Figure 9-38 ■ *A*, Sagittal MR image, T2 fast spin echo. Mild disc degeneration of L3-4 and L4-5 is seen as decreased disc signal intensity. Small foci of increased signal intensity involve the posterior disc margins at L3-4 and L4-5, compatible with annular tears (*arrows*). *B*, Lateral radiograph. Contrast medium is seen centrally in the disc, and curvilinear contrast bridges the posterior disc margin (*arrows*), compatible with annular tear.

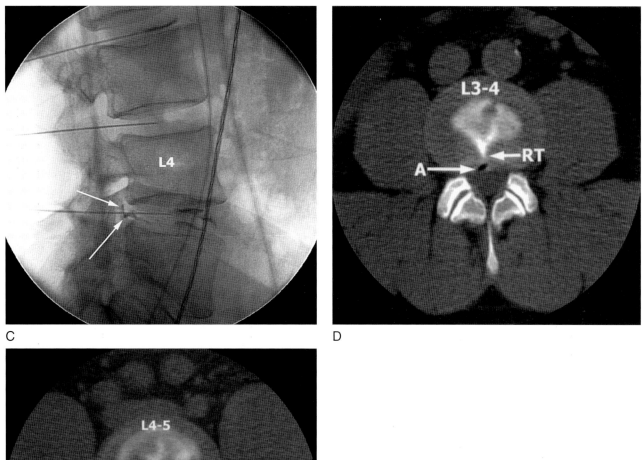

C

D

E

Figure 9-38 *(Cont'd)* ■ *C*, Lateral radiograph. Contrast medium outlines the disc, with extension posteriorly (*arrows*). *D*, Post-discography axial CT image, L3-4. Contrast medium extends posteriorly from the central nucleus toward the disc margin. Note the small focus of air (A) in the posterior central annulus, likely iatrogenically injected. Grade 3 radial tear (RT). *E*, Post-discography axial CT image, L4-5. Contrast medium extends posteriorly from the central nucleus to the disc margin, with bilateral posterolateral spread, compatible with a grade 4 tear (*arrows*).

CASE 3

Clinical Presentation

The patient is a 45-year-old woman with an 8-month history of bilateral central neck pain and pain radiating into both shoulders. The precipitating event was a car accident in which her car was rear-ended while stationary. The pain is worse with flexion and extension. The patient's strength is normal.

Imaging and Therapy

Lateral cervical discography demonstrated contrast medium extending to the posterior disc margins at C3-4, C4-5, and C5-6, compatible with tears, with contrast medium extending into a disc protrusion at C5-6 (Fig. 9-39*A*). Axial post-discography CT demonstrated contrast medium extending posteriorly into a focal central disc herniation, which caused mild central spinal canal narrowing (see Fig. 9-39*B*).

Results

Injection of the C5-6 disc with 0.5 mL of injection mixture (contrast material and antibiotic) reproduced the patient's neck and shoulder pain. Injection of the C3-4 and C4-5 discs produced neck discomfort that was discordant with her usual pain.

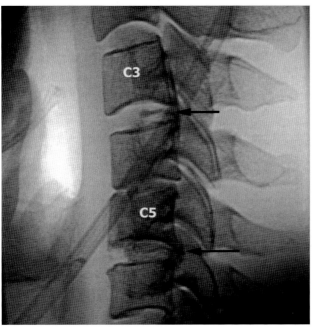

A

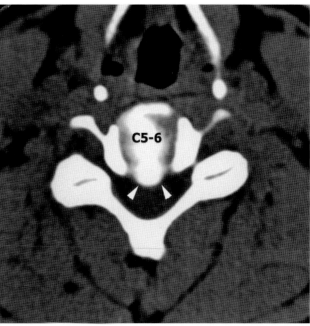

B

Figure 9-39 ■ *A*, Lateral radiograph, cervical discogram. Contrast medium is seen in the C3-4, C4-5, and C5-6 discs. There is mild disc bulging and the contrast agent extends slightly posteriorly at C3-4 and more so at C5-6 (*arrows*). *B*, Post-discography axial CT image, C5-6. Contrast medium extends from the central nucleus to the anterior and posterior disc margin and enters a small central disc herniation (*arrowheads*). (Courtesy of William Greenlee, Jr., MD.)

CURRENT PROCEDURAL TERMINOLOGY (CPT) CODES

CPT codes change often and sometimes are valid only for certain states or regions. It is best to consult with coding experts to make sure that coding for one's procedures is legitimate and complete. Below is a sample of codes that are being used for discography at this writing.[20]

Lumbar Spine

72295   Discography, lumbar, radiological supervision and interpretation

62290   Injection procedure for discography, each level; lumbar

72131   Computerized axial tomography, lumbar spine; without contrast material

Cervical or Thoracic Spine

72285   Discography, cervical or thoracic, radiological supervision and interpretation

62291   Injection procedure for discography, each level; cervical or thoracic

72125   Computerized axial tomography, **cervical** spine; without contrast material

72128 Computerized axial tomography, **thoracic** spine; without contrast material

76375 Coronal, sagittal, multiplanar, oblique, 3-dimensional and/or holographic reconstruction of computerized tomography, magnetic resonance, or other tomographic modality

(Can add **76375** if performing orthogonal reformatted images from the axial CT images)

99141 Sedation with or without analgesia (conscious sedation); intravenous, intramuscular or inhalation

References

1. Guyer RD, Ohnmeiss DD. Contemporary concepts in spine care lumbar discography. Position Statement from the North American Spine Society Diagnostic and Therapeutic Committee. Spine 1995; 20:2048–2059.
2. Bogduk N. The innervation of the lumbar spine. Spine 1983; 8:286–293.
3. Aprill CN, Bogduk N. High-intensity zone: A diagnostic sign of painful lumbar disc on magnetic resonance imaging. Br J Radiol 1992; 65:361–369.
4. Schellhas KP, Pollei SR, Gundry CR, et al. Lumbar disc high-intensity zone. Spine 1996; 21:79–86.
5. Bogduk N, Windsor M, Inglis A. The innervation of the cervical intervertebral discs. Spine 1988; 13:2–8.
6. Lindblom K. Diagnostic puncture of intervertebral disks in sciatica. Acta Orthop Scand 1948; 17:213–239.
7. Holt EP. The question of lumbar discography. J Bone Joint Surg Am 1968; 50:720–726.
8. Simmons JW, Aprill CN, Dwyer AP, et al. A reassessment of Holt's data on: "The Question of Lumbar Discography." Clin Orthop 1988; 237:120–124.
9. Physicians' Desk Reference, 56th ed. Montvale, NJ: Medical Economics Company, 2002.
10. Schellhas KP. Diskography. Neuroimaging Clin North Am 2000; 10:579–596.
11. Connor PM, Darden BV. Cervical discography complications and clinical efficacy. Spine 1993; 18:2035–2038.
12. Zeidman SM, Thompson K, Ducker TB. Complications of cervical discography: Analysis of 4400 diagnostic disc injections. Neurosurgery 1995; 37:414–417.
13. Sachs BL, Vanharanta H, Spivey MA, et al. Dallas discogram description: A new classification of CT/discography in low-back disorders. Spine 1987; 12:287–298.
14. Fraser RD, Osti OL, Vernon-Roberts B. Iatrogenic discitis: The role of intravenous antibiotics in prevention and treatment. Spine 1989; 14:1025–1032.
15. Lang R, Saba K, Folman Y, et al. Penetration of ceftriaxone into the intervertebral disc. J Bone Joint Surg Am 1994; 76:689–691.
16. Fraser RD, Osti OL, Vernon-Roberts B. Discitis after discography. J Bone Joint Surg Br 1987; 69:26–35.
17. Zeidman SM, Thompson K, Ducker TB. Complications of cervical discography: Analysis of 4400 diagnostic disc injections. Neurosurgery 1995; 37:414–417.
18. Adams MA, Dolan P, Hutton WC. The stages of disc degeneration as revealed by discograms. J Bone Joint Surg Br 1986; 68:36–41.
19. Fenton DS, Czervionke LF. Discography. In Williams AL, Murtagh FR (eds). Handbook of Diagnostic and Therapeutic Spine Procedures. St. Louis: CV Mosby, 2002, pp 187–188.
20. CPT 2002, CPT Intellectual Property Services. Chicago: American Medical Association, 2002.

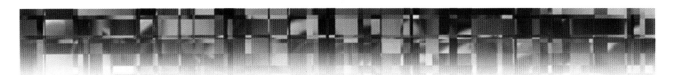

A Spine Surgeon's Perspective

Discography

Joseph T. Alexander, MD

Few areas in spinal medicine are as likely to cause controversy as the role of discography. Standard imaging techniques (other than flexion and extension radiographs) generate a static image of the spine, and it is generally recognized that these images do not provide "functional" information about the relationships of the spinal elements to the nerves during activity. Although not widely available, dynamic imaging in special open magnetic resonance (MR) imagers has demonstrated disc bulging and nerve compression when patients assume certain postures. Discography, on the other hand, can provide additional information, in certain cases, to link radiographic findings with clinical signs and symptoms. The patient's response to the injection of the disc can be qualitatively assessed in terms of the pain response as well as quantitatively evaluated in terms of the injection pressure. The internal disc morphology can be assessed after injection of contrast medium by plain radiographs or computed tomography, although the role of this additional information in the era of routine MR evaluation of the spine is in evolution. At least for surgeons, the debate over discography has centered on the value of a positive result in terms of predicting outcome after spinal fusion for axial pain.

In my practice, I typically use discography in only a small number of patients who have already failed to respond to conservative treatment, usually to evaluate patients for a specific treatment such as IntraDiscal ElectroThermal therapy (IDET) or in preoperative planning. I am more interested in the nature of the pain response than in the morphology of the disc. I believe that it is best if an independent proceduralist conducts the test, although this would be disputed by some who believe that only the surgeon/clinician, who knows the patient, can accurately assess the pain response. This test has been useful to help me sort out whether a disc with mild degenerative changes seen on MR at a level adjacent or noncontiguous to that of a planned fusion procedure is contributing to the patient's pain pattern. It can also be useful to exclude a mildly degenerated disc as the specific pain generator in selected cases in which there is concern for issues of secondary gain.

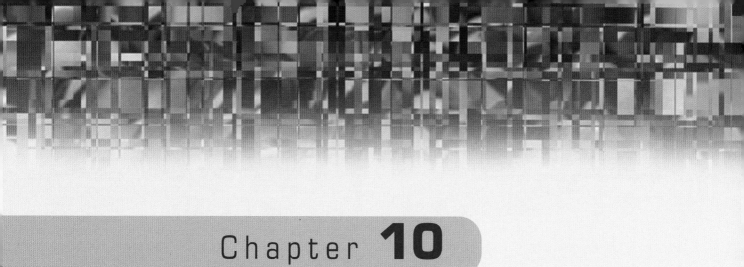

Chapter 10

IntraDiscal ElectroThermal Therapy (IDET™)

- Douglas S. Fenton, MD
- Leo F. Czervionke, MD

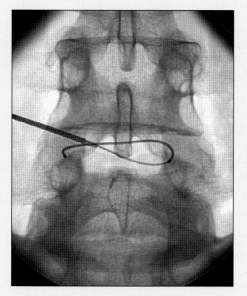

BACKGROUND

Low back pain cuts across all races, religions, and creeds. It strikes without regard to wealth or fame. It is estimated that 70% to 90% of all persons will experience low back pain at some time in their lives.[1, 2] Eighty to 90 percent will recover within about 3 months with physical therapy, medication, exercise, rest, and change in diet. However, some of these persons will go on to have chronic low back pain. In some of them, pain is caused by internal disc derangement. Until recently, it was not widely accepted that the intervertebral disc could be a pain generator.[3] However, several studies have demonstrated nerve fibers in the annulus fibrosis of the disc[4–6]; furthermore, there is ingrowth of new nerves into degenerated discs in persons with chronic back pain.[7] The exact cause of discogenic pain remains elusive. It is generally accepted that disc pain is not caused solely by mechanical stretching of the disc; there is evidence that other factors, including chemical mediators such as phospholipase A2 and prostaglandin E, also play a role.[8–10] Discogenic pain elicited with low-pressure discography may be caused by a chemically sensitive disc, and pain caused at higher pressures may be related to mechanoreceptive pain.

Treatment of "discogenic" back pain can be medical or surgical. The usual course of medical therapy for the patient with degenerative disc disease includes physical therapy, rest, narcotic and non-narcotic analgesia, pain injections, activity modification, and diet. When medical therapy fails, surgical treatment such as fusion is sometimes considered. In patients with chronic low back pain, many surgeons rely on discography to find the symptomatic disc levels and thus limit the length of the fusion.

A new and promising outpatient therapy has been introduced that may offer some of these patients an alternative to surgical fusion. This treatment is called IntraDiscal ElectroThermal therapy (IDET™). The theory of IDET™ is straightforward. If discogenic pain is caused by small nerves within the annulus fibrosis, destruction of these nerves should relieve the patient's pain. It has been demonstrated that permanent nerve blocks occur in the brain at a temperature at or above 45°C.[11] During the IDET™ procedure, radiofrequency energy is converted into heat in a thermal-resistive coil that is percutaneously placed into the disc with fluoroscopic guidance. The heating of the disc is performed in a controlled fashion. Heat is delivered at a specific temperature for a specific length of time to thermocoagulate the intradiscal nerves. Because the disc is a relatively avascular structure, heat is retained within it. If the catheter is placed properly, significant heating of the intraspinal, foraminal, or other paradiscal structures should not occur, because there exists a rich vascular plexus that acts as a heat sink and quickly removes heat from these areas. Heating of the disc also thermomodulates the disc collagen, breaking some of the heat-sensitive triple-helix bonds and causing the collagen to retract and thicken. The overall volume of the disc is said to decrease by approximately 10% after IDET™ therapy. Therefore, there may be some utility for IDET™ in treating patients who have compressive symptoms, owing to very small disc protrusions, although this is not recommended by the manufacturer. It has been postulated that the thickening of the collagen may enhance the structural integrity of the disc and possibly stabilize intradiscal fissures and decrease the chance of new nerve ingrowth, although no formal studies have been performed to prove or disprove this claim.[12]

The use of heat is not new in the treatment of the intervertebral disc. Laser thermal energy and radiofrequency-generated heat have also been attempted. Laser thermal energy is difficult to target and is not temperature controlled (temperatures achieved are around 250°C).[13] At this extreme temperature, the tissues are actually burned, and scar tissue and an intense inflammatory reaction will ensue.[13] Furthermore, lasers are expensive and require much technical expertise.[13]

Radiofrequency procedures, on the other hand, provide a well-controlled spherical lesion around an electrode tip. Although radiofrequency lesioning can provide temperatures sufficient to thermocoagulate nervous tissue, it is limited by the distance it can transmit heat. One cadaveric study demonstrated that intradiscal thermocoagulation from radiofrequency energy destroyed only a portion of the disc around the electrode probe.[14] Another study demonstrated that intradiscal radiofrequency therapy was unable to raise annular tissue to the temperature necessary to cause neuronal destruction.[15] Furthermore, the change in annular temperature 11 mm from the radiofrequency probe was only 1°C above baseline. Therefore, radiofrequency energy alone could not supply enough heat through the annulus fibrosis to destroy all the nerves. If the radiofrequency probe was in the annulus fibrosis, destruction would occur in that local region. One would have to make a radiofrequency probe with a tip long enough to be within and extend across the length of the posterior annular wall. This would likely be technically impossible. However, studies like these brought about the idea of having a temperature-controlled, thermal-resistive coil catheter that could be percutaneously placed and navigated throughout the nucleus pulposus so that the thermal element would lie along the posterior nucleus. Then, radiofrequency energy could be supplied to the catheter and be converted into thermal energy. By conduction, this heat would transfer throughout the annulus fibrosis at temperatures sufficient to thermocoagulate the nerves but below temperatures that would cause tissue burning, an inflammatory reaction, and scar formation.

No procedure is without potential complications. Strict adherence to technique, patient positioning, and selection is mandatory. There has been a reported case of cauda equina syndrome in a patient after IDET™,[16] and discitis always remains a potential complication with any invasive disc procedure. Although IDET™ may appear rather simple to perform, given the potential risks to the patient this procedure should be performed by physicians who have had significant training and experience with fluoroscopically guided procedures with respect to anatomy, patient positioning and monitoring, needle placement, and catheter manipulation.

PATIENT SELECTION

Persistent low back pain for at least 6 months
No definitive radicular component to the pain

- There can be some referred proximal lower extremity pain.
- No nerve root distribution weakness
- No evidence of reflex abnormality

History is consistent with discogenic back pain

- Back pain
- Cumulative loading intolerance (can stand for only a short period of time)
- Sitting intolerance (can sit for only a short period of time)
- ± vague/mild radicular-like symptoms
- Equivocal positive straight-leg raise (low back pain without leg pain)

Patient has failed at least 3 months of aggressive nonoperative therapy such as:

- Medications (nonsteroidal anti-inflammatory drugs, nonnarcotic analgesics, narcotic analgesics, neural-stabilizing medications)
- Injection therapies such as epidural and facet injections
- Activity modification and physical therapy

Imaging within the past 6 months has consisted of standing neutral, flexion, and extension radiographs of the lumbar spine to evaluate for segmental instability and high-quality magnetic resonance (MR) imaging or computed tomography (CT) if contraindication to MR imaging demonstrating:

- At least 40% to 50% of disc height remains.
- Detecting an annular tear (bright T2-weighted signal in

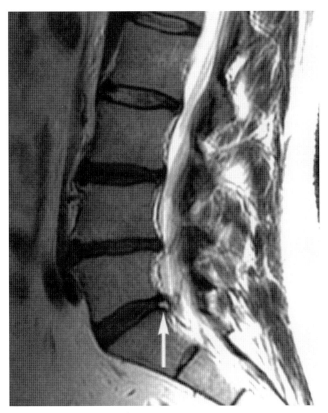

Figure 10-1 ■ Sagittal T2-weighted fast spin echo MR image. The small focus of increased signal intensity ("high intensity zone") in the posterior annulus of the L5-S1 disc (*arrow*) is compatible with an annular tear.

posterior annulus, also called "high-intensity zone") (Fig. 10-1)
- No significant compressive lesion
- No significant central canal, neural foraminal, or lateral recess stenosis at the symptomatic level
- Small, contained disc herniations may still remain a candidate

Other selection criteria include:

- Concordant pain during discography involving 1 or more discs
- When surgical fusion is the only other therapeutic alternative
- Complete history and physical examination within 30 days of the procedure
- Motivated patient with realistic expectations

Within our institution, physicians from the departments of neuroradiology, neurosurgery, pain management, and physical medicine and rehabilitation evaluate each candidate. Each specialist must conclude that the patient is a candidate for IDET™.

CONTRAINDICATIONS

- Coagulopathy (International Normalized Ratio [INR] >1.5 or platelets <50,000/mm^3)
- Severe radicular symptoms

- Previous disc surgery at the suspect level (relative contraindication)
- Imaging studies suggestive of nondiscogenic pathology. This may include a compressive pathologic process caused by central canal, foraminal, or lateral recess stenosis or by disc herniation (a patient with a small, subligamentous disc herniation or protrusion can usually receive IDET™ therapy); segmental instability (need to evaluate with lateral neutral, flexion and extension radiographs of the lumbar spine); and severe loss of disc height (<40% to 50% of disc height remaining). The less the disc height, the more difficult it becomes to successfully navigate the thermal catheter into proper position.
- Psychologic impairment that may interfere with the patient's ability to follow post-procedure rehabilitation instructions
- Inflammatory arthritides
- Pregnancy (to prevent fetal radiation exposure)
- Infection (either systemic or local involving the skin of the puncture site or sites)
- An extensive, solid posterior bone fusion, which may not allow percutaneous disc access
- A "high" iliac crest, which may not allow percutaneous access to the L5-S1 disc level (although, if necessary, a surgical defect can be made in the crest to gain access to an otherwise inaccessible L5-S1 disc)

PROCEDURE

Equipment/Supplies

Procedural

Generator (ORA-50S™), foot pedal, and generator power cord
SpineCATH™ Intradiscal Catheter (2 available for each disc level to be treated)
Smith & Nephew Introducer Needle, 17-gauge, 6-inch (15 cm) (2 available for each disc level to be treated)
Smith & Nephew sterile connecting cable
SpineCATH™ XL Intradiscal Catheter with corresponding 17-gauge, 9-inch (23 cm) Introducer Needle XL available for larger patients
Styleted spinal needles, 22-gauge, 6-inch, for deep local anesthesia (Monoject Special Technique Needle With Stylet, Diamond Point, Sherwood Medical, St. Louis, MO)
Luer-lock syringe, 3 mL (1 for each disc level)
Control syringe, 12 mL with 25-gauge, 1.5-inch needle containing 9.5 mL 1% lidocaine for local anesthesia and 0.5 mL 8.4% sodium bicarbonate injectable (1 mEq/mL) to alleviate burning pain associated with anesthetic
Luer-lock syringe, 3 mL, containing 3 mL of antibiotic (1 mL for each disc level)
Povidone-iodine (Betadine) scrub
Alcohol scrub
Sterile drapes
Sterile gauze
Adhesive bandages
Hats, masks, sterile gloves and gowns, lead apron

Medications

Lidocaine-MPF 1% (Xylocaine-MPF 1%, AstraZeneca LP, Wilmington, DE)

Cefazolin (Ancef, SmithKline Beecham, Philadelphia, PA), 1 g intravenously within 1 hour before procedure

Cefazolin (Ancef), 10 mg/5 mL normal saline

Clindamycin (Cleocin Phosphate, Pharmacia & Upjohn, Peapack, NJ), 600 mg intravenously if patient is allergic to cephalosporin or penicillin

Clindamycin, 6 mg/5 mL normal saline if patient is allergic to cephalosporin or penicillin

Precautions

Preservative-free medications should be used:

- MPF means methylparaben free.
- The MPF form is preferable for use in spine intervention procedures because steroid is often given at the same time.
- Many steroid suspensions, when mixed with certain preservatives (e.g., paraben, phenol), may cause flocculation of the steroid.[17]
- Some preservatives, if they are inadvertently injected intrathecally, have been implicated as causing arachnoiditis.

Discitis is a known complication of discography and should be prevented.

- It is recommended that an antibiotic be given to decrease the risk of infection.
- One gram of intravenous cefazolin (Ancef) is given routinely within 1 hour of the procedure.
- Two milligrams of cefazolin is injected into each disc through the introducer needle after IDET therapy. If a bilateral approach is performed, only the last needle placed into **each** disc is injected with antibiotic.
- If the patient has a known cephalosporin or penicillin allergy, 600 mg of clindamycin can be given intravenously with 0.6 mg (6 mg/5 mL) added to each disc injection syringe.

All medications used should not contain epinephrine, because vasocontrictive properties are neither needed nor desired because of the risk of vasospasm.

Methodology

IDET is usually performed as an outpatient procedure. Patients are instructed to have a driver with them after the procedure as well as someone who can be responsible for their well-being for the remainder of the day because sedation is usually given during the examination. Discography is always performed at least 2 weeks or more before IDET to identify the disc level or levels to be treated. A post-discogram CT is important to identify the precise location of the annular fissures for planning optimal IDET catheter placement. Annular tears are quite often posterior or posterolateral, although symptomatic tears can occur laterally and rarely even anteriorly. The IDET procedure should not be performed at the same time as the diagnostic discogram. The fluid injected into the disc during discography will act

as a heat sink during IDET; therefore, sufficient heating to the outer annulus may not be achieved, and, as a result, the outcome may be suboptimal. We prefer to wait approximately 2 weeks between the diagnostic discogram and IDET. This waiting period is usually not a problem because precertification for IDET can take 3 to 4 weeks.

Checking the Generator

There are two types of generators. The newer-generation model has the AutoTemp™ mode, and the older model does not. The on/off switch on the back of the generator turns on the generator. The thumbwheel on the back of the generator is set to 2. The mode button is pressed once for AutoTemp mode or twice for Temperature Control mode. In the AutoTemp mode, the Set Power indicator should read P90 and the Set Temperature and Preset indicators should show dashes.[12]

With the older model of generator or when one is not using the AutoTemp mode, the Temperature Control mode is used. The starting Set Temperature should read 65°C, and the Set Power should be 5 watts. The Preset Selector thumbwheel on the back of the generator is at setting 2, and the Preset display on the front of the generator will show 002.[12]

For more information about the generator and how to use the various modes, we suggest that the physician attend a formal IDET course and/or contact a vendor.

Checking the Thermal Catheter

Each thermal catheter should be inspected and tested before its use. A sterile thermal catheter is placed on the sterile working table. A connecting cable is used to attach the catheter to the generator to test the catheter's proper functioning before it is placed in the patient. A white mark on the connecting cable should align with the white mark on the thermal catheter hub for proper connection. A click is heard when the connections to the catheter are properly made. The catheter, when attached to the generator outside the patient's body, should read room temperature. Also, the impedance reading **must** be in the range of 120 to 200 ohms before and during the procedure. If it is not, another catheter must be used and/or the connections and generator should be checked. **Each thermal catheter should be heated only once.** The catheter is then detached from the connecting cable and placed back on the sterile working table.[12]

Patient Positioning and Other Considerations

The IDET procedure is performed in a fashion similar to that for discography. Informed consent is obtained. The patient is placed prone on the fluoroscopy table. Unlike the positioning for discography, the patient is placed flat prone on the table. Ideally, the IDET procedure is performed from a unilateral approach. However, to achieve adequate catheter coverage over the entire posterolateral annulus, it may be necessary to perform bilateral disc punctures. Therefore, if one side is up, it becomes difficult not only to keep the contralateral side sterile but also to perform a contralateral skin puncture. We opt to keep the patient flat prone throughout the entire therapy. In addition, a pillow or sponge is placed

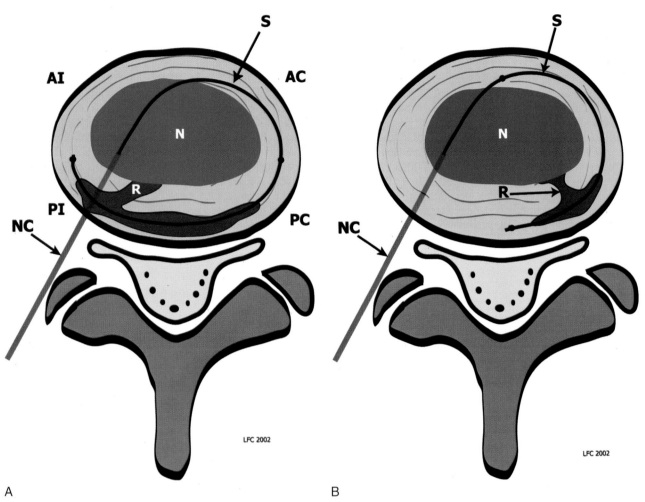

A   B

Figure 10-2 ■ *A,* Ipsilateral catheter placement. The needle cannula (NC) enters the posterolateral disc (PI) ipsilateral to the radial tear (R). The thermal catheter (S) courses through the nucleus (N) anteriorly toward the contralateral side (AC), then turns posteriorly (PC), and finally crosses the posterior nucleus back to the posterior ipsilateral disc. The heating portion of the catheter is demarcated by the small black balls on the catheter extending from the 3 o'clock to the 9 o'clock position of the disc. AI = anterior ipsilateral disc. *B,* Contralateral catheter placement. The needle cannula (NC) enters the posterolateral disc contralateral to the radial tear (R). The thermal catheter (S) courses through the nucleus (N) anteriorly toward the contralateral side, turns posteriorly, crosses the radial tear, and terminates in the posterior midline. The heating portion of the catheter is demarcated by the small black balls on the catheter extending from the 12 o'clock to the 6 o'clock position of the disc.

symmetrically under the patient's lower abdomen/upper pelvis. This not only facilitates lower lumbar disc puncture but, by decreasing lumbar lordosis, also facilitates navigation of the catheter in the posterior annulus.

The patient's lower back is prepared and draped in a sterile fashion. Monitored anesthetic care is suggested, with the patient monitored by electrocardiography, pulse oximetry, and blood pressure readings. Anesthesia is usually limited to a mild sedative and analgesic (midazolam, 1 to 3 mg; fentanyl, 100 to 200 μg). **It is extremely important that the patient not be sedated to the point that he or she is not able to fully understand questions or feel pain. When the heating protocol begins, the patient's pain response is the earliest warning that the catheter may not be in a satisfactory position.**

Three basic conditions determine how much of the annulus needs to be treated:

1. In patients with central or bilateral back pain, the entire posterior annulus needs to be treated.
2. In patients with unilateral back pain and an annular tear only on the side of the back pain, only the annulus on that side needs to be treated.
3. In patients with unilateral back pain with annular tears on both sides of the disc, we recommend treating both sides of the annulus.

Proper positioning is the key to a successful IDET procedure. In the case of central or bilateral back pain and in patients with unilateral back pain with bilateral disc tears, our initial, and perhaps only, disc puncture is usually performed on the patient's more affected side. This approach is used because the patient's pain often lateralizes to the side of the radial tear and it is easier for the catheter to cross the tear from an approach at an acute angle to the tear, although many times a contralateral puncture also allows adequate catheter placement. This will be discussed in more detail later in the chapter. The navigable catheter enters the nucleus pulposus and is directed toward the contralateral anterior aspect of the nucleus (Fig. 10-2A). The catheter is then navigated to the posterior annulus on the contralateral side and is turned across the posterior annulus back toward the side of entry (see Fig. 10-2*A*). Ideally, the heating portion of the thermal catheter lies across the posterior annulus from the 3 o'clock to the 9 o'clock position (see Fig. 10-2*A*). If the catheter is not navigated into this position, a contralateral puncture may have to be performed to cover that portion of the annular fissure not adequately treated. If one is absolutely certain that the annular tear has been crossed, a unilateral approach may be all that is necessary. In the case of a patient with unilateral back pain, a concordant discogram, and a tear ipsilateral to the back pain, a contralateral approach can be taken and the catheter need only be positioned with its tip to the midline of the posterior annulus (see Fig. 10-2*B*). Regardless of the situation, the opposite approach should be used to place the catheter if the catheter cannot be successfully navigated across the annular tear with the initial approach.

C-Arm Positioning

Fluoroscopic positioning is nearly identical to that used in discography, with very minor differences. The introducer needle is positioned slightly lateral to midline, ipsilateral to the needle approach, in the anteroposterior (AP) plane and slightly in the mid to anterior aspect of the disc on the lateral plane. In this position, there is enough room for the thermal catheter to be maneuvered inside the nucleus. The actual working position of the introducer needle should be decided on before the procedure. The pre-IDET™ discogram and

post-discogram CT provide valuable information about the size and shape of the nucleus pulposus and the location and direction of annular tears. From the pre-procedure discogram, one can see the boundaries of the nucleus pulposus. We use the vertebral pedicles as our landmarks for the AP plane (Fig. 10-3). The pre-IDET™ discogram and CT are also used to demarcate the posterior aspect of the nucleus (Fig. 10-4*A* and *B*) and annulus (see Fig. 10-4*C* through *E*) in relation to bone landmarks. We find this method extremely valuable because with posterior disc protrusions it is difficult to assess whether the catheter is in the posterior annulus of the disc or in the ventral epidural space. Lastly, the pre-IDET™ CT demonstrates the entire extent of the tear including both radial and concentric components. The authors believe that the concentric portions of the tear, even anteriorly, are pathologic and should be treated in addition to the radial portion (e.g., grade 4 tears).

L1-2 THROUGH L4-5

The C-arm (image intensifier above the patient) is rotated in an ipsilateral oblique angle with respect to the side of puncture. The C-arm is rotated until the ventral aspect of the superior articulating process (ear of the "Scotty dog"), which has the same number as the inferior vertebrae of the disc space to be injected, is 35% to 40% of the distance from the anterior aspect of the vertebral body. For optimal needle placement, the superior end plates of the same vertebral body should superimpose (Fig. 10-5).

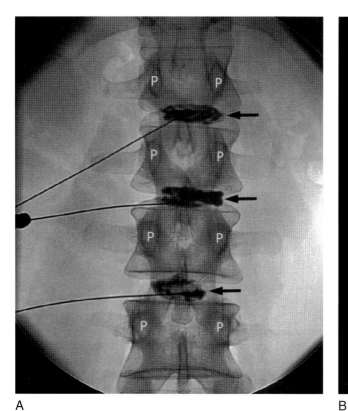

A

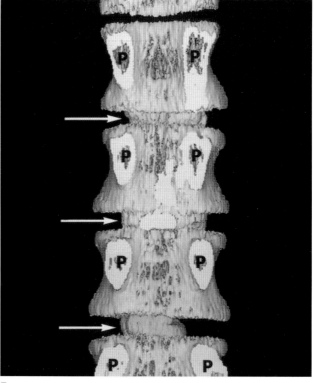

B

Figure 10-3 ■ AP discography radiograph (*A*) and three-dimensional CT surface rendering with posterior elements electronically removed (*B*). Contrast medium is seen within the nuclei of the L1-2, L2-3, and L3-4 discs (*black arrows, A; white arrows, B*). The lateral extent of each nucleus is visualized in relation to the pedicles (P).

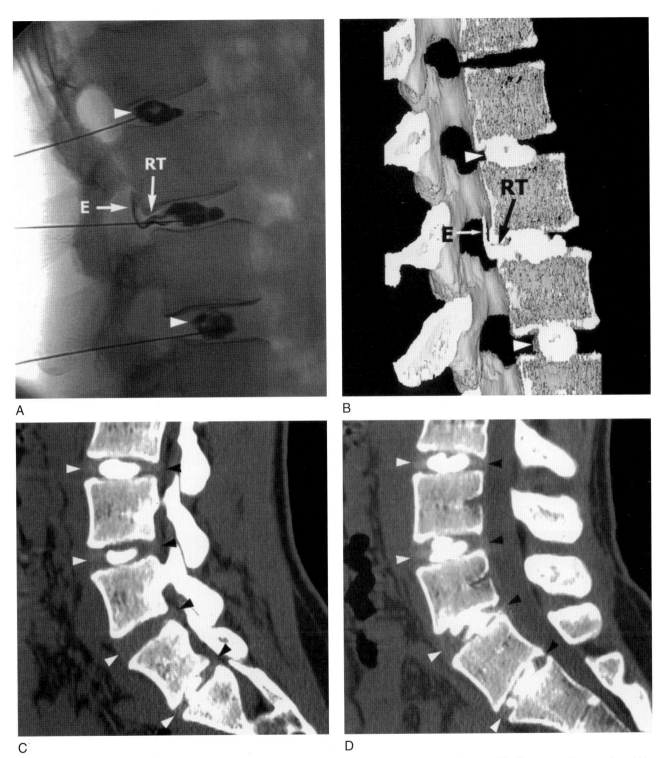

Figure 10-4 ■ Lateral radiograph (*A*) and sagittal three-dimensional CT, midline slice, three-level discogram (*B*). Contrast medium remains within the central disc contained by the posterior nucleus (*arrowheads*) in the superior and inferior disc levels. It extends through a radial tear (RT) with epidural extension (E) superiorly. Left paramidline (*C*), central (*D*).

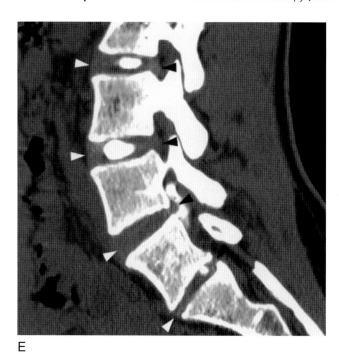

E

Figure 10-4 (*Cont'd*) ■ Right paramidline (*E*) three-dimensional sagittal reconstructed images demonstrate the anterior (*white arrowheads*) and posterior (*black arrowheads*) boundaries of the disc (outer annulus fibrosis).

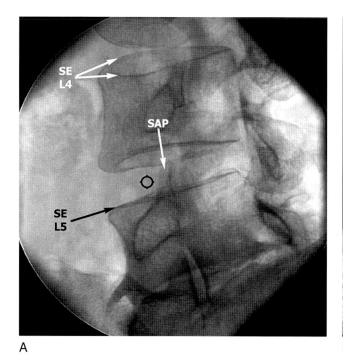

A

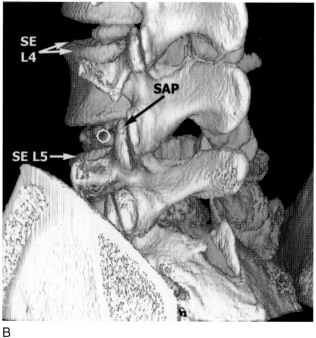

B

Figure 10-5 ■ Proper positioning for L4-5 IDET, left-sided approach. RAO radiograph (*A*) and three-dimensional CT image (*B*). The left superior articular process of L5 (SAP) is positioned 35% to 40% from the anterior aspect of the L5 vertebral body. Anterior and posterior aspects of the L5 superior end plate (SE L5) superimpose. The needle puncture should be just ventral to the L5 superior articular process (*black target*, A; *white target*, B). Note that the anterior and posterior superior end plates of L4 (SE L4) are not superimposed.

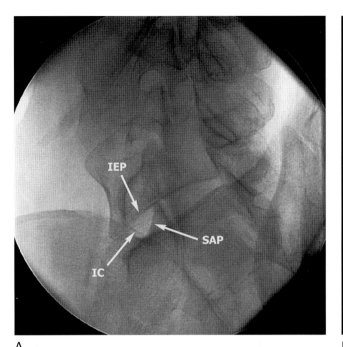

A

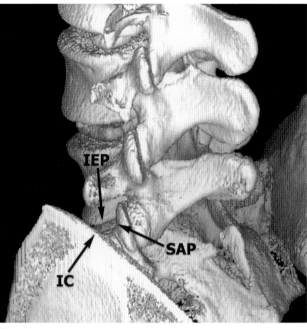

B

Figure 10-6 ■ Proper positioning for L5-S1 IDET, left-sided approach. RAO radiograph (*A*) and three-dimensional CT image (*B*). The left superior articular process of S1 (SAP) is positioned 35% to 40% from the anterior aspect of the S1 segment. The anterior and posterior aspects of the S1 superior end plate superimpose. The needle puncture target is a triangle formed by the left S1 superior articular process, iliac crest (IC), and left L5 inferior end plate (IEP).

L5-S1

The L5-S1 level can be highly challenging because of a patient's anatomy. For needle insertion into the L5-S1 level, significant caudal beam angulation (image intensifier above the patient, obliqued toward the patient's head) may be required for optimal visualization. The C-arm is rotated in a fashion that is similar to that for the upper lumbar discs. Many times, the area through which one has to pass the needle through appears at fluoroscopy as a small upside-down triangle formed by the inferior end plate of L5, the superior articulating process of S1, and the iliac crest (Fig. 10-6). However, the iliac crest may obstruct one's approach (Fig. 10-7*A*). If one is unable to achieve a position that places the superior articular process 35% to 40% across the vertebral body, one obtains the best possible angle that allows visualization of the upside-down triangle but still allows intranuclear placement of the introducer needle (see Fig. 10-7*B*). Despite this C-arm angulation, the iliac crest may still prove to be an obstacle to optimal needle placement. Sometimes, the L5-S1 disc can be entered by using a somewhat steeper approach. However, if too steep an approach is taken, the needle may not enter the nucleus and remain within the annulus. One possible solution may be to slightly bend the distal aspect of the introducer needle by placing the styleted introducer needle a few millimeters into the small opening of a plastic syringe and bending it 5 to 10 degrees. If these maneuvers are unsuccessful, we find that if the patient brings his or her knee (the one contralateral to the side of puncture) up toward the chest, the iliac crest on the side of the puncture moves slightly inferiorly, which might be just enough to allow safe passage of the introducer

needle. If all these methods fail, a decision has to be made whether to abandon the procedure or to make a small surgical window in the iliac crest with a nonthreaded drill bit or bone biopsy needle. The bit or needle must be larger than the outer diameter of the introducer needle. Of course, only experienced persons should perform this maneuver. If it is to be performed, the L5-S1 disc should be positioned as if the iliac crest did not obstruct access and the drill bit or biopsy needle should be placed along the path that allows for optimal disc access. Once the bit or needle contacts the iliac crest, a surgical defect is made in the iliac crest. If a drill bit is used, it is removed and the introducer needle is placed through the trephine and into the disc. If a bone biopsy needle is used, before its removal a guidewire can be placed through the bone biopsy needle and trephine. The needle is removed and the wire is left in place. The stylet of the introducer needle is removed, and the introducer needle is advanced over the wire through the trephine. Once it is through, the wire is removed and the needle is re-styleted before the disc is entered.

Introducer Needle and Insertion

As of the writing of this chapter, there were two types of introducer needles. The original needle had a bevel/scoop distally to aid in controlling the direction the catheter enters the nucleus. This needle has been phased out because of the potential of shearing the thermal catheter on withdrawal. The most recent introducer needle, Gen II, is a two-piece needle with a 17-gauge, 6-inch cannula and a diamond-point stylet. The stylet and cannula are connected by a clockwise

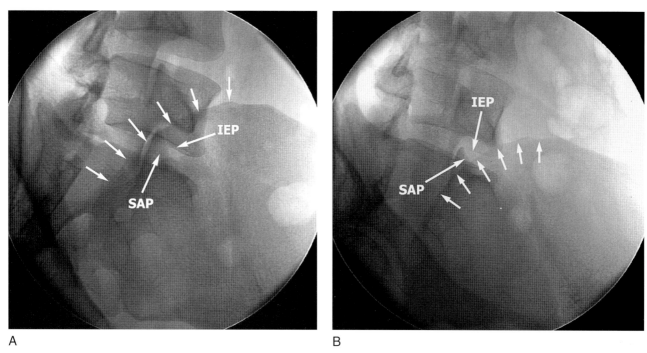

A   B

Figure 10-7 ■ *A,* Obstructed approach to L5-S1 IDET, right-sided approach. With proper S1 vertebral positioning, the iliac crest (*arrows*) obstructs entrance into the disc. *B,* In the same patient, more caudocranial x-ray beam angulation allows the iliac crest (*arrows*) to drop, opening the target. Note that the target is not optimal because the superior end plate of S1 does not superimpose. SAP = right S1 superior articular process; IEP = right L5 inferior end plate.

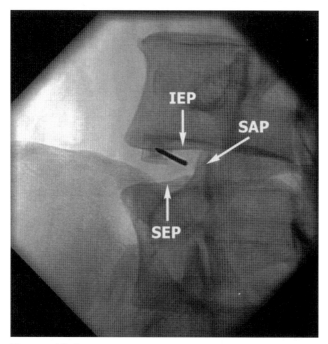

Figure 10-8 ■ RAO radiograph during L4-5 IDET, left-sided approach. The needle tip is just ventral to the left L5 superior articular process (SAP). IEP = left L4 inferior end plate; SEP = left L5 superior end plate.

turn. It is recommended that a small skin incision be made to aid in the insertion of the new introducer needle.

Local anesthesia is given along the path of the puncture. The introducer needle is then inserted parallel to the x-ray beam and advanced, using intermittent fluoroscopy, so that the needle tip remains just ventral to the superior articulating process and midway between the vertebral end plates (Fig. 10-8). Similar to discography, if this course is strictly followed, the chance of contacting the exiting nerve root or other vital structure is virtually eliminated. The introducer needle will enter the posterolateral margin of the disc. The patient often describes a brief sharp pain as the needle contacts and courses through the outer annular fibers. The annular fibers have a firm gritty feel. As the needle passes into the nucleus pulposus, one experiences a decrease in resistance to needle penetration. The introducer needle is advanced until it comes to rest in the middle third of the disc in the lateral plane, and at the junction of the lateral and middle thirds of the disc ipsilateral to the needle puncture in the AP plane (Fig. 10-9).

Thermal Catheter and Placement

The SpineCATH wire is 30 cm long. It has a gray plastic hub to facilitate catheter advancement and rotation and a slightly angled distal tip to aid in controlling direction (Fig.

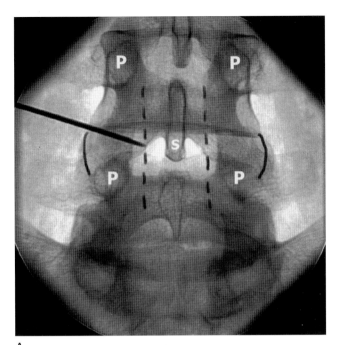

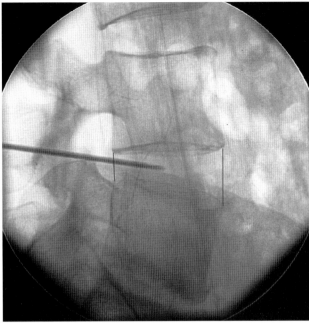

A   B

Figure 10-9 ■ AP (*A*) and lateral (*B*) radiographs with introducer needle positioned. The needle is at the junction of the ipsilateral lateral and middle thirds of the disc in the AP plane and within the middle third of the disc in the lateral plane. P = pedicle; S = spinous process. *Lines* demarcate the anterior, posterior, and lateral extents of the annulus.

10-10*A*). There are 12 external hash marks on the proximal aspect of the thermal catheter, each separated by 1 cm, 2 of which are thicker than the others (see Fig. 10-10*B*). The first thick mark is the distalmost one, and the other is 5 cm proximal. There are also two radiopaque markers, separated by approximately 5.5 cm, on the distal aspect of the thermal catheter, which are the boundaries of the heating element (see Fig. 10-10*C*). When the distalmost external mark enters a few millimeters into the needle hub (Fig. 10-11*A*), the distal radiopaque marker has exited the introducer needle and has entered the nucleus (see Fig. 10-11*B*). The proximal radiopaque marker does not exit the needle when the proximal external hash mark enters the needle hub, because there is a 5-mm discrepancy between distal and proximal external hash marks and distal and proximal radiopaque marks. The proximal external mark must be advanced farther into the hub (see Fig. 10-11*C*) to allow the proximal radiopaque mark to exit the needle tip (see Fig. 10-11*D*). However, one should not use the external markings on the catheter to decide whether heating can commence. **The catheter should not be heated unless both radiopaque distal markers have exited the needle, which should be confirmed fluoroscopically.**

The stylet is removed from the introducer needle. The thermal catheter is then inserted through the introducer needle. Using lateral fluoroscopy, the catheter is visualized entering the nucleus pulposus and coursing anteriorly (Fig. 10-12*A*). The catheter is viewed crossing the anterior midline to the contralateral anterior corner of the disc (see Fig. 10-12*B*). The catheter is then manipulated until it courses posteriorly. Fluoroscopy is switched back to the lateral plane, and the catheter is followed until it begins to bend at the contralateral posterior corner of the disc (see Fig. 10-12*C*). Fluoroscopy is once again changed to the AP plane, and the catheter is viewed coursing across the posterior aspect of the nucleus pulposus across the midline and back to the ipsilateral posterolateral disc margin (see Fig. 10-12*D*). The catheter is then viewed in both AP and lateral planes to ensure that it has remained within the confines of the disc, which was predetermined on the pre-IDET discogram (see Fig. 10-12*D* and *E*). The heating element should also be observed in various views to ensure that no part of the heating element is in contact with the introducer needle, because heat could be transmitted down the needle (Fig. 10-13). If there is contact between the heating element and the introducer needle, the needle should be withdrawn until contact is no longer made. Once the proper catheter position is achieved, the heating protocol can begin.

Heating Protocol

The thermal catheter is connected to the generator once again. The actual temperature before the heating protocol should register body temperature. Delivery of thermal energy commences when the generator's RF power button is

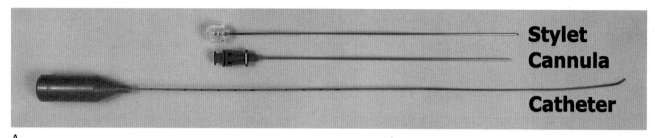

A

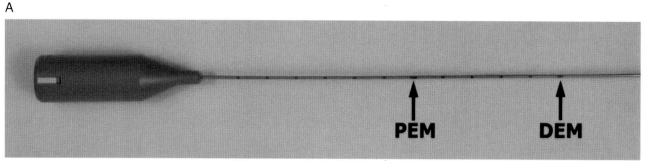

B

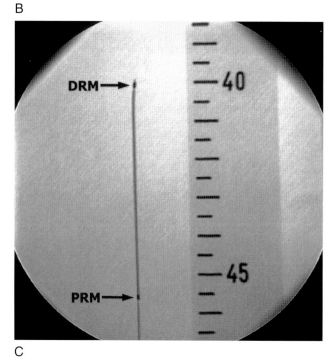

C

Figure 10-10 ■ *A*, IDET spinal system: SpineCATH catheter, with gray hub, 12 external 1-cm markers, slightly bent distal tip for navigation, and 17-gauge cannula and stylet. *B*, SpineCATH proximal shaft. Note the 12 external hash marks, each separated by 1 cm. Two hash marks, the proximal external mark (PEM) and the distal external mark (DEM), are thicker and are separated by 5 cm. *C*, Radiograph, SpineCATH distal shaft. The thermal portion of the catheter is bound by the distal radiopaque mark (DRM) and the proximal radiopaque mark (PRM), which are separated by 6 cm. (IDET™ system photographed with permission of Smith & Nephew, Menlo Park, CA.)

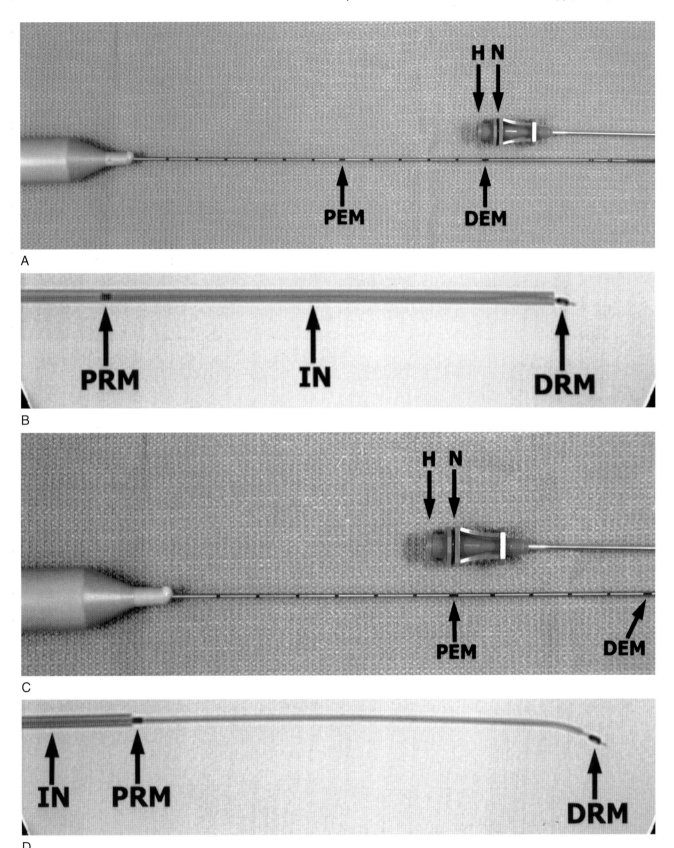

Figure 10-11 ▪ Photograph of proximal portions (*A*) and radiograph of distal portions (*B*) of SpineCATH and introducer needle. When the distal external mark (DEM) of the catheter enters the needle hub opening (H) a few millimeters, the distal radiopaque mark (DRM) exits the introducer needle (IN). N = notch on needle hub; PEM = proximal external mark; PRM = proximal radiopaque mark. Photograph of proximal portions (*C*) and radiograph of distal portions (*D*) of SpineCATH and introducer needle. When the proximal external mark (PEM) of the catheter is within the needle hub at approximately the level of the notch (N), the proximal radiopaque mark (PRM) exits the introducer needle (IN). H = needle hub opening; DEM = distal external mark; DRM = distal radiopaque mark. (IDET™ system photographed with permission of Smith & Nephew, Menlo Park, CA.)

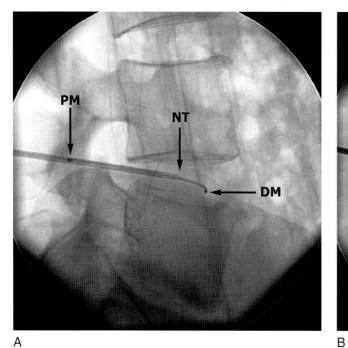

A

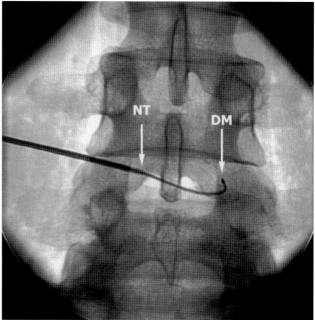

B

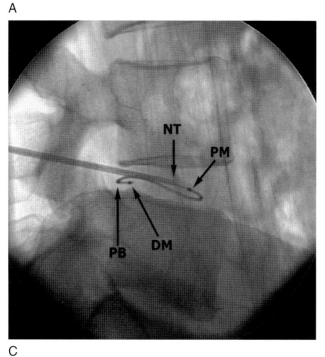

C

Figure 10-12 ■ *A*, Lateral fluoroscopy during L4-5 IDET. Introducer needle is seen with the needle tip (NT) in the center of the disc. The distal marker on the SpineCATH (DM) has exited the needle tip. The proximal marker (PM) remains within the needle shaft. *B*, Anterior view demonstrates the SpineCATH thermal catheter crossing the anterior midline. The catheter begins to bend posteriorly at the contralateral anterior corner of the nucleus. The proximal marker remains within the needle. *C*, Lateral fluoroscopy. The SpineCATH has been advanced and has navigated across the posterior nucleus. Note that the proximal marker has exited the needle tip. PB = posterior bend of SpineCATH.

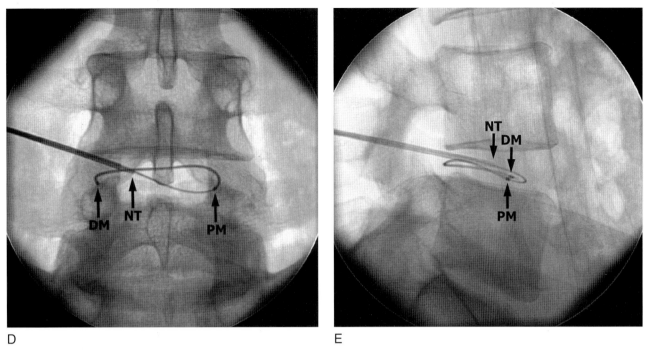

D   E

Figure 10-12 (*Cont'd*) ■ *D*, Final AP position. The SpineCATH has successfully navigated across the posterior midline back to the ipsilateral posterolateral corner and within the lateral confines of the disc. The distal and proximal markers have exited the needle tip. *E*, Final lateral position. The anterior bend of the catheter is within the disc confines. The posterior bend of the catheter is slightly posterior to the vertebral margin but is within the disc when compared with the pre-procedure discogram.

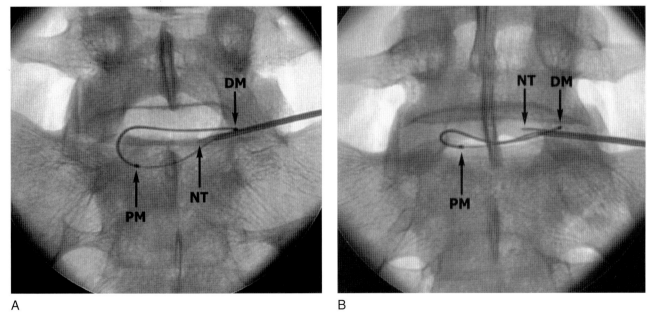

A   B

Figure 10-13 ■ *A*, AP radiograph with caudocranial x-ray beam angulation. The proximal marker (PM) and the distal marker (DM) have exited the needle tip (NT). There is questionable contact of the distal catheter with the needle. *B*, AP radiograph with craniocaudal x-ray beam angulation. The distal marker is projected off the needle and is therefore not in contact with it.

pressed. The generator will emit a tone, and a blue light will light on the front panel of the generator as the thermal energy is delivered. The standard heating protocol (P90) takes the catheter from a temperature of 65°C to 90°C over 12.5 minutes, increasing by 1° increments every 30 seconds. The catheter then remains at 90°C for an additional 4 minutes. The newer generators perform this function automatically.

During the beginning of the heating protocol, when the patient is the most lightly sedated, he or she is monitored for any signs of paresthesia, neuritis, or any other symptom that may suggest that the heating element of the catheter is not in the optimal position. If the patient has any unusual discomfort or signs of pain different from his or her typical pain, the heating protocol should be paused or discontinued. It is not unusual for the patient to experience his or her typical pain. Heat delivery can be paused by pressing the foot pedal or RF power button once. The catheter may then need to be placed more anteriorly within the nucleus, or a different pathway through the nucleus may have to be sought (Fig. 10-14). If during the first 10° of the heating protocol the patient does not have any symptoms aside from his or her typical pain, additional sedation can be given if needed.

Once the heating protocol has been completed, the generator will shut off. The thermal catheter should be removed slowly with minimal back-and-forth rotational movement, using fluoroscopy to ensure that the catheter remains intact. If a one-sided approach is all that is necessary, 2 mg of cefazolin is instilled through the introducer needle into the disc before needle removal. If a two-sided disc approach is necessary, the cefazolin is not instilled until after the contralateral needle puncture, because additional fluid in the disc may decrease the amount of thermal heat dissipated throughout the disc during the heating protocol. If there is any difficulty with catheter removal, the needle should be withdrawn a few millimeters and then catheter removal should again be attempted. If there is still resistance, the catheter **and** the introducer needle should be removed together as a single unit. If this was to occur and the procedure was a one-sided approach, a 22-gauge, 6-inch spinal needle should be inserted into the disc to deliver the antibiotic.

Additional Methodology

Proper Catheter Positioning

Navigating the thermal catheter across the entire posterior annulus is of utmost importance. We will describe several different methods that have helped us achieve this goal.

We find quite often that the thermal catheter navigates smoothly to the contralateral anterior annulus and usually turns smoothly to the contralateral posterior annulus. The point where the catheter needs to turn from the contralateral posterior annulus toward midline is usually the most difficult, and most crucial, part of the technique. In this regard, we find that any method that decreases the patient's lumbar lordosis serves to decrease pressure on the posterior annulus and thus provides more space in the posterior annulus, which facilitates catheter advancement. For each patient, a pillow or cushion is placed under the lower abdomen/upper pelvis to decrease lumbar lordosis.

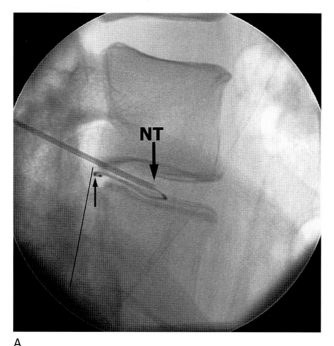
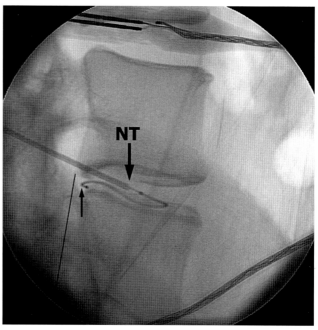

A   B

Figure 10-14 ■ *A*, Lateral radiograph demonstrates that the posterior aspect of the SpineCATH (*arrow*) is in close contact with a line connecting the posteroinferior aspect of the vertebral bodies above and below the disc level. The needle tip (NT) projects over the middle of the disc. *B*, The needle tip is repositioned more posteriorly, and the posterior aspect of the SpineCATH is positioned more ventrally.

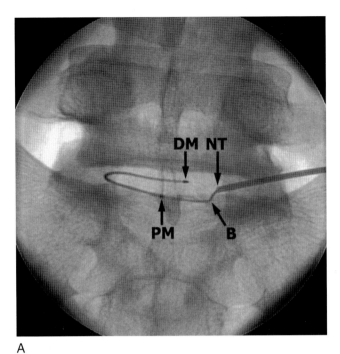

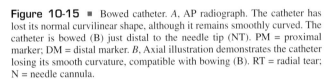

A

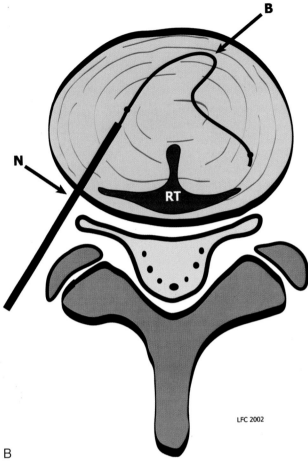

B

Figure 10-15 ▪ Bowed catheter. *A*, AP radiograph. The catheter has lost its normal curvilinear shape, although it remains smoothly curved. The catheter is bowed (B) just distal to the needle tip (NT). PM = proximal marker; DM = distal marker. *B*, Axial illustration demonstrates the catheter losing its smooth curvature, compatible with bowing (B). RT = radial tear; N = needle cannula.

It is important to use frequent, intermittent fluoroscopy during any catheter manipulation. Often during each attempt at passing the catheter, it enters and reenters the same pathway. Using fluoroscopy, one can see where the catheter enters into the same position. The catheter can then be withdrawn to that position and turned slightly to take a different pathway, which may be more successful. Also, frequent fluoroscopy can virtually eliminate the catheter's kinking, exiting the disc, and entering the spinal canal, neural foramen, or other paradiscal structures.

Often the catheter advances smoothly. However, if resistance is met, the catheter **should not be forced**. Again, it is of utmost importance that one not cause injury to the patient. If one cannot safely perform the procedure, it should be abandoned. The thermal catheter, like any other catheter, can bow (Fig. 10-15), kink (Fig. 10-16), or even break if too much force is applied. If resistance is met, withdrawing the catheter somewhat and re-advancing it, possibly with the catheter tip at a slightly different orientation, becomes necessary. Sometimes it is necessary to withdraw the catheter entirely within the introducer needle and start the catheter on a different pathway. A different pathway can be achieved by several different methods. The introducer needle can be left in place and the catheter can be turned various degrees as it exits the needle tip. The introducer needle can also be

advanced or withdrawn slightly within the nucleus so that the catheter takes a different pathway.

If there is resistance to catheter advancement, one should always check for catheter bowing or kinking in two planes. The catheter can also be viewed in the AP plane with steep cranial or caudal angulation of the C-arm to visualize the entire length of the catheter (Fig. 10-17). If the catheter is bowed or kinked but is in position for heating, then heating should commence. One must be sure that the impedance and catheter temperatures are within normal operating levels. If the operating levels are not normal, or if the catheter is not in proper heating position, the catheter should be withdrawn. **It is very important that continuous fluoroscopy be used during withdrawal of a kinked or bowed catheter to ensure that stretching or breaking of the catheter does not occur.** If there is any resistance to withdrawing the bowed or kinked catheter, one should proceed as follows. The introducer needle should be withdrawn a few millimeters, keeping the needle within the nucleus, and then one can gently attempt to withdraw the catheter. If there is still resistance to catheter withdrawal, the catheter **and** the introducer needle should be removed as a single unit. A catheter that was bowed can be reinserted; however, a catheter that was kinked should be discarded. **Note that if a decision is made to abandon electrothermal therapy**

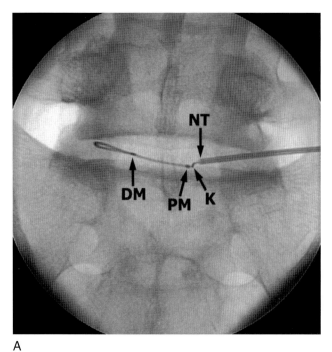

A

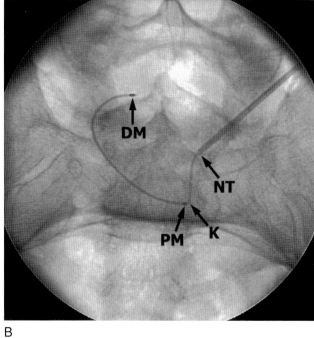

B

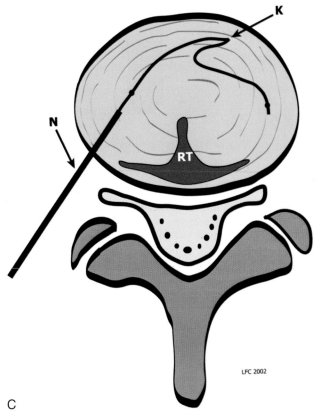

C

Figure 10-16 ■ Kinked catheter. *A*, AP radiograph. The catheter has been repositioned, and there is now a sharp bend in the catheter, compatible with a kink (K). PM = proximal marker; DM = distal marker; NT = needle tip. *B*, AP radiograph with caudocranial x-ray beam angulation confirms the catheter kink. *C*, Axial illustration demonstrates a sharp angle in the mid catheter, compatible with a kink (K). RT = radial tear; N = needle.

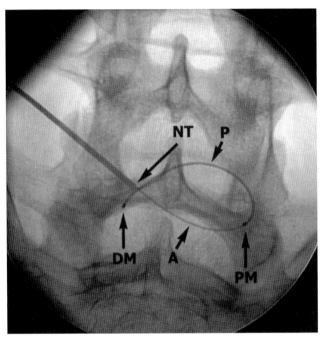
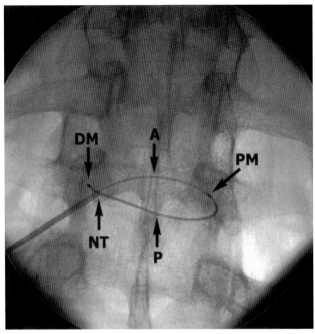

A   B

Figure 10-17 ■ *A*, AP radiograph with caudocranial x-ray beam angulation performed to evaluate the length of the SpineCATH for bowing, kinking, and breakage. The distal marker (DM) and the proximal marker (PM) have exited the needle tip (NT). *B*, AP radiograph with craniocaudal x-ray beam angulation serves the same purpose but allows easier reporting of positioning of the active thermal portion of the SpineCATH by the use of o'clock coordinates (e.g., 2 to 10 o'clock). A = catheter along anterior nucleus; P = catheter along posterior nucleus.

after placement of the needle in the disc, an antibiotic should still be instilled in the disc. A spinal needle should be inserted into the nucleus pulposus to introduce the antibiotic.

Redirecting the catheter tip is a skill that comes with practice. Small rotations of the catheter hub can cause significant changes in where the catheter tip will go. One should not turn the catheter more than half a turn in either direction during the first 90 degrees of catheter navigation and thereafter limit catheter turning to no more than a quarter turn. Excessive catheter turning can cause the catheter to break. The catheter would likely break at the point of least resistance, which would be where the catheter wire is attached to the plastic hub.

We have found that when an approach is made contralateral to the radial tear, the catheter can enter the radial tear and follow it back into the nucleus (Fig. 10-18*A*) or enter and remain within a disc protrusion on the symptomatic side (see Fig. 10-18*B*). It is of utmost importance to cross the disc pathology with the thermal catheter to provide adequate therapy. We found in our bilateral approaches that it was easier to cross a fissure when the catheter contacted the fissure at an acute angle as opposed to an obtuse angle (Fig. 10-19). Therefore, anecdotally, it may be easier to get complete posterior annular coverage from an approach ipsilateral to the patient's more symptomatic side when a radial tear is seen on post-discogram CT, and we often use an ipsilateral approach as our primary method.

Care must be taken when inserting the catheter through the introducer needle. If catheter advancement is smooth, catheter manipulation can occur from the gray plastic hub. However, if resistance is met and there is still significant catheter wire external to the needle hub, the catheter should be advanced by gripping the catheter wire like a pencil between the thumb and the index and ring fingers as close to the introducer needle hub as possible and attempting to advance the catheter in small steps. This is sometimes helped by rhythmically jiggling the catheter a few millimeters in and out while trying to advance a small amount at a time. It is important to perform this maneuver under fluoroscopy because the catheter can bend or kink. If the catheter is held at the gray hub when resistance is met, the catheter wire will likely bend or kink inside the disc or external to the needle hub.

When heating is activated, the heating element of the catheter should not be in contact with the introducer needle, because of a theoretical risk that heat could be transmitted along the metal introducer needle and cause significant damage to structures near the needle, including the dorsal root ganglion, thecal sac, and vascular structures. Angulating the C-arm several degrees craniad and caudad will allow optimal visualization of the thermal catheter element with respect to the needle cannula (see Fig. 10-13). If the catheter is in satisfactory position but is in contact with the needle, the needle should be withdrawn a few millimeters until the catheter and needle no longer make contact.

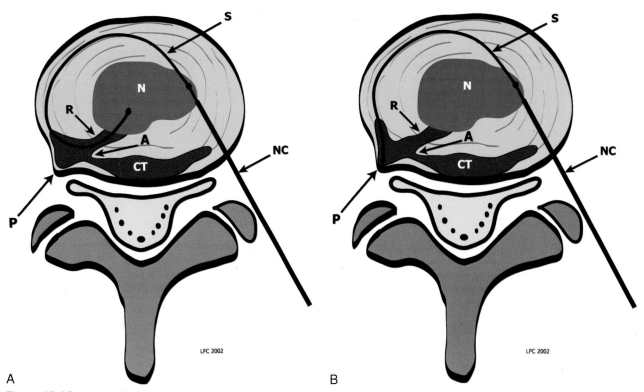

Figure 10-18 ■ Axial illustration with needle cannula (NC) approach contralateral to radial tear (R) and disc protrusion (P). *A*, The thermal catheter (S) follows the radial tear back toward the nucleus (N). *B*, The thermal catheter lodges in the disc protrusion. A = acute angle of radial tear; CT = concentric tear.

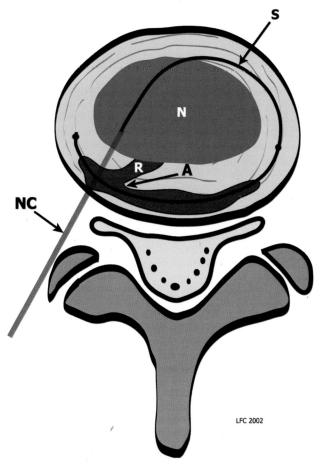

Figure 10-19 ■ Axial illustration with needle cannula (NC) approach ipsilateral to radial tear (R). The thermal catheter (S) crosses the radial tear at an acute angle (A). N = nucleus.

TABLE 10–1 ■ Heating Protocols

Heating Protocol	Peak Temp. (°C)	Time to Peak Temp. (min)	Time at Peak Temp. (min)	Total Therapy Time (min)
P80	80	7.5	6.0	13.5
P81	81	8.0	5.7	13.7
P82	82	8.5	5.5	14
P83	83	9.0	5.5	14.5
P84	84	9.5	5.2	14.7
P85	85	10.0	5.0	15
P86	86	10.5	4.7	15.2
P87	87	11.0	4.5	15.5
P88	88	11.5	4.5	16
P89	89	12.0	4.2	16.2
P90	90	12.5	4.0	16.5
P91	91	13.0	4.0	17
P92	92	13.5	4.0	17.5
P93	93	14.0	4.0	18
P94	94	14.5	4.0	18.5
P95	95	15.0	4.0	19

Modified with permission from Smith & Nephew IDET Training Course Syllabus. Smith & Nephew, Menlo Park, CA.

It is recommended that no more than two disc levels be treated at any one sitting. If more levels need to be treated, an 8- to 10-week wait is recommended for IDET™ at additional levels.

Alternate Heating Protocols

The recommended heating protocol (P90) begins at 65°C. The catheter temperature is increased by 1° every 30 seconds over the next 12.5 minutes, ultimately reaching 90°C (194°F). If the patient cannot tolerate this protocol despite sedation and analgesia, a lower temperature profile can be used. The comfort of the patient is important, and he or she should not have to endure severe discomfort or pain that is different than his or her usual pain. The overall temperature achieved is not as important as the amount of heat delivered over a period of time. It is strongly suggested that the temperature reach at least 80°C. The physician can choose to follow any of the following heating protocols or can opt to modify a heating protocol during the case. The general recommendation is not to exceed the P90 protocol. **Note that if the patient has symptoms of nerve root stimulation, the heating should be immediately terminated and the patient should be carefully evaluated before continuing heating or repositioning the catheter.** Table 10–1 depicts several different heating protocols.

POTENTIAL COMPLICATIONS

Procedural

* Bleeding
* Inadvertent puncture of the dura
* Headache
* Anesthesia-related allergic reactions
* Damage to the thecal sac and its contents, ranging from mild transient paresthesia to permanent cauda equina syndrome

Post-procedural

* Infection, specifically discitis
* Traumatic disc herniation due to weakened state of annulus during the first month post procedure

POST-PROCEDURE CARE/FOLLOW-UP

Immediate[18]

1. The patient should be observed for 2 to 3 hours after IDET.
2. The patient is placed at bed rest.
3. Blood pressure, pulse, heart rate, and respiration are evaluated every 30 minutes.

Discharge[18]

1. The patient is discharged into the care of a responsible person.
2. The patient is instructed not to drive or perform any other tasks that require clear thought and quick reactions for the remainder of the day, especially if sedation was given.
3. A 2- to 3-day nonrenewable prescription for a narcotic pain reliever and/or a muscle relaxant is given to the patient.
4. Multiple adhesive bandages may be on the patient's back. These should remain dry for at least 24 hours, at which point they can be removed.
5. The patient is instructed to continue to take his or her prescription medication, although pain medication may be tapered as indicated.
6. A discharge sheet should be given to the patient outlining the following:
   a. Which procedure was performed and at what levels
   b. Procedurally related symptoms that typically resolve in 7 to 10 days
      * Pain at the needle puncture site(s)
      * Mild increased back stiffness
      * Deep back pain
   c. Treatment for mild post-procedure symptoms
      * Rest the affected area for 3 to 4 days.
      * Avoid movements that aggravate the pain.
      * Apply cold compresses to the area that hurts.
   d. Signs and symptoms of infection
      * Fever
      * Chills
      * Swelling or drainage from the puncture sites
      * New back pain that is different from the usual pain
   e. Signs and symptoms of possibly more serious problems
      * Stiff neck
      * Increasing pain
      * Motor dysfunction such as difficulty walking or lifting
      * Bowel or bladder dysfunction
   f. Physician name and contact number if the patient has any concerns or if any problems arise as a result of the procedure

After IDET, it is common for the patient to experience an increase in back pain symptoms for 7 to 10 days. This pain will gradually subside, but it may take up to 6 weeks before improvement is noticed. We frequently find that in patients with back and leg pain, the leg pain gets better before the back pain after IDET. However, the pain will continue to subside over the next 6 to 9 months. The following is a basic chart that we use for our patients after IDET therapy, but such follow-up should be tailored specifically to each person.

First 24 Hours after IDET

1. Rest in a reclining or lying-down position.
2. Limit walking or sitting to 15 minutes at a time.
3. Apply ice to the procedure area to reduce local swelling and soreness.
4. Continue taking anti-inflammatory and pain medications as needed.
5. **Back support (e.g., soft back brace, Cybertec) must be worn for the first 6 weeks.**

First Week after Procedure

1. Rest 1 to 3 days.
2. Limit vertical sitting and walking to 20 to 30 minutes for the first 6 weeks.
3. Avoid bending, twisting, and sexual activity.
4. Driving may begin after 3 to 5 days.

Second Week after Procedure

1. Keep lifting within 10-pound limit.
2. Daily walking is allowed; increase to 20 minutes twice daily as tolerated.
3. Return to sedentary work with sitting and lifting restrictions.
4. Resume light housework.
5. Avoid bending, strenuous activity, and twisting.
6. Gentle stretching may be started (as instructed by the physical therapist).

Third Week after Procedure

1. Keep lifting to a 20- to 50-pound limit for the next 3 months.
2. Avoid strenuous activity or twisting.
3. Abdominal strengthening exercises may be started (as instructed by the physical therapist).
4. Make follow-up appointment with physician.

Fourth Week to 3 Months after Procedure

1. More aggressive strengthening exercises may be started (as instructed by the physical therapist).

2. Exercises may include supervised aerobic exercises, bicycling, and swimming.

When to Re-treat?

Before any re-treatment, formal diagnostic discography is performed as well as a complete history and physical examination. Re-treatment is considered in the following circumstances:

1. If the patient sustains a new injury (we usually wait at least 8 months after IDET before re-treating)
2. If there is reason to believe there was suboptimal catheter positioning during initial IDET
3. In cases in which there are no surgical options and the patient's only pain relief is through narcotics
4. We usually do not re-treat patients who receive only partial improvement, as long as numbers 1 through 3 do not apply.
5. Possibly in cases of late recurrence of similar symptoms (>1 year)

SAMPLE DICTATION

Procedure:	IDET (Intradiscal ElectroThermal therapy and decompression)
Date of Procedure:	Month/date/year
Facility:	Name of facility
Level Treated:	L4-5
Approach:	Bilateral
Supplies:	2 SpineCATH Intradiscal Catheters 2 Introducer needles

The procedure, potential complications, and treatment options were explained to the patient and voluntary informed, signed consent was obtained and placed in the patient's chart. Intravenous access was established in the right antecubital fossa. The patient received 1 g of intravenous cefazolin 1 hour before the procedure. Electrocardiography, pulse oximetry, and blood pressure checks were performed throughout the procedure. Conscious sedation was administered by members of the anesthesiology department through the intravenous access.

The patient's lower back was prepped and draped in usual sterile fashion, and the image intensifiers were covered in sterile fashion. The image intensifier was positioned over the L4-5 disc and aligned so that the left superior articulating facet of the L5 vertebral body was approximately one third of the distance from the ventral aspect of the vertebral body. The image intensifier was also rotated so that the superior end plates of L5 superimposed. Superficial local anesthesia was obtained with 1% lidocaine. A 22-gauge, 6-inch spinal needle was advanced directly ventrolateral to the superior articulating facet and deep anesthesia was given. A 17-gauge, 6-inch styleted introducer needle was placed to the left posterolateral margin of the L4-5 disc without complication. The disc was entered, and the location of the needle tip was confirmed with AP and lateral fluoroscopy. A SpineCATH® Intradiscal Catheter was connected and pretested to be certain its parameters were within normal range. The thermal treatment catheter was placed through the introducer needle. The catheter was advanced, using biplane fluoroscopy, and navigated into the proper antero-posterior and cephalocaudal location. The heater coil of the thermal catheter was seen to be intradiscal and out of the introducer needle. The heating portion of the catheter was seen to extend from the right anterolateral aspect of the nucleus pulposus to the posterior midline (1 o'clock to 6 o'clock position).

Delivery of thermal energy was initiated at 65°C. The Smith & Nephew generator (ORA-50S) was utilized, and the catheter temperature was raised 1°C every 30 seconds to 90°C over 12.5 minutes with continuous monitoring of the patient for symptoms. The catheter temperature was maintained at 90°C for an additional 4 minutes, at which point heating was terminated. The catheter was removed under fluoroscopic guidance and inspected. The left entry to the disc permitted only partial access to the posterior annular wall. Therefore, the image intensifier was repositioned and the disc was entered on the right side with a new introducer needle and SpineCATH Intradiscal Catheter. The heating portion of the catheter was seen to extend from the left posterolateral aspect of the nucleus pulposus across the posterior midline to the right lateral margin of the disc (9 o'clock to 4 o'clock position). Thermal treatment was performed in a similar fashion. The catheter was removed and inspected. Two milligrams of cefazolin was instilled through the introducer needle into the disc.

During the procedure, the patient experienced pain that was concordant with his usual pain, and at no time did he experience dissimilar pain. No complications were observed during or immediately after the procedure.

CASE REPORTS

CASE 1

Clinical Presentation

The patient is a 45-year-old man with long-standing low back pain. At times, he has vague pain in both proximal lower extremities without a radicular component. The pain is worse with standing and walking, but it is not completely relieved with sitting or lying down. The patient has had only minimal benefit from physical therapy and medication. His gait and strength are normal. Straight-leg raising is weakly positive at 75 degrees bilaterally. Reflexes are intact.

Imaging and Therapy

MR imaging demonstrated mild loss of signal of the L5-S1 disc without significant loss of height. Flexion/extension lumbar radiographs showed no evidence of instability. Post-discography axial CT at L5-S1 demonstrated a band of contrast medium extending from the central nucleus to the posterior paramidline annulus, compatible with a grade 3 radial tear (Fig. 10-20A). AP (see Fig. 10-20B) and lateral (see Fig. 10-20C) radiographs during IDET™ demonstrated introducer needle placement from a left

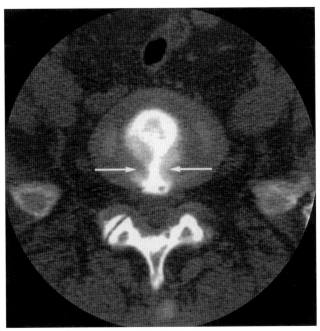

Figure 10-20 ∎ A, Post-discography axial CT image of L5-S1. Contrast medium extends from the central nucleus to the posterior annular margin, compatible with a grade 3 tear (*arrows*).

A

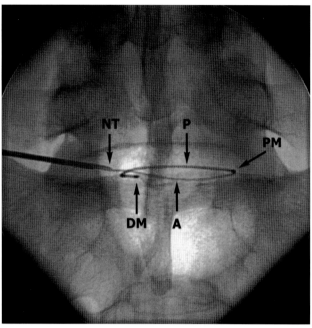

B

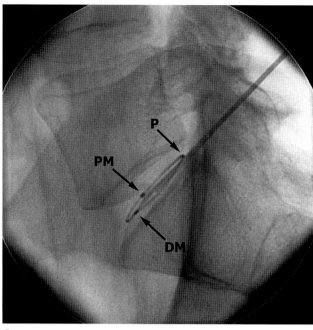

C

Figure 10-20 (*Cont'd*) ■ AP (*B*) and lateral (*C*) radiographs during L5-S1 IDET, left-sided approach. The catheter has been navigated across the midline, and both the distal marker (DM) and the proximal marker (PM) have exited and are not in contact with the needle tip (NT). The anterior (A) and posterior (P) portions of the SpineCATH are within the margins of the outer annulus as seen on the post-discography CT.

posterolateral approach, with excellent intradiscal positioning of the thermal catheter (3 o'clock to 10 o'clock positions).

Results

During discography, injection of 0.7 mL of injection mixture at L5-S1 (myelographic contrast material and antibiotic) produced severe concordant low back pain and mild proximal leg pain. Injection at other levels produced no pain. Given the patient's clinical history, positive discogram, and preserved disc height, he was an excellent candidate for IDET. The procedure was uneventful. One year after IDET, the patient is relieved of approximately 90% of his pre-procedure pain.

CASE 2

Clinical Presentation

The patient is a 35-year-old man with 1½ years of low back pain. The pain spreads diffusely across the low back and buttocks without any radiating or referred pain into the lower extremities. It is most severe when moving from sitting to standing. The patient has had no significant benefit from 6 months of physical therapy, oral medication, and pain injections. His gait and strength are normal. Straight-leg raising is negative to 90 degrees bilaterally. Reflexes are intact.

Imaging and Therapy

MR imaging demonstrated mild loss of signal of the L4-5 disc without significant loss of height. Flexion/extension lumbar radiographs showed no evidence of instability. A post-discography CT at the L4-5 level demonstrated a narrow band of contrast medium extending to the posterior central annulus with bilateral spread along annular tissue planes, compatible with a grade 4 tear (Fig. 10-21*A*). The distal catheter could be navigated only to the right posterolateral annulus (the 4 o'clock position) during

IDET from a left posterolateral (see Fig. 10-21*B*) approach. Because the entire tear was not crossed, a second puncture was performed from a right posterolateral approach (see Fig. 10-21*C*). From this approach, the thermal catheter from the right posterolateral approach was successfully navigated across the annulus to its right posterolateral margin, overlapping the treatment performed from the contralateral puncture.

Results

During discography, injection of 0.8 mL of injection mixture at L4-5 (myelographic contrast material and antibiotic) produced severe concordant low back pain. Injection at other levels produced no pain. Given the patient's clinical history, positive discogram, and preserved disc height, he was an excellent candidate for IDET. Aside from the need to perform a bilateral approach to cover the entire annular tear, the procedure was uneventful. One year after IDET, the patient is relieved of approximately 90% of his pre-procedure pain.

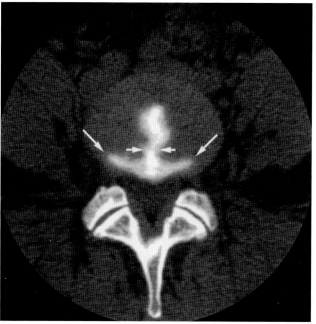

A

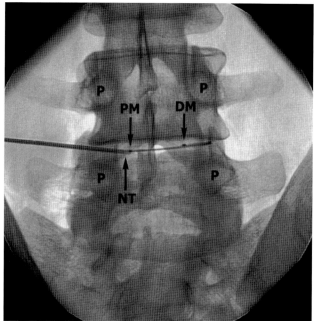

B

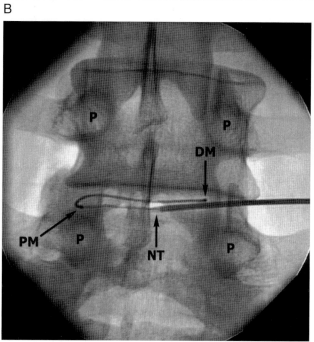

C

Figure 10-21 ■ *A*, Post-discography axial CT image of L4-5. Contrast medium extends from the central nucleus to the posterior central annular margin (*short white arrows*) with bilateral posterolateral spread (*long white arrows*), compatible with a grade 4 tear. *B*, AP radiograph during L4-5 IDET, left-sided approach. SpineCATH could be navigated only to the contralateral posterolateral nucleus. The distal marker (DM) is approximately 5 mm medial to the medial border of the right-sided pedicles (P). The proximal marker (PM) has not exited the needle tip (NT); therefore, the needle was slightly retracted before thermal therapy. *C*, AP radiograph during L4-5 IDET, right-sided approach. The SpineCATH has been successfully navigated across the midline. The distal marker (DM) has reached the medial border of the right-sided pedicles (P). The entire posterior and bilateral posterolateral annulus has been treated by the two-sided approach. PM = proximal marker; NT = needle tip.

Clinical Presentation

The patient is a 47-year-old man with long-standing low back pain. His pain is low in the center of the back and radiates into both buttocks, with no radicular component. The pain is most severe with prolonged standing or sitting. The patient has had no significant benefit from 3 months of aggressive physical therapy, oral medication, and pain injections. His gait and strength are normal. Straight-leg raising is negative to 90 degrees bilaterally. Reflexes are intact.

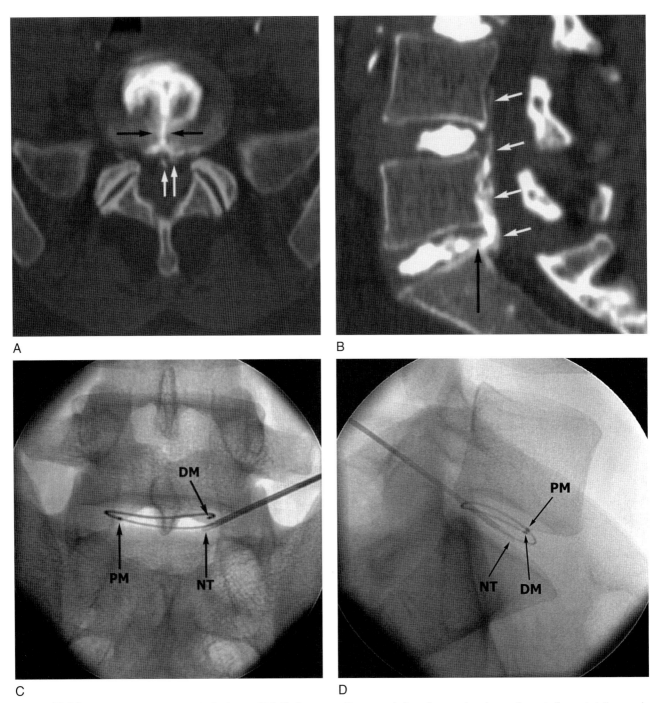

Figure 10-22 ■ *A,* Post-discography axial CT image of L5-S1. Contrast medium extends from the central nucleus to the posterior central disc margin (*black arrows*). Note extra-annular spread of contrast agent (*white arrows*), compatible with a grade 5 tear. *B,* Midline sagittal reconstructed lumbar spine L3-S1. Contrast medium at L5-S1 extends through the posterior annulus (*black arrow*), with cephalad extra-annular spread to mid-L4 level (*white arrows*). AP (*C*) and lateral (*D*) radiographs during L5-S1 IDET, right-sided approach. The catheter has been navigated across the midline, and both the distal marker (DM) and the proximal marker (PM) have exited and are not in contact with the needle tip (NT). The anterior and posterior portions of the SpineCATH are within the confines of the annulus as seen on the post-discography CT.

Imaging and Therapy

MR imaging demonstrated a focal region of increased signal intensity in the posterior annulus of L5-S1, compatible with an annular tear with preserved disc height. The disc height at L5-S1 was seen to be preserved. Axial (Fig. 10-22A) and reformatted sagittal (see Fig. 10-22B) post-discography CT images demonstrated contrast medium extending posteriorly to the L5-S1 annular margin, with extravasation of contrast agent in the ventral epidural space superior to the level of L4, compatible with a grade 5 tear. AP (see Fig. 10-22C) and lateral (see Fig. 10-22D) radiographs during L5-S1 IDET from a right posterolateral approach demonstrated excellent intradiscal positioning of the thermal catheter (10 o'clock to 2 o'clock positions).

Results

During discography, injection of 1.0 mL of injection mixture at L5-S1 (myelographic contrast material and antibiotic) produced severe concordant low back and bilateral buttock pain. Injection at other levels produced discordant pain. Given the patient's clinical history, positive discogram, and preserved disc height, he was an excellent candidate for IDET. The procedure was uneventful. One and a half years after IDET, the patient is relieved of 75% to 85% of his pre-procedure pain.

CURRENT PROCEDURAL TERMINOLOGY (CPT) CODES

No specific CPT code is available for IDET at this writing, but this situation is expected to change in the near future. CPT codes change often and sometimes are valid only for certain states or regions. It is best to consult with coding experts to make sure that coding for one's procedures is legitimate and complete. Below is a sample of codes that are being used for the IDET procedure at this writing.[19]

The American Medical Association (AMA) currently suggests using 64999 (Unlisted procedure, nervous system) for IDET.

Other potential CPT codes are as follows:

62287 Aspiration or decompression procedure, percutaneous, of nucleus pulposus of intervertebral disc, any method, single or multiple levels, lumbar (e.g., manual or automated percutaneous discectomy, percutaneous discectomy, percutaneous laser discectomy)

64640 Destruction by neurolytic agent, chemical, thermal, electrical of peripheral nerve or branch

72295 Discography, lumbar, radiological supervision and interpretation

76005-26 Fluoroscopic guidance and localization of needle or catheter tip for spine or paraspinous diagnostic or therapeutic injection procedures (epidural, transforaminal epidural, subarachnoid, paravertebral facet joint, paravertebral facet joint nerve or sacroiliac joint), including neurolytic agent destruction

99141 Sedation with or without analgesia (conscious sedation), intravenous, intramuscular or inhalation

Single-Level Unilateral Approach	Single-Level Bilateral Approaches
62287	62287-22
64640	64640
72295-26*	72295-26*,†
76005-26	76005-26†

Two-Level Unilateral Approach	Two-Level Bilateral Approaches
62287	62287-22
64640-51	64640-51
72295-26*,†	72295-26*,†
76005-26†	76005-26†

*Drop the -26 charge if the physician owns the equipment.
†Multiply this by the number of catheters used to perform the IDET procedure.

The **72295** code is for supervision and evaluation of proper catheter placement.

The **99141** code can be submitted if the physician performing the IDET procedure is also performing the sedation with appropriate charting.

References

1. Kennedy M. IDET: A new approach to treating lower back pain. WMJ 1999; 98:18–20.
2. Andersson GBJ. Epidemiological features of chronic low-back pain. Lancet 1999; 354:581–585.
3. Holt EP. The question of lumbar discography. J Bone Joint Surg Am 1968; 50:720–726.
4. Bogduk N. The innervation of the lumbar spine. Spine 1983; 8:286–293.
5. Bogduk N, Tynan W, Wilson AS. The nerve supply to the human lumbar intervertebral discs. J Anat 1981; 132:39–56.
6. McCarthy PW, Carruthers B, Martin D, et al. Immunohistochemical demonstration of sensory nerve fibers and endings in lumbar intervertebral discs of the rat. Spine 1991; 16:653–655.
7. Freemont AJ, Peacock TE, Goupille P, et al. Nerve ingrowth into diseased intervertebral disc in chronic back pain. Lancet 1997; 350:178–181.
8. Derby R, Howard MW, Grant JM, et al. The ability of pressure-controlled discography to predict surgical and nonsurgical outcomes. Spine 1999; 24:364–372.

9. Coppes MH, Marani E, Thomeer RTWM, et al. Innervation of "painful" lumbar discs. Spine 1997; 22:2342–2350.

10. Roberts S, Eisenstein SM, Menage J, et al. Mechanoreceptors in intervertebral discs: Morphology, distribution and neuropeptides. Spine 1995; 20:2645–2651.

11. Brodkey JS, Miyazaki Y, Ervin FR, et al. Reversible heat lesions with radiofrequency current. J Neurosurg 1964; 21:49–53.

12. IntraDiscal ElectroThermal (IDET) Therapy Training Course Syllabus. Menlo Park, CA: Oratec Interventions, Inc.

13. Derby R, Eek B, Chen Y, et al. Intradiscal Electrothermal Annuloplasty (IDET): A novel approach for treating chronic discogenic back pain. Neuromodulation 2000; 3:82–88.

14. Troussier B, Lebas JF, Chirossel JP, et al. Percutaneous intradiscal radio-frequency thermocoagulation: A cadaveric study. Spine 1995; 20:1713–1718.

15. Houpt JC, Conner ES, McFarland EW. Experimental study of temperature distributions and thermal transport during radiofrequency current therapy of the intervertebral disc. Spine 1996; 21:1808–1813.

16. Hsia AW, Issac K, Katz JS. Cauda equina syndrome from intradiscal electrothermal therapy. Neurology 2000; 55:320.

17. Physicians' Desk Reference, 56th ed. Montvale, NJ: Medical Economics Company, 2002.

18. Fenton DS, Czervionke LF. Discography. In Williams AL, Murtagh FR (eds). Handbook of Diagnostic and Therapeutic Spine Procedures. St. Louis: CV Mosby, 2002, pp 187–188.

19. CPT 2002, CPT Intellectual Property Services. Chicago: American Medical Association, 2002.

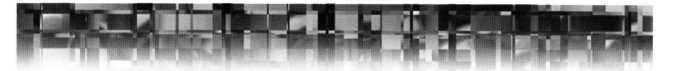

A Spine Surgeon's Perspective

IntraDiscal ElectroThermal Therapy (IDET™)

Joseph T. Alexander, MD

Patients with intractable mechanical back pain and radiographic evidence of mild or early disc degeneration continue to present a major management problem for spine care specialists. Although most such patients will improve with anti-inflammatory medications, therapeutic modalities, spine stabilization exercises, work modification, and time, there remain a large number who have disabling symptoms. Evaluation of these patients is often more challenging because issues of litigation and/or disability may further cloud the picture. Traditional surgical techniques have been relatively less successful for patients who have failed to respond to conservative treatment regimens. There have been a number of previous attempts at minimally invasive procedures designed to shrink or reduce a bulging disc, none of which gained lasting acceptance once they spread into the wider medical community.

The preliminary published clinical data on the efficacy of IDET has been mixed but is generally encouraging. Several large, prospective, randomized trials currently under way have yet to be reported. Little morbidity has been documented to date, and use of IDET does not preclude later surgical intervention. Until definitive studies are available, I will continue to refer for IDET a small, select group of patients with severe subjective symptoms and modest radiographic findings who have not responded to extensive conservative treatment and who I believe do not represent good candidates for surgery.

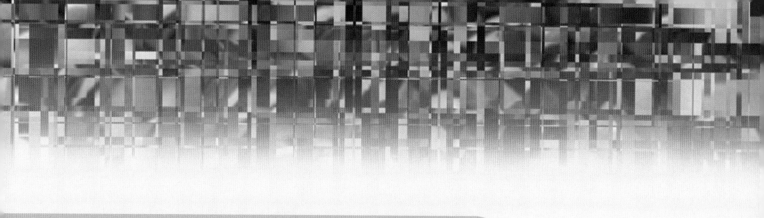

Chapter 11

Pharmacology for the Spine Injectionist

■ B. Todd Sitzman, MD, MPH

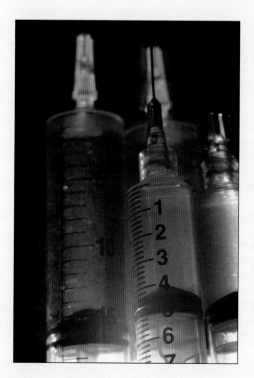

Drugs used for diagnostic and therapeutic spine injections fall into one of three broad categories: radiocontrast agents, local anesthetics, and corticosteroids. It is imperative that the spine injectionist has a firm understanding of each drug administered in his or her practice. Although it is beyond the scope of this chapter to provide a comprehensive review of all drugs within these three categories, a number of commercially available examples from each category are presented. This overview consists of a brief description of drug pharmacology, pharmacokinetics, possible side effects, and cautions. Before using any of these drugs, clinicians should refer to the official prescribing information for each drug, including approved indications, contraindications, and warnings. These can be found within published manufacturer product information as well as a current Physicians' Desk Reference.[1]

Drug dosage information for specific injections or therapies is not covered in this chapter but can be found within this book's respective chapters. Because inherent risks are associated with any medication, the injectionist should administer drugs only when there is a clear clinical indication and when the prospects of patient benefit outweigh the risks. Additionally, drugs should be administered in the smallest dose that will reliably produce the desired effect. An increased total dose or volume should not be used to compensate for inadequate injection technique.

287

TABLE 11–1 ■ Common Radiocontrast Agents Used for Spinal Injections

Agent	Concentration (w/v%)	Ionic Concentration (mg iodine/mL)	Osmolality (mOsm/kg H₂O)
Isovue-M			
Isovue-M 200	Iopamidol 41%	200	300
Isovue-M 300	Iopamidol 61%	300	616
Omnipaque			
Omnipaque 180	Iohexol 39%	180	360
Omnipaque 240	Iohexol 52%	240	510
Omnipaque 300	Iohexol 65%	300	672

TABLE 11–2 ■ Potential Adverse Reactions Associated with Contrast Agents

Chemotoxic
1. Thyrotoxicosis—rare with second-generation contrast agents containing a minimal amount of free iodine atoms
2. Nephrotoxicity

Hyperosmolality—rare when used at concentrations that approximate physiologic osmolality, 300 mOsm/kg H₂0
1. Erythrocyte damage
2. Endothelial damage and thrombosis
3. Vasodilation of arteriolar and capillary vasculature (feeling of warmth, discomfort)
4. Hypervolemia
5. Cardiac depression

Allergic
1. Vasomotor (warmth, flush)
2. Cutaneous (scattered hives, severe urticaria)
3. Bronchospasm (wheezing)
4. Cardiovascular (hypotension)
5. Vasovagal (bradycardia, hypotension, nausea)
6. Anaphylactoid reaction (angioedema, urticaria, bronchospasm, hypotension).

Data from Grainger RG. Intravascular contrast media. In Grainger RG, Allison DJ (eds). Diagnostic Radiology, 2nd ed. New York: Churchill Livingstone, 1992, pp 11–22.

TABLE 11–3 ■ Pretreatment Regimen for Previous Radiocontrast Allergic Reactions

12 Hours before Contrast Medium Exposure
1. Prednisone, 20 to 50 mg orally
2. Ranitidine, 50 mg orally
3. Diphenhydramine, 25 to 50 mg orally

2 Hours before Contrast Medium Exposure
1. Prednisone, 20 to 50 mg orally
2. Ranitidine, 50 mg orally
3. Diphenhydramine, 25 to 50 mg orally

Immediately before Contrast Medium Injection
Diphenhydramine, 25 mg intravenously

RADIOCONTRAST AGENTS

Radiographic contrast agents, in themselves, serve no therapeutic purpose in spinal injections. Their role is diagnostic, by aiding in the localization of anatomic structures and needle placement under x-ray guidance (i.e., fluoroscopy). As an x-ray beam passes through the body, it is attenuated by the various structures through which it passes. Each structure has an attenuation coefficient that is dependent on its thickness and the energy level of the x-ray radiation source.[2] Iodine atoms within contrast agents provide greater x-ray attenuation relative to tissue and bone and thus decrease the amount of radiation reaching the detector (e.g., fluoroscopic image intensifier). Although conventional "iodinated" contrast agents provide radiopacity by way of a tri-iodinated benzoate anion, their use is clinically limited by their extremely high osmolar concentration–up to eight times the physiologic level. Osmolality depends on the number of particles of solute in solution. Additionally, the hyperosmolality of a conventional contrast agent is directly related

to its toxicity (e.g., more hemodynamic effects as well as patient discomfort). This led to the development of "second-generation" radiocontrast agents. Although labeled as "nonionic," these agents still contain iodine atoms that are tightly bound to a benzene ring, with a minimal amount of free iodine. Their higher iodine-to-particle ratio (over conventional agents) leads to comparable attenuation of radiation with a lower osmolality. Because of their more physiologic properties, approaching an osmolality of 300 mOsm/kg water, these second-generation contrast agents are more commonly used in spine injections.

Examples of two commonly used radiocontrast agents are iopamidol (Isovue-M) and iohexol (Omnipaque). Each agent is commercially available in preparations of varying ionic concentration and osmolality[3, 4] (Table 11-1). Both iopamidol and iohexol are absorbed rapidly into the bloodstream from intrathecal, epidural, and paraspinal tissues. There are measurable plasma levels within 1 hour of injection, with nearly the entire remaining drug reaching the systemic circulation within 24 hours.[3, 4] Both agents undergo minimal, if any, metabolism, deiodination, or biotransformation. Excretion is primarily renal (>90%), with minimal fecal excretion (<1%).

Adverse reactions associated with radiocontrast agents may be chemotoxic, osmolar related, or allergic (Table 11-2).

Ninety percent of severe adverse reactions occur within 15 minutes of exposure to the contrast agent.[6] For this reason, it is imperative that all patients be observed for a minimum of 30 to 60 minutes after any type of injection using radiocontrast agents. When an allergic reaction is suspected, treatment should be prompt and aggressive, using current basic and advanced life support therapies established by the

Agent	Available Concentrations (%)	Onset	Duration (hr)	pKa (25°C)	pH of Plain Solutions	Recommended Maximal Single Dose (mg) without Epinephrine
Lidocaine	0.5, 1, 1.5, 2, 5	Fast	1–2	7.7	6.5	300
Bupivacaine	0.25, 0.5, 0.75	Slow	2–4	8.1	4.5–6	175

TABLE 11-4 ■ Physiochemical Properties of Local Anesthetic Agents Used in Spinal Injections

Data from Covino BG, Wildsmith JAW. Clinical pharmacology of local anesthetic agents. In Cousins MJ, Bridenbaugh PO (eds). Neural Blockade in Clinical Anesthesia and Management of Pain, 3rd ed. Philadelphia: Lippincott-Raven, 1998, pp 97–128.

American Heart Association.[7] These measures include oxygen, intravenous fluids, antihistamines (H$_1$ and H$_2$ blockers), adrenergic drugs (epinephrine), and corticosteroids.

In patients with a known previous allergic reaction to radiocontrast agents, pretreatment options to minimize a subsequent reaction should be exercised. The regimen used at our institution is a modification of previously published regimens[8, 9] (Table 11-3).

LOCAL ANESTHETICS

A local anesthetic reversibly interrupts nerve impulse conduction by blocking sodium channels located on internal neuronal membranes. This results in inhibition of sodium permeability necessary for action potential propagation.[10] Local anesthetics are weak bases classified according to their ester- or amide-type chemical structures. Because of the more popular and widespread use of amide-type local anesthetics over ester-type agents for spinal diagnostic and therapeutic purposes, the focus here is on the amide-type local anesthetics lidocaine and bupivacaine.[11, 12]

The clinical action of a local anesthetic is often described in terms of its potency, speed of onset, and duration of action. It is simplistic to state that a local anesthetic's potency is related to lipid solubility, its speed of onset to pKa, and its duration of action to protein binding without fully understanding the physiochemical properties of local anesthetics (Table 11-4). This is especially true when these agents are used for diagnostic and or prognostic purposes.

The **potency** of a local anesthetic is related to its lipid solubility, which is often described by its in vitro octanol:water partition coefficient.[13] The more lipophilic a local anesthetic, the more readily it permeates neuronal membranes, resulting in greater affinity for sodium channel binding. For example, bupivacaine is more potent than lidocaine, with a ninefold greater octanol:water partition coefficient (27.5 vs. 2.9).

The **speed of onset** of most local anesthetics depends on their dissociation constants (pKa) and the pH of the local tissue. The pKa is the pH at which a given drug is half ionized (i.e., local anesthetic protonated form) and half in its neutral, unionized form (i.e., local anesthetic base form). It is the un-ionized form that more readily diffuses across the nerve membrane; therefore, a local anesthetic whose pKa approximates physiologic tissue pH will have a faster onset of action. Another factor affecting speed of onset is the pH of the local anesthetic preparation itself. Commercially available local anesthetic preparations containing a vasoconstrictor (i.e., epinephrine) are often adjusted to an acidic pH with the addition of hydrochloric salts to enhance the stability of added vasoconstrictors. For this reason, clinicians are advised to note the pH of the local anesthetic preparation they are using. If the pH is acidic, and a more rapid onset of action is desired, small amounts of sodium bicarbonate may be added.[14, 15] Care should be taken to add only small amounts of bicarbonate (NaHCO$_3$-to-anesthetic volume ratio of 1:20). Adjusting to a pH greater than 7 will render the local anesthetic less soluble in aqueous solution and thereby increase the risk of drug precipitation.

The **duration of action** is dependent on multiple factors: the site of injection, the presence of vasoconstrictors, the lipid solubility of the agent itself, and the dose administered. It is erroneous to state that the duration of local anesthetic action is primarily a function of its protein binding. Protein binding is strictly the mode by which local anesthetics are transported in the blood. Longer-duration local anesthetics are more lipid soluble and hence are more slowly "washed out" from neural membranes, both in vitro and in vivo. The duration of local anesthetic action depends on the absorption from the site of injection, and it is therefore dependent on the blood supply to that site. The more vascular the location (subcutaneous > intercostal > caudal > epidural > peripheral nerve > intrathecal), the more rapidly the agent is absorbed into the bloodstream, distributed, metabolized, and excreted.

The metabolism of a local anesthetic is dependent on its chemical structure: ester or amide. Ester-type agents (e.g., procaine, benzocaine) undergo rapid metabolism via plasma pseudocholinesterase, yielding para-aminobenzoic acid (PABA) as a metabolic byproduct. PABA has been implicated as an allergenic source with ester-type local anesthetics. Amide-type local anesthetics (e.g., lidocaine and bupivacaine) undergo oxidative dealkylation via the hepatic cytochrome P450 enzyme system as well as conjugation. Because nearly all metabolism is via the liver, clearance of lidocaine and bupivacaine is highly dependent on hepatic blood flow, extraction, and enzyme function. For this reason, caution should be used in patients with liver dysfunction.

Adverse reactions associated with local anesthetics may result from toxicity, reaction to an added vasoconstrictor or preservative, or an allergic reaction (Table 11-5). Toxicity results from high blood levels of local anesthetic, usually as a consequence of accidental intravascular injection, increased uptake from perivascular areas, or overdosage.

TABLE 11-5 ■ Adverse Rections Associated With Local Anesthetic

Central Nervous System (CNS) Toxicity
CNS toxicity is proportional to the potency of the local anesthetic and to the serum blood level. Initial symptoms are usually excitatory and result from blockade of central inhibitory pathways. In order of appearance, CNS symptoms include the following:
1. Numbness of the tongue or a foreign taste (initial symptom)
2. Lightheadedness
3. Auditory disturbances
4. Muscular twitching
5. Unconsciousness
6. Convulsions
7. Coma
8. Respiratory arrest
9. Cardiovascular depression

Cardiovascular Toxicity
Most local anesthetics will not produce cardiovascular toxicity until blood levels are twice that needed to produce seizures.[17] Local anesthetics bind to and inhibit cardiac sodium channels, with bupivacaine binding more avidly and for a longer duration than lidocaine.[18]

Neuronal Toxicity[19, 20]
1. Preservative related (i.e. sodium metabisulfite)
2. Local anesthetic concentration related—5% lidocaine

Vasoconstrictor
These types of reactions are caused by inadvertent injection or uptake of epinephrine. They are commonly misdiagnosed as allergic rections.
1. Tachycardia
2. Elevated blood pressure
3. Headache
4. Apprehension

Allergic Reaction
Allergic reactions are more common with ester-type local anesthetics than with amide-type agents.[21]
1. Vasomotor (warmth, flush)
2. Cutaneous (scattered hives, severe urticaria)
3. Bronchospasm (wheezing)
4. Cardiovascular (hypotension)
5. Vasovagal (bradycardia, hypotension, nausea)
6. Anaphylactoid reaction (angioedema, urticaria, bronchospasm, hypotension

Data from Covino BG, Wildsmith JAW. Clinical pharmacalogy of local anesthetic agents. In Cousins MJ, Bridenbaugh PO (eds). Neural Blockade in Clinical Anesthesia and Management of Pain, 3rd ed. Philadelphia: Lippincott-Raven, 1998, pp 97–128.

Prevention of local anesthetic–related adverse reactions requires both appropriate dosage administration (dependent on concentration and volume) and clinical vigilance for early detection of toxic reactions. Treatment of an adverse reaction should be prompt and aggressive, based on the severity of symptoms. Central nervous system toxicity necessitates supportive therapies (i.e., airway, breathing, circulation, supplemental oxygen) but may also require pharmacologic intervention. Seizures may be terminated with an intravenous benzodiazepine (midazolam, 0.05 to 0.1 mg/kg) or with an intravenous short-acting barbiturate (thiopental, 1 to 2 mg/kg). Signs and symptoms of cardiovascular toxicity should be treated as aggressively as possible, using advanced cardiac life-support guidelines.[7] Note that in the setting of local anesthetic–induced ventricular dysrhythmias, amiodarone rather than lidocaine should be used. Lastly, allergic reactions to amide-type local anesthetics are rare. If one is suspected, treatment should include administration of

Agent (Trade Name)	Biologic Half-Life (hr)	Anti-inflammatory Potency*	Salt-Retaining Potency*
Hydrocortisone (Hydrocortone[23,24])	8–12	1	1
Triamcinolone (Kenalog-40,[25] Aristocort Forte[26])	12–36	5	0
Methylprednisolone (Depo-Medrol[27])	12–36	5	0.5
Dexamethasone (Decadron Phosphate[28])	36–72	25	0
Betamethasone (Celestone Soluspan[29])	36–72	25	0

*These are relative potencies based on an equivalent milligram dose (i.e., with regard to their anti-inflammatory potency, 6 mg Celestone Soluspan is equivalent to 30 mg of Kenalog-40).

intravenous fluids, antihistamines (H_1 and H_2 blockers), adrenergic drugs (epinephrine), and corticosteroids.

CORTICOSTEROIDS

Naturally occurring corticosteroids are classified into three functional groups: mineralocorticoids, glucocorticoids, and adrenal androgens. Glucocorticoids, originally named for their role in glucose metabolism, are the corticosteroids clinically used in the management of pain disorders. Although frequently classified by their duration of action (biologic half-life), it is equally important to recognize their relative mineralocorticoid (sodium retaining) and anti-inflammatory potencies (Table 11-6).

Several therapeutic mechanisms of action for corticosteroids have been proposed. They include anti-inflammatory effects, direct neural membrane stabilization, and modulation of peripheral nociceptor neurons and spinal cord dorsal horn cells.

The anti-inflammatory effects of glucocorticoids are primarily attributable to their inhibition of the production of inflammatory mediators at both the local tissue and the systemic immune response levels. With any type of spinal tissue trauma (e.g., disc, spinal nerve, dura, muscle, fascia, ligament, or facet joint), inflammatory mediators are released. Corticosteroids injected in the area of injury may inhibit the production of local inflammatory mediators, including arachidonic acid and its metabolites (prostaglandins, leukotrienes), various cytokines (interleukins 1 and 6, tumor necrosis factor-α), and other acute-phase reactants.[22, 30]

Other mechanisms of action for injected corticosteroids include a reduction in the spontaneous ectopic discharge rate seen after nerve injury, including neuromas.[31] Reversible inhibition of nociceptive C-fiber transmission, but not of A-B–fiber transmission, has been shown after corticosteroid administration.[32] Similar effects were obtained by the use of methylprednisolone in a peripheral mononeuropathy nerve injury animal model.[33] These studies confirm that locally

TABLE 11-7 ■ Adverse Reactions Associated with Corticosteroids

1. Fluid retention
2. Elevated blood pressure
3. Hyperglycemia
4. Generalized erythema/facial flushing
5. Menstrual irregularities
6. Gastritis/peptic ulcer disease
7. Hypothalamic-pituitary-adrenal axis suppression
8. Cushing syndrome
9. Bone demineralization
10. Steroid myopathy
11. Allergic reaction

Data from references 23 through 29.

applied corticosteroids suppress afferent ectopic discharges at the site of nerve injury and thus support a direct membrane-stabilizing effect. Lastly, glucocorticoid receptor sites have been located on norepinephrine and 5-hydroxytryptamine neurons within the dorsal horn substantia gelatinosa, known pathways of pain transmission.[34,35] This finding suggests that corticosteroids may modulate nociceptive input from peripheral nociceptors by a direct action on the spinal cord.

Chemical modifications to the parent four-ringed hydrocortisone (cortisol) molecule have made possible synthetic glucocorticoids with a vast array of anti-inflammatory potencies, mineralocorticoid activities, durations of action, and rates of metabolic transformation. A commercially available form of betamethasone provides an example of how a minor chemical modification can change the pharmacokinetic profile of a glucocorticoid. Each milliliter of Celestone Soluspan injectable suspension contains equal amounts of betamethasone sodium phosphate (freely water soluble) and betamethasone acetate (highly lipophilic).[29] The more soluble betamethasone sodium phosphate provides rapid activity, whereas the microcrystalline betamethasone acetate provides sustained activity. In general, the efficacy and duration of activity are greater with less soluble corticosteroid preparations.

After systemic absorption, the majority of corticosteroid is reversibly bound to two plasma proteins: corticosteroid-binding globulin and albumin.[22] Note that only the unbound fraction of a corticosteroid is responsible for its cellular-mediated anti-inflammatory effects. The protein-bound corticosteroid undergoes sequential oxidative-reduction reactions yielding inactive compounds. This is followed by hepatic-mediated conjugation (sulfate or glucuronide), resulting in water-soluble metabolites that are excreted in the urine.

The majority of corticosteroid-related adverse reactions are mild and transient when the drug is administered as an intermittent injection-type therapy (as opposed to long-term daily use) (Table 11-7).

Several other purported adverse reactions have been reported after corticosteroid injection. Sterile meningitis and arachnoiditis has been reported after intrathecal injection of methylprednisolone, although this was possibly related to the polyethylene additive of the preparation.[36] Brief euphoric or manic reactions have been reported after high-dose corticosteroid therapy.[37,38] Although rare, anaphylactoid reactions have been reported with intravenous, intramuscular, and soft tissue injection of corticosteroids.[39-41] The "succinate" salts of hydrocortisone and methylprednisolone have most often been implicated; allergic-type reactions are absent after use of the acetate or phosphate salts of the same corticosteroid. Any type of anaphylactic reaction should be treated promptly and aggressively with supportive therapies (i.e., airway, breathing, circulation, supplemental oxygen), including advanced cardiac life support guidelines when indicated.[7]

Lastly, co-administration of corticosteroids with preservative-containing local anesthetics (e.g., methylparaben-, propylparaben-, and phenol-containing local anesthetics) may result in flocculation of the steroid.[29] Injection of a steroid precipitate imposes a theoretical risk of mechanical damage to soft tissue (cartilage, tendon, joint), neural, and vascular structures. Inadvertent injection of a steroid precipitate into the artery of Adamkiewicz during a thoracic or upper-lumbar–level transforaminal epidural steroid injection or selective nerve root block could result in spinal cord ischemia or infarction, leading to profound lower extremity motor deficits and even paraplegia. For this reason, the injectionist should always visually inspect the injectate for compatibility if a corticosteroid is mixed with a preservative-containing local anesthetic.

References

1. Physicians Desk Reference, 56th ed. Montvale, NJ: Medical Economics Company, 2002.
2. Morris TW, Katzberg RW. Intravenous contrast media: Properties and general effects. In Katzberg RW (ed). The Contrast Media Manual. Baltimore: Williams & Wilkins, 1992, pp 1–18.
3. Product Information: Isovue, iopamidol. Princeton, NJ: Bracco Diagnostics, revised August 1999.
4. Product Information: Omnipaque, iohexol. Princeton, NJ: Nycomed Inc., revised July 1996.
5. Grainger RG. Intravascular contrast media. In Grainger RG, Allison DJ (eds). Diagnostic Radiology, 2nd ed. New York: Churchill Livingstone, 1992, pp 11–22.
6. Grainger RG. Annotation: Radiological contrast media. Clin Radiol 1987; 38:3–5.
7. American Heart Association in collaboration with International Liaison Committee on Resuscitation. Guidelines 2000 for Cardiopulmonary Resuscitation and Emergency Cardiovascular Care: International Consensus on Science. Anaphylaxis. Circulation 2000; 102(Suppl I):I241–243.
8. Lasser EC, Berry CC, Talner LB, et al. Pre-treatment with corticosteroids to alleviate reactions to intravenous contrast media. N Engl J Med 1987; 317:845–849.
9. Bush WH. Treatment of acute reactions to contrast media. In Katzberg RW (ed). The Contrast Media Manual. Baltimore: Williams & Wilkins, 1992, pp 19–27.
10. Butterworth JF, Strichartz GR. Molecular mechanisms of local anesthesia: A review. Anesthesiology 1990; 72:711–734.
11. Product Information: Lidocaine Hydrochloride Injection. North Chicago, IL: Abbott Laboratories, revised January 2001.
12. Product Information: Bupivacaine Hydrochloride Injection. North Chicago, IL: Abbott Laboratories, revised September 1999.
13. Strichartz GR, Sanchez V, Arthur GR, et al. Fundamental properties of local anesthetics: II. Measured octanol:buffer partition coefficients and pKa values of clinically used drugs. Anesth Analg 1990; 71:158–70.
14. Ririe DG, Walker FO, James RL, et al. Effect of alkalinization of lidocaine on median nerve block. Br J Anaesth 2000; 84:163–168.
15. DiFazio CA, Carron H, Grosslight KR, et al. Comparison of pH-adjusted lidocaine solutions for epidural anesthesia. Anesth Analg 1986; 65:760–764.
16. Covino BG, Wildsmith JAW. Clinical pharmacology of local anesthetic agents. In Cousins MJ, Bridenbaugh PO (eds). Neural Blockade in

Clincal Anesthesia and Management of Pain, 3rd ed. Philadelphia: Lippincott-Raven, 1998, pp 97–128.

17. Reiz S, Nathan S. Cardiotoxicity of local anaesthetic agents. Br J Anaesth 1986; 58:736–746.

18. Chernoff DM. Kinetic analysis of phasic inhibition of neuronal sodium currents by lidocaine and bupivacaine. Biophys J 1990; 58:53–68.

19. Gissen AJ, Datta S, Lambert D. The chloroprocaine controversy. Is chloroprocaine neurotoxic? Reg Anesth 1984; 9:135–145.

20. Lambert LA, Lambert DH, Strichartz GR. Irreversible conduction block in isolated nerve by high concentrations of local anesthetics. Anesthesiology 1994; 80:1082–1093.

21. deShazo RD, Nelson HS. An approach to the patient with a history of local anesthetic hypersensitivity: Experience with 90 patients. J Allergy Clin Immunol 1979; 63:387–394.

22. Schimmer BP, Parker KL. Adrenocortical steroids. In Hardman JG, Gilman AG, Limbird LE (eds). Goodman and Gilman's The Pharmacologic Bass of Therapeutics, 9th ed. New York: McGraw-Hill, 1996, pp 1465–1481.

23. Product Information: Hydrocortone Acetate, hydrocortisone acetate. West Point, PA: Merck & Co., February 1997.

24. Product Information: Hydrocortone Phosphate, hydrocortisone phosphate. West Point, PA: Merck & Co., February 1997.

25. Product Information: Kenalog-40 Injection, triamcinolone acetonide. Princeton, NJ: Bristol-Myers Squibb, revised April 2001.

26. Product Information: Aristocort Forte, triamcinolone diacetate. Carolina, Puerto Rico: Lederle Parenterals, April 1999.

27. Product Information: Depo-Medrol, methylprednisolone acetate. Kalamazoo, MI: Pharmacia & Upjohn, revised March 1999.

28. Product Information: Decadron Phosphate Injection, dexamethasone sodium phosphate. West Point, PA: Merck & Co., October 1996.

29. Product Information: Celestone Soluspan, betamethasone sodium phosphate and betamethasone acetate. Kenilworth, NJ: Schering, revised October 1999.

30. Saal JS, Franson RC, Dobrow R, et al. High levels of inflammatory phospholipase A2 activity in lumbar disc herniations. Spine 1990; 15:674–678.

31. Devor M, Govrin-Lippman R, Raber P. Corticosteroids suppress ectopic neural discharge originating in experimental neuromas. Pain 1985; 22:127–137.

32. Johansson A, Hao J, Sjolund B. Local corticosteroid blocks transmission of normal nociceptive C-fibres. Acta Anaesthesiol Scand 1990; 34:335–338.

33. Johansson A, Bennett GJ. Effect of local methylprednisolone on pain in a nerve injury model. Reg Anesth 1997; 22:59–65.

34. Fuxe K, Harfstrand A, Agnati LF, et al. Immunocytochemical studies on the localization of glucocorticoid receptor immunoreactive nerve cells in the lower brain stem and spinal cord of the male rat using monoclonal antibody against rat liver glucocorticoid receptor. Neurosci Lett 1985; 60:1–6.

35. Hua SY, Chen YZ. Membrane receptor-mediated electrophysiological effects of glucocorticoid on mammalian neurons. Endocrinology 1989; 124:687–691.

36. Nelson DA. Dangers from methylprednisolone acetate therapy by intraspinal injection. Arch Neurol 1988; 45:804–806.

37. Krauthammer C, Klerman GL. Secondary mania. Arch Gen Psychiatry 1978; 35:1333–1339.

38. Patten SB, Neutel CI. Corticosteroid-induced adverse psychiatric effects: Incidence, diagnosis and management. Drug Safety 2000; 22:111–122.

39. Goldstein DA, Zimmerman B, Spielberg S. Anaphylactic response to hydrocortisone in childhood: A case report. Ann Allergy 1985; 55:599–600.

40. Freedman MD, Schocket AL, Chapel N, et al. Anaphylaxis after intravenous methylprednisolone administration. JAMA 1981; 245:607–608.

41. Peller JS, Bardana EJ. Anaphylactoid reaction to corticosteroid: Case report and review of the literature. Ann Allerg 1985; 54:302–305.

Index

Note: Page numbers followed by the letter f refer to figures; those followed by t refer to tables.

293